D0152865

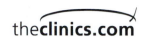

CLINICS IN PERINATOLOGY

Congenital Heart Disease: Impact on the Fetus, Pregnancy, Neonate, and Family

GUEST EDITORS
Gil Wernovsky, MD
Stuart Berger, MD
S. David Rubenstein, MD

December 2005 • Volume 32 • Number 4

SAUNDERS

An Imprint of Elsevier, Inc.
PHILADELPHIA   LONDON   TORONTO   MONTREAL   SYDNEY   TOKYO

W.B. SAUNDERS COMPANY
A Division of Elsevier Inc.

Elsevier, Inc., 1600 John F. Kennedy Blvd., Suite 1800, Philadelphia, PA 19103-2899

http://www.theclinics.com

CLINICS IN PERINATOLOGY	**Volume 32, Number 4**
December 2005	**ISSN 0095-5108**
Editor: Carin Davis	**ISBN 1-4160-3226-6**

Copyright © 2005 by Elsevier Inc. All rights reserved. No part of this publication may be reproduced or transmitted in any form or by any means, electronic or mechanical, including photocopy, recording, or any information retrieval system, without written permission from the Publisher.

Single photocopies of single articles may be made for personal use as allowed by national copyright laws. Permission of the publisher and payment of a fee is required for all other photocopying, including multiple or systematic copying, copying for advertising or promotional purposes, resale, and all forms of document delivery. Special rates are available for educational institutions that wish to make photocopies for non-profit educational classroom use. Permissions may be sought directly from Elsevier's Rights Department in Philadelphia, PA, USA: phone: (+1) 215 239 3804, fax: (+1) 215 239 3805, e-mail: healthpermissions@elsevier. com. Requests may also be completed on-line via the Elsevier homepage (http://www.elsevier. com/locate/permissions). In the USA, users may clear permissions and make payments through the Copyright Clearance Center, Inc., 222 Rosewood Drive, Danvers, MA 01923, USA; phone: (978) 750-8400, fax: (978) 750-4744, and in the UK through the Copyright Licensing Agency Rapid Clearance Service (CLARCS), 90 Tottenham Court Road, London W1P 0LP, UK; phone: (+44) 171 436 5931; fax: (+44) 171 436 3986. Other countries may have a local reprographic rights agency for payments.

Reprints. For copies of 100 or more, of articles in this publication, please contact the Commercial Reprints Department, Elsevier Inc., 360 Park Avenue South, New York, New York 10010-1710. Tel. (212) 633-3813, Fax: (212) 462-1935, e-mail: reprints@elsevier.com.

The ideas and opinions expressed in *Clinics in Perinatology* do not necessarily reflect those of the Publisher. The Publisher does not assume any responsibility for any injury and/or damage to persons or property arising out of or related to any use of the material contained in this periodical. The reader is advised to check the appropriate medical literature and the product information currently provided by the manufacturer of each drug to be administered, to verify the dosage, the method and duration of administration or contraindications. It is the responsibility of the treating physician or other health care professional, relying on independent experience and knowledge of the patient, to determine drug dosages and the best treatment for the patient. Mention of any product in this issue should not be construed as endorsement by the contributors, editors, or the Publisher of the product or manufacturers' claims.

Clinics in Perinatology (ISSN 0095-5108) is published quarterly by Elsevier, Inc., Corporate and editorial offices: Elsevier, Inc., 1600 John F. Kennedy Blvd., Suite 1800, Philadelphia, PA 19103-2899. Accounting and circulation offices: 6277 Sea Harbor Drive, Orlando, FL 32887-4800. Periodicals postage paid at Orlando, FL 32862, and additional mailing offices. Subscription prices are $165.00 per year (US individuals), $250.00 per year (US institutions), $195.00 per year (Canadian individuals), $310.00 per year (Canadian institutions), $225.00 per year (foreign individuals), $310.00 per year (foreign institutions), $80.00 per year (US students), and $110.00 per year (foreign students). Foreign air speed delivery is included in all Clinics subscription prices. All prices are subject to change without notice. POSTMASTER: Send address changes to *Clinics in Perinatology*, W.B. Saunders Company, Periodicals Fulfillment, Orlando, FL 32887-4800. **Customer Service: 1-800-654-2452 (US). From outside of the US, call 1-407-345-4000.** E-mail: hhspcs@harcourt.com.

Clinics in Perinatology is also published in Spanish by McGraw-Hill Interamericana Editores S.A., P.O. Box 5-237, 06500 Mexico D.F., Mexico.

Clinics in Perinatology is covered in *Index Medicus, Current Contents, Excerpta Medica, BIOSIS,* and *ISI/BIOMED.*

Printed in the United States of America.

GUEST EDITORS

GIL WERNOVSKY, MD, FACC, FAAP, Staff Cardiologist, Cardiac Intensive Care Unit; Director of Program Development, Cardiac Center; The Children's Hospital of Philadelphia; Professor of Pediatrics, University of Pennsylvania School of Medicine, Philadelphia, Pennsylvania

STUART BERGER, MD, Children's Hospital of Wisconsin; Department of Pediatrics, Medical College of Wisconsin, Milwaukee, Wisconsin

S. DAVID RUBENSTEIN, MD, Division of Neonatal-Perinatal Medicine, Children's Hospital of New York; College of Physicians and Surgeons, Columbia University, New York, New York

CONTRIBUTORS

ANNE ADES, MD, Clinical Associate of Neonatology; Associate Medical Director, Newborn Infant Center; Division of Neonatology, The Children's Hospital of Philadelphia, Philadelphia, Pennsylvania

STUART BERGER, MD, Children's Hospital of Wisconsin; Department of Pediatrics, Medical College of Wisconsin, Milwaukee, Wisconsin

ULRICH BROECKEL, MD, Associate Professor, Department of Pediatrics, Medical College of Wisconsin, Milwaukee, Wisconsin

MATTHEW D. BROWN, MD, Division of Cardiology, Children's Hospital of Wisconsin; Department of Pediatrics, Medical College of Wisconsin, Milwaukee, Wisconsin

MERYL S. COHEN, MD, Assistant Professor of Pediatrics, Division of Cardiology, The Children's Hospital of Philadelphia, Philadelphia, Pennsylvania

KATHRYN M. DODDS, RN, MSN, CRNP, Clinical Liaison Nurse Practitioner, Cardiac Center, The Children's Hospital of Philadelphia, Philadelphia, Pennsylvania

MICHAEL G. EARING, MD, Director, Adult Congenital Heart Disease Program, Herma Heart Center, Medical College of Wisconsin, Milwaukee, Wisconsin

MICHELE A. FROMMELT, MD, Associate Professor of Pediatrics, Children's Hospital of Wisconsin, Milwaukee, Wisconsin

ELIZABETH GOLDMUNTZ, MD, Associate Professor of Pediatrics, Division of Cardiology, The Children's Hospital of Philadelphia; University of Pennsylvania School of Medicine, Philadelphia, Pennsylvania

PETER J. GRUBER, MD, PhD, Cardiac Center, The Children's Hospital of Philadelphia; The Molecular Cardiology Research Center, University of Pennsylvania School of Medicine, Philadelphia, Pennsylvania

ROBERT D.B. JAQUISS, MD, Associate Professor of Surgery, Medical College of Wisconsin; Children's Hospital of Wisconsin, Milwaukee, Wisconsin

BETH ANN JOHNSON, MD, MA, FAAP, Instructor, Neonatology and Pediatric Cardiology, Medical College of Wisconsin; Fellow, Herma Heart Center, Children's Hospital of Wisconsin, Milwaukee, Wisconsin

RALPH A. LUGO, PharmD, Associate Professor, Vice-Chair, Department of Pharmacotherapy, University of Utah College of Pharmacy; Adjunct Associate Professor of Pediatrics, University of Utah School of Medicine, Salt Lake City, Utah

CHRISTINE MERLE, RN, MSN, PNP, Faculty Nurse Practitioner, Morgan Stanley Children's Hospital of New York-Presbyterian; Assistant Professor of Clinical Nursing, Columbia University, New York, New York

KATHY A. MUSSATTO, BSN, Division of Cardiology, Children's Hospital of Wisconsin; Department of Pediatrics, Medical College of Wisconsin, Milwaukee, Wisconsin

ANDREW N. PELECH, MD, Associate Professor, Department of Pediatrics, Medical College of Wisconsin, Milwaukee, Wisconsin

BARBARA PICK, RD, CSP, CD, Nutritional Services; Children's Hospital of Wisconsin, Medical College of Wisconsin, Milwaukee, Wisconsin

NANCY RUDD, RN, MS, CPNP, Division of Pediatric Cardiology, Children's Hospital of Wisconsin, Medical College of Wisconsin, Milwaukee, Wisconsin

JACK RYCHIK, MD, Director, Fetal Heart Program, Cardiac Center, The Children's Hospital of Philadelphia; Associate Professor of Pediatrics, University of Pennsylvania School of Medicine, Philadelphia, Pennsylvania

MICHELLE STELTZER, RN, MS, CPNP, Division of Pediatric Cardiology, Children's Hospital of Wisconsin, Medical College of Wisconsin, Milwaukee, Wisconsin

JANETTE F. STRASBURGER, MD, Professor of Pediatrics, Medical College of Wisconsin, Milwaukee; Division of Cardiology, Children's Hospital of Wisconsin, Milwaukee; Director of Cardiac Services, Children's Hospital of Wisconsin–Fox Valley, Neenah, Wisconsin

ANITA SZWAST, MD, Cardiology Fellow, The Children's Hospital of Philadelphia; Instructor in Pediatrics, University of Pennsylvania School of Medicine, Philadelphia, Pennsylvania

JAMES S. TWEDDELL, MD, Professor of Surgery and Chief, Division of Cardiothoracic Surgery, Medical College of Wisconsin; S. Bert Litwin Chair in Cardiothoracic Surgery, Children's Hospital of Wisconsin, Milwaukee, Wisconsin

ROBERT M. WARD, MD, Professor of Pediatrics; Director, Pediatric Pharmacology Program, Division of Neonatology, University of Utah, Salt Lake City, Utah

GARY D. WEBB, MD, Director, Philadelphia Adult Congenital Heart Center, The Children's Hospital of Philadelphia and University of Pennsylvania Health System, Philadelphia, Pennsylvania

GIL WERNOVSKY, MD, FACC, FAAP, Staff Cardiologist, Cardiac Intensive Care Unit; Director of Program Development, Cardiac Center; The Children's Hospital of Philadelphia; Professor of Pediatrics, University of Pennsylvania School of Medicine, Philadelphia, Pennsylvania

CONTENTS

> Congenital heart disease remains a significant cause of morbidity and mortality. In recent years, significant advances in molecular genetics, improved understanding of morphogenesis, recognition of specific patterning of abnormalities within and between species, and the impact of the Human Genome Project have accounted for these advances. Continued rapid developments in genomics and proteomics are anticipated. Epidemiologic investigations continue to be necessary to assess the influence of the environment on genetics. We are on the threshold of influencing the occurrence of congenital heart diseases.

> Understanding normal development is a prerequisite to unraveling the mechanisms that underlie congenital heart disease, a critical step if one is to design rational new therapies. Over the past 20 years, human molecular genetics and developmental biology have provided a group of powerful tools to uncover a number of now well-defined pathways. There is now a confluence of new technologies and experimental systems that may allow for a more profound understanding in the near future.

poor functional class, however, pregnancy poses significant risk for cardiovascular complications, including premature death. As result, preconception counseling and risk stratification are mandatory and should be done in all women of childbearing age with CHD.

Delivery Room and Early Postnatal Management of Neonates Who Have Prenatally Diagnosed Congenital Heart Disease

Beth Ann Johnson and Anne Ades

Advances in fetal echocardiography are providing highly accurate diagnoses of congenital heart disease prior to delivery, making it possible to plan the delivery-room management of these newborns. Knowledge of the expected transitional circulation occurring with birth and the pathophysiologic implications of congenital heart disease increases the likelihood of providing efficient and effective therapies. The majority of neonates who have congenital heart disease will not require delivery room resuscitation in excess of routine care; however, a small number of prenatally diagnosed cardiac lesions are more likely to require urgent postnatal intervention immediately following delivery. These cardiac lesions include transposition of the great arteries with intact ventricular septum and restrictive atrial septum, hypoplastic left heart syndrome with intact atrial septum, obstructed total anomalous pulmonary venous return, and complete congenital heart block. Prenatal diagnosis allows for coordination of care surrounding delivery and during the early postnatal hours.

The Neonate with Congenital Heart Disease: What the Cardiac Surgeon Needs to Know from the Neonatologist and the Cardiologist

Robert D.B. Jaquiss and James S. Tweddell

To plan and accomplish a successful operation for a neonate with congenital heart disease, the cardiac surgeon requires a complete anatomic description of the cardiovascular malformation. For optimum outcome, this information must be supplemented by a complete report of the prenatal and postnatal course of the newborn as well as by a thorough summary of any noncardiac congenital or acquired abnormalities. In the most favorable circumstance, the neonate arrives in the operating room completely diagnosed, fully resuscitated, well nourished, and with appropriate monitoring devices in place. Unique perioperative considerations attach to each cardiac anomaly and are briefly reviewed, and the importance of continuity of care for the patient and family is emphasized.

DiGeorge Syndrome: New Insights

Elizabeth Goldmuntz

Most patients with the clinical features of DiGeorge, velocardiofacial, and conotruncal anomaly face syndromes share a common genetic cause, namely, a deletion of chromosome 22q11, and define the most common deletion syndrome known at this time. The clinical features of the 22q11 deletion syndrome are highly variable between individuals; some have subtle findings, whereas others are severely affected. The most common clinical features include specific types of congenital heart disease, hypocalcemia, immunodeficiency, facial dysmorphia, palate anomalies, velopharyngeal dysfunction, renal anomalies, and speech and feeding disorders as well as neurocognitive, behavioral, and psychiatric disorders. A significant number of patients with tetralogy of Fallot, truncus arteriosus, an interrupted aortic arch, isolated aortic arch anomalies, and perimembranous ventricular septal defects have a 22q11 deletion. Routine testing for a 22q11 deletion in this subset of patients should be considered to provide anticipatory medical intervention and appropriate family counseling.

Cardiovascular Drugs for the Newborn 979
Robert M. Ward and Ralph A. Lugo

This article reviews the various cardiovascular drugs for newborns, including antiarrhythmics, antihypertensives, inotropes, and pulmonary vasodilators. Antiarrhythmic drugs are classified according to their mechanisms of action, such as effects on ion channels, duration of repolarization, and receptor interaction, which help with understanding the effects of individual antiarrhythmic drugs and selection of drugs for specific arrhythmias. Drug treatement for hypertension should start with a single drug from one of the following classes: ACE inhibitors, angiotensin-receptor antagonists, beta-receptor antagonists, calcium channel blockers, or diuretics. The inotropic drug should be selected according to its specific pharmacologic properties and the specific cardiovascular abnormality to be corrected. An effective pulmonary vasodilator must dilate the pulmonary vasculature more than the systemic vasculature.

Management of Low Birth Weight Infants with Congenital Heart Disease 999
Anne Ades, Beth Ann Johnson, and Stuart Berger

Low birth weight infants with congenital heart disease (CHD) have a higher mortality risk and likely a higher morbidity risk than their preterm or appropriate for gestational age counterparts without CHD and term counterparts with CHD. As our understanding of the pathophysiology and treatment of the diseases associated with prematurity and growth restriction improves, the outcomes for these infants should continue to improve. In addition, as more of these infants survive and are referred for surgery, operative techniques and strategies are likely to continue to improve. At this time, there is no adequate evidence that mortality is improved by delaying surgery for weight gain or performing palliative operations initially. Given the challenging physiology in this population, optimal management includes early referral to a tertiary or quaternary facility and a multidisciplinary team approach consisting of cardiologists, neonatologists, surgeons, nurses, perfusionists, and anesthesiologists.

Those health care professionals entrusted with the care of infants with congenital heart disease require an understanding of the unique nutritional needs of this population. This article defines the congenital, physiologic, and nutritional variables encountered in this population. The nutritional needs, multi-factorial sources of undernutrition, and consequences of inadequate nutrition in infants with congenital heart disease are discussed, as well as medical and nutritional management strategies intended to optimize growth and reduce morbidity.

Discharging neonates to home after cardiac surgery takes time, effective communication, and a commitment to continuity of care. The efforts of all members of a multidisciplinary team are necessary and valuable to ensure success. The discharge process involves many steps beginning at the time of admission and continuing past the actual discharge date. Discharge planning is an evolving process rather than a single event.

As short-term survival of complex congenital heart disease continues to improve dramatically with advances in medical and surgical treatment, further efforts must be made to understand the long-term outcomes of our efforts. As survival continues to improve, cardiovascular morbidity and, equally importantly, neurodevelopmental and social outcomes must be a continual focus in our treatment of these complex patients. Further study of these effects is underway, and more is certainly warranted. Understanding should lead to modification of current techniques and management strategies, all with the ultimate goal of improving our patients' quality of life.

GOAL STATEMENT

The goal of *Clinics in Perinatology* is to keep practicing neonatologists and maternal-fetal medicine specialists up to date with current clinical practice in perinatology by providing timely articles reviewing the state of the art in patient care.

ACCREDITATION

The *Clinics in Perinatology* is planned and implemented in accordance with the Essential Areas and Policies of the Accreditation Council for Continuing Medical Education (ACCME) through the joint sponsorship of the University of Virginia School of Medicine and Elsevier. The University of Virginia School of Medicine is accredited by the ACCME to provide continuing medical education for physicians.

The University of Virginia School of Medicine designates this educational activity for a maximum of 60 category 1 credits per year, 15 category 1 credits per issue, toward the AMA Physician's Recognition Award. Each physician should claim only those credits that he/she actually spent in the activity.

The American Medical Association has determined that physicians not licensed in the US who participate in this CME activity are eligible for AMA PRA category 1 credit.

Category 1 credit can be earned by reading the text material, taking the CME examination online at http://www.theclinics.com/home/cme, and completing the evaluation. After taking the test, you will be required to review any and all incorrect answers. Following completion of the test and evaluation, your credit will be awarded and you may print your certificate.

FACULTY DISCLOSURE/CONFLICT OF INTEREST

The University of Virginia School of Medicine, as an ACCME accredited provider, endorses and strives to comply with the Accreditation Council for Continuing Medical Education (ACCME) Standards of Commercial Support, Commonwealth of Virginia statutes, University of Virginia policies and procedures, and associated federal and private regulations and guidelines on the need for disclosure and monitoring of proprietary and financial interests that may affect the scientific integrity and balance of content delivered in continuing medical education activities under our auspices.

The University of Virginia School of Medicine requires that all CME activities accredited through this institution be developed independently and be scientifically rigorous, balanced and objective in the presentation/ discussion of its content, theories and practices.

All authors/editors participating in an accredited CME activity are expected to disclose to the readers relevant financial relationships with commercial entities occurring within the past 12 months (such as grants or research support, employee, consultant, stock holder, member of speakers bureau, etc.). The University of Virginia School of Medicine will employ appropriate mechanisms to resolve potential conflicts of interest to maintain the standards of fair and balanced education to the reader. Questions about specific strategies can be directed to the Office of Continuing Medical Education, University of Virginia School of Medicine, Charlottesville, Virginia.

The authors/editors listed below have identified no professional or financial affiliations for their spouse/ partner:

Anne Ades, MD; Stuart Berger, MD; Ulrich Broeckel, MD; Matthew D. Brown, MD; Meryl S. Cohen, MD; Carin Davis, Acquisitions Editor; Kathryn M. Dodds, RN, MSN, CRNP; Michael G. Earing, MD; Michele A. Frommelt, MD; Elizabeth Goldmuntz, MD; Peter J. Gruber, MD, PhD; Robert D. B. Jaquiss, MD; Beth Ann Johnson, MD, MA, FAAP; Ralph A. Lugo, PharmD; Christine Merle, RN, MSN, PNP; Kathleen A. Mussatto, BSN; Andrew N. Pelech, MD; Barbara Pick, RD, CSP, CD; S. David Rubenstein, MD; Nancy A. Rudd, RN, MS, CPNP; Jack Rychik, MD, FACC; Michelle M. Steltzer, RN, MS, CPNP; Janette F. Strasburger, MD; Anita L. Szwast, MD; James S. Tweddell, MD; and Gil Wernovsky, MD, FACC, FAAP.

The author listed below identified the following professional or financial affiliations for himself, his spouse/ partner:

Richard A. Polin, MD is a consultant for Discovery Laboratories and General Electric.

Robert M. Ward, MD is an independent contractor for Abbot Pharmaceuticals, Wyeth Pharmaceuticals, and Medimmune; and is also a consultant for Wyeth.

Gary D. Webb, MD is the vice-president of research for GlaxoSmithKline.

Disclosure of Discussion of non-FDA approved uses for pharmaceutical products and/or medical devices: The University of Virginia School of Medicine, as an ACCME provider, requires that all faculty presenters identify and disclose any "off label" uses for pharmaceutical and medical device products. The University of Virginia School of Medicine recommends that each physician fully review all the available data on new products or procedures prior to instituting them with patients.

TO ENROLL

To enroll in the *Clinics in Perinatology* Continuing Medical Education program, call customer service at 1-800-654-2452 or visit us online at www.theclinics.com/home/cme. The CME program is available to subscribers for an additional fee of $195.00

FORTHCOMING ISSUES

RECENT ISSUES

THE CLINICS ARE NOW AVAILABLE ONLINE!

Access your subscription at
http://www.theclinics.com

Cardiology 2006

Ninth Annual
Update on Pediatric Cardiovascular Disease

State-of-the-Art Management of the
Neonate and Infant with Cardiac Disease

February 8-12, 2006
Hyatt Regency Scottsdale Resort
and Spa at Gainey Ranch
Scottsdale, Arizona

Sponsored by

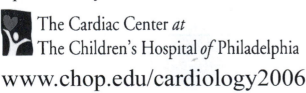

The Cardiac Center *at*
The Children's Hospital *of* Philadelphia

www.chop.edu/cardiology2006

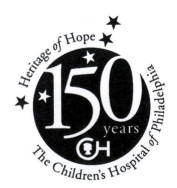

RECEIPT

CENTRAL OHIO PRIMARY
CARE PHYSICIANS, INC.

Date 2/15/06

512560

RECEIVED FROM Snyder

$ 20 00

FOR copay - Laura

DOLLARS

BY

THANK YOU

ELSEVIER
SAUNDERS

CLINICS IN
PERINATOLOGY

Clin Perinatol 32 (2005) xv–xvi

Foreword

Congenital Heart Disease: Impact on the Fetus, Pregnancy, Neonate, and Family

It is rare in one's lifetime to witness the kind of progress that has been made in the care of infants who have congenital heart disease. The specialty of pediatric cardiology has transformed from a predominantly descriptive one with various palliative operations to one in which most heart defects are totally or partially corrected in the neonatal period.

In the 1970s, echocardiography was in its infancy and cardiac catheterizations were common. With the widespread use of cardiac MRI and improved echocardiographic technology, only in unusual circumstances do infants require invasive diagnostics. The availability of prostaglandin E1 now permits operative procedures to be scheduled electively rather than emergently. Most importantly, with advancements in antenatal diagnostic techniques the diagnosis of congenital heart disease is rarely a surprise. As the mortality rate for many common congenital heart lesions has plummeted to single digits, the attention of neonatologists and cardiologists has been appropriately redirected to find ways to improve neurologic outcomes in infants who have complex congenital heart disease. Improvements in developmental outcomes will probably not come from changes in surgical techniques or advances in life support technology (although both are important); it will likely come from attention to the minute details of cardiac and neonatal intensive care and better ways of assessing central nervous system function in the preoperative, intraoperative, and postoperative periods. This will require the expertise of cardiac intensivists, anesthesiologists, neonatologists, and experienced nurses working in close collaboration.

This issue of the *Clinics in Perinatology*, edited by Gil Wernovsky, Stuart Berger, and David Rubenstein focuses on the coming frontiers in the subspecialty of pediatric cardiology. Although the articles do not provide all the answers, they clearly outline the way the problems will be solved. Drs. Wernovsky, Berger, and

0095-5108/05/$ – see front matter © 2005 Elsevier Inc. All rights reserved.
doi:10.1016/j.clp.2005.11.001
perinatology.theclinics.com

Rubenstein are to be congratulated on their foresight and for organizing an outstanding issue.

Richard A. Polin, MD
Professor of Pediatrics
College of Physicians and Surgeons
Columbia University
630 West 168th Street
New York, NY 10032, USA

Director
Division of Neonatology
Morgan Stanley Children's Hospital of New York-Presbyterian
New York, NY, USA
E-mail address: rap32@columbia.edu

CLINICS IN
PERINATOLOGY

Clin Perinatol 32 (2005) xvii–xviii

Preface

Congenital Heart Disease: Impact on the Fetus, Pregnancy, Neonate, and Family

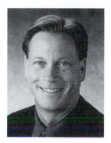 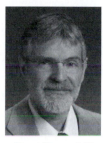 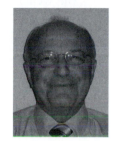

Gil Wernovsky, MD   Stuart Berger, MD   S. David Rubenstein, MD
Guest Editors

Dr. Wernovsky would like to thank all of the contributors to this issue of Clinics in Perinatology, and the medical and nursing staffs of the Children's Hospital of Philadelphia for their ongoing support and daily challenge to improve the outcomes for our patients. I would also like to acknowledge the tolerance and love from my wife Lauren (who really gets all the work done) and my children Simon and Jenna; without them, nothing would ever be accomplished. Finally, the editors wish to thank Carin Davis, Donald Mumford, and the staff at Elvesier for putting together yet another terrific issue of *Clinics in Perinatology* and for their tireless work on the project.

With tremendous gratitude, Dr. Berger would like to thank his colleagues at the Children's Hospital of Wisconsin and the Medical College of Wisconsin for their contributions to this issue of the *Clinics in Perinatology* and for the great care and hard work that they put forth on a daily basis. It is that hard work—along with a cooperative, multidisciplinary team approach to our complex patients—that allows for the advancement of knowledge and progressive improvement in outcomes that we have realized and will continue to realize. This team approach includes all who are involved in the care of the fetus, neonate, child, adolescent, and adult with congenital heart disease. In addition, I would like to thank and acknowledge the coeditors of this issue, Drs. Wernovsky and

0095-5108/05/$ – see front matter © 2005 Elsevier Inc. All rights reserved.
doi:10.1016/j.clp.2005.10.001

Rubenstein. It has been great fun working with them and with our colleagues at Children's Hospital of Philadelphia and Columbia University. Without this cooperative effort, this issue would not have been possible. I would also like to thank Carin Davis, Donald Mumford, and the staff at Elsevier for their support with this project and for their untiring dedication in coordinating the efforts between three institutions—not an easy task. Last but not least, I thank my wife Julie, and my children Jake, Leah, and Mollie for their love, support, and perspective on life.

Dr. Rubenstein would like to thank all those who helped produce this issue of the *Clinics in Perinatology*, in particular the authors and coeditors. A special thanks goes to Gil Wernovsky, whose unyielding committment to the project helped ensure its creation and completion. Additionally, I want to thank Carin Davis and Donald Mumford of Elsevier for their persistence in helping us produce this issue.

Gil Wernovsky, MD
Pediatric Cardiology
The Children's Hospital of Philadelphia
34th Street and Civic Center Boulevard
Philadelphia, PA 19104, USA
E-mail address: wernovsky@email.chop.edu

Stuart Berger, MD
Children's Hospital of Wisconsin
Department of Pediatrics
Medical College of Wisconsin
9000 W. Wisconsin Avenue
Milwaukee, WI 53226, USA
E-mail address: sberger@mcw.edu

S. David Rubenstein, MD
Division of Neonatal-Perinatal Medicine
Children's Hospital of New York
3959 Broadway, BHN 1201
New York, NY 10032, USA
E-mail address: sdr26@columbia.edu

ELSEVIER
SAUNDERS

CLINICS IN
PERINATOLOGY

Clin Perinatol 32 (2005) 825–844

Toward the Etiologies of Congenital Heart Diseases

Andrew N. Pelech, MD*, Ulrich Broeckel, MD

*Department of Pediatrics, Medical College of Wisconsin, Milwaukee, PO Box 26509,
8701 Watertown Plank Road, Milwaukee, WI 53266–0509, USA*

In 1898, Sir William Osler urged the young assistant curator of the pathology collection at McGill University in Montreal to reorganize the specimens as a teaching and instructional tool. As written by Dr. Maude Abbott, "And so he quietly dropped the seed that dominated all my future work for very many years" [1]. Dr. Abbott's contributions included a detailed redescription of the original double-inlet left ventricle or "Holmes" heart [2], the original chapter on congenital heart disease in Osler and McCrae's *Modern Medicine* [3], and, most importantly, the *Atlas of Congenital Heart Disease* [4]. This was the first systematic analysis of congenital heart disease, based on the 750 specimens in the McGill collection, and included detailed diagrams and descriptions of most congenital heart anomalies. She was first to quote the oft-heard parental concern, "What has caused this problem to occur?" Subsequent pathologic descriptions have formed the basis for our understanding of cardiac morphology and physiology [5].

The desire to understand heart formation and the creation of congenital malformations has motivated the study of cardiac embryology. Initial work included the observation of the beating chick hearts [6], detailed microscopic work [7], and detailed wax plate reconstruction methods [8]. These early techniques established the time lines of appearance of different cardiac structures in the developing embryo. Two scales of morphologic development, the Carnegie scales [9] and the "horizon scales" of Streeter [10–12], provide the temporal landmarks enabling sequencing of cardiac embryonic events [13].

Investigational techniques, including scanning microscopy [14], marker studies [15], cinemicrophotography [16], radioisotope labeling studies [17], and

* Corresponding author.
E-mail address: apelech@chw.org (A.N. Pelech).

0095-5108/05/$ – see front matter © 2005 Elsevier Inc. All rights reserved.
doi:10.1016/j.clp.2005.09.005

histochemical methods [18], have enabled functional studies of the cardiac embryo, including study of intracardiac flow, cell migration, and cellular proliferation and death. Patterns of development have been found to be similar between species, enabling comparison of parallel developmental events in various experimental animals.

Recent advances in medical genetic analysis, including cluster analysis [19], animal knockout experiments [20], and the impact of the Human Genome Project [21], have facilitated significant advances in the past decade (see article in this issue on new concepts of cardiac development by Gruber).

Several factors have accounted for delays in the search for the causes of congenital heart disease, including primarily the low incidence of hemodynamically significant congenital heart defects, 0.8% to 1% of live births. This number may significantly underestimate the true incidence of anomalies, because many minor abnormalities, such as bicuspid aortic valves, left-sided superior vena cavae, and right-sided aortic arches, are not included in these frequency studies. The failure to recognize the concept and significance of variable penetrance and the absence of comprehensive phenotypic descriptions have resulted in an underestimation of the incidence of inheritable anomalies. Additional encumbrances include lack of consensus on a standardized nomenclature, lack of automatic or structured reporting tools, and federal governmental restrictions on cooperative epidemiologic communications (Health Insurance Portability and Accountability Act [HIPAA]). Recently, a consensus nomenclature has been developed and accepted by the international pediatric cardiology community [22]. In conjunction with these developments, improved databasing and computer communications have enabled the development of several regional epidemiologic databases, including the Wisconsin Pediatric Cardiac Registry [23], the National Center on Birth Defects and Developmental Disabilities [24], and the Baltimore-Washington Infant Study [25], which serve as genetic and environmental research resources.

Genetic approaches to identify genes for cardiac malformations

From the beginning, it was apparent that cardiac malformations cluster in families. This focused the research direction on improving the understanding of how genetic factors influence susceptibility of families for developing congenital cardiac malformations. In the recent past, identification of a genetic or environmental causal etiology included initial recognition of a phenotypic population, determination of the inheritance pattern, identification of an altered protein or enzyme or substrate, and, finally, identification of the genetic defect if at all possible. With regard to the mode of inheritance, diseases have been categorized according to the classic Mendelian inheritance mode or based on a more complex polygenic pattern. The distinction between the two categories is made by careful evaluation of the family history and establishing the mode of inheritance by analysis of pedigree information. The underlying genetic basis for Mendelian diseases, caused by single gene mutations, follows a dominant or recessive mode of inheritance. In some cases, the development of the disease might not always be observed because of incomplete penetrance of the mutation causing the disease. For diseases entities that do not follow clear Mendelian inheritance patterns, it is assumed that sporadic mutations or multiple genes determine the disease phenotype. Initially, as the methods for localizing genes were developed for Mendelian diseases, some success was achieved in identifying single gene mutations. For example with regard to congenital cardiac malformations, the identification of GATA4 mutations associated with the autosomal dominant form of secundum atrial septal defect (ASD) represents a landmark finding [26].

Current approaches focus initially on localization of the chromosomal regions harboring the disease-causing gene using genome-scanning techniques. Subsequent fine-mapping procedures narrow the region to a gene or limited number of genes, and, finally, direct mutation detection with sequencing is used to identify causal mutations. With the availability of current genetics technologies, this approach has been successfully used for a broad variety of monogenic diseases, although this approach has been less successful with regard to diseases that do not follow Mendelian inheritance patterns.

Approaches for complex polygenic diseases

Identification of genes for cardiac malformations not following a clear Mendelian pattern or sporadic cases has presented significant challenges. Depending on the disease of interest, affected sibling pairs, affected relative pairs, or extended pedigrees can be used. Linkage analysis identifies chromosomal regions harboring potential disease-causing genes. This analytic approach requires a large number of families, and, often, the linkage signal does not provide substantial statistical evidence. In addition, the identified regions may be rather large with a large number of genes localized in the identified chromosomal region, making the subsequent fine mapping and gene identification difficult. Despite these challenges, this approach is promising and has been used recently for some common cardiac malformations [27]. Based on the theoretic analyses by Risch and Merikangas [28], which indicate that an association study design can be sufficiently powerful, there has been growing interest in an association approach using case-control, nuclear [29], or extended families. The family-based association approach requires testing of the affected individual, siblings, and parents to estimate the preferential transmission of affected alleles from the parents to the offspring. Novel statistical tests have been developed to correct and account for population stratification in the analysis of unrelated individuals [30–32]. Using these methodologies and with the availability of the human genome sequence generated by the Human Genome Project, new interest has been focused toward the use of association studies for polygenic diseases. Finally, high-throughput genotyping technologies are now available to analyze hundreds of thousands of polymorphisms at the same time for a reasonable cost. Currently, the Affymetrix (Santa Clara, California) 500,000–single-nucleotide genotyping chip allows for the analysis of 500,000 polymorphisms at the same time [33]. It is conceivable that this technology can be used in studies that include a number of children with congenital cardiac malformations to identify chromosomal regions and disease-causing polymorphisms. To date, only a limited number of studies on noncardiac diseases have been published using high-density genotyping methodologies for the identification of genes of polygenic diseases. Most recently, this approach has been used successfully to identify genes for macular degeneration [34,35]. The goal of these studies is to improve our understanding of how genetic variation contributes to the more common forms of cardiac malformation and, ultimately, to develop a genetic test that can identify and describe susceptibility.

Cardiogenesis

The cardiovascular system is the first functioning organ in the embryo. Studies of other species have revealed an evolutionarily conserved program of heart development triggered by specific signaling molecules and mediated by tissue-specific transcription factors. The heart begins as mesodermal cells in the early embryo, coalesces as a linear heart tube, and then proceeds through a series of morphologic events culminating in a wondrous and complicated organ system. Recent advances and influences on cardiac growth during different stages of development have been reviewed [36] and are summarized. A genetic blueprint or flow chart (Fig. 1), originally conceived by Srivastava and Olson [37], provides a guide to follow developments in this area but requires constant revision and updates as new genes are implicated.

Cardiomyocyte origin

By day 15 of life, cardiac progenitor cells can be defined. To this point in gestation, the embryo is a two-layered disk of endodermal and ectodermal cells termed a *blastocyst*. A structure arises on the surface of the ectoderm known as the primitive streak, which is the site of a new cell layer. Cells of the ectoderm migrate toward this streak, detaching from neighboring cells and slipping beneath the ectodermal layer to become the intraembryonic mesoderm. These cardiac progenitor cells can be labeled experimentally with tritiated thymidine which allows identification with radioautography [38,39] enabling observance of cell migration on either side of the primitive streak to coalesce cephalad as the cardiogenic plate (Fig. 2). Experimentally, if cells from this area are moved to different regions of the embryo, they should continue to develop myofibrils and have rhythmic contractions [40].

It seems that these cardiomyocytes originate in response to paracrine signaling molecules, including bone morphogenetic proteins (BMP, a member of the transforming growth factor-β [TGFβ] family), which are secreted from adjacent endoderm [41]. In *Drosophila* flies, the protein *tinman* is necessary for speci-

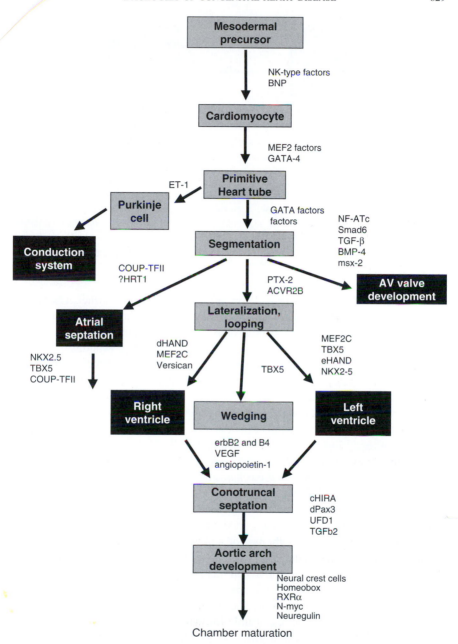

Fig. 1. A genetic blueprint for heart development. A simplified schematic shows the steps in cardiac morphogenesis. The formation of valves, ventricles, atria, and the conduction system is under the control of groups of regulatory proteins that may act independently or in a common pathway. Factors necessary for distinct steps during cardiogenesis in model organisms or human beings are indicated beside the arrows. AV, atrioventricular; NK, natural killer. (*Adapted from* Srivastava D, Olson E. A genetic blueprint for cardiac development. Nature 2000;407:224; with permission.)

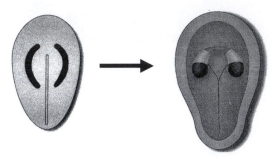

Fig. 2. Cardiomyocyte origin. At the time of gastrulation, widespread cell migration and reor-ganization in the two-layered blastocyst occur, with an identifiable groove termed the *primitive streak* defining the cranial-caudal axis. This primitive groove is the site of entry for ectodermal cells to form the future mesoderm. Cardiac myocytes arise within the lateral mesoderm in response to signals secreted from the adjacent endoderm and migrate cephalad to form the "cardiac plate." (*Modified from* Schultheiss TM, Lassar AB. Vertebrate heart induction. In: Harvey RP, Rosenthal N, editors. Heart development. San Diego (CA): Academic Press; 1999. p. 52; with permission.)

fication of the cardiac lineage and formation of the dorsal cardiac vessel and directly activates transcription of the Mef2 gene, which controls myocyte differentiation. In *Drosophila*, *tinman* and Nkx2-5 interact with GATA family genes to activate cardiac gene expression. Dominant negative versions of Nkx2-5 are also known to block cardiogenesis in frog and zebrafish embryos [42,43]. The same is not true for the homologous Nkx2 through 5 in mammals. Master regulators of the cardiac muscle lineage are still under investigation. Identi-fication of a transcriptional factor, which determines cardiac commitment, is confined to GATA-4 at this point, which is a tissue-restricted transcription factor expressed in early myocardial and endocardial cells [44].

Cell movement is an essential component of early cell migration and sub-sequent organ formation. Several mechanisms and theories of cellular movement have been postulated [45]. Most plausibly, cell movement in a given direction is described as a consequence of a modification of the general mechanism of en-docytosis [46]. This involves cell membrane invagination of an appropriate molecule or ligand that is brought into the cell cytoplasm, with subsequent renewal of the leading cell membrane. The leading edge of the cell is continually being expanded with unbound receptors and recycled membrane, enabling forward "crawling" of the leading edge. Fibronectins are a family of glycoproteins in the cellular basement membranes and extracellular matrix involved in the interactions of the receptor and substrate responsible for this cell movement. Fibronectin is a polypeptide 2500 amino acid with a relatively small recognition site of 3 and 4 amino acids (Arg-Gly-Asp-Ser), which is essential as a cell attachment rec-ognition signal. Fibronectin is present on the surfaces of many bacteria and viruses and may have a role in this form of attachment in mammalian cells [47]. Disruption of embryonic cell migration in many species may be accomplished by injection of the tripeptide recognition site analogue Arg-Gly-Asp, demonstrating the importance of these receptors throughout the animal kingdom [48].

Primitive heart tube

Cords and clusters of angioblastic cells in the mesoderm form two strands, which lie on either side of the developing foregut. When these two areas become confluent, they form a lumen, the endocardial tube or the primitive heart tube. The primitive heart has begun contracting by this stage. The primitive heart tube consists of an outer layer, the epimyocardium, and an inner layer, the endocardium, separated by an extracellular matrix termed the *cardiac jelly* [49,50]. The primitive linear heart tube is made up in sequence of the sinus venosus, the primitive atria, the future left ventricle, the future right ventricle, the bulbus cordis, the truncus arteriosus, and the aortic sac, which is connected by paired branchial arches to the dorsal aorta (Fig. 3). Subsequently, characteristic en-

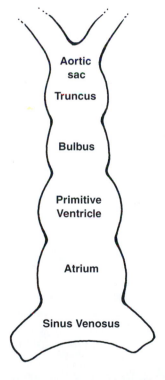

Fig. 3. The primitive heart tube. A ventral view of the primitive straight heart tube demonstrates the early delineation of cardiac segments, beginning caudally with the sinus venosus (site of entrance of the six systemic venous channels), the primitive atrium, the primitive ventricle, the bulbus cordis, the truncus arteriosus, and the aortic sac. Subsequently, the smooth sinus venarum is divided from the trabeculated atrium by the crista terminalis. The atria are separated from the ventricles by the atrioventricular canal. The fetal right and left ventricles remain in communication via the bulboventricular foramen. The bulbus cordis becomes separated from the truncus arterious by the semilunar valves. (*Modified from* Colwin EV. Cardiac embryology. In: Garson A, Bricker JT, McNamara DG, editors. The science and practice of pediatric cardiology. Philadelphia: Lea & Febiger; 1990. p. 81; with permission.)

largement and narrowing of each of these cardiac segments (segmentation) becomes evident as differentiation of cell types occurs [51]. Each chamber has distinguishing anatomic, structural, and functional differences that likely involve specific transcription factors. The mechanisms establishing chamber identity are largely unknown.

Lateralization and looping

At this stage, a signaling system results in differential growth of the cardiac segments, giving rise to characteristic asymmetry or "looping." The midportion of the straight heart tube is allowed to bend ventrally, bringing the caudal sinus venous cephalad, and the primitive right ventricle is seen to enlarge and position itself anterior and rightward with respect to the left ventricle (Fig. 4). The mechanisms by which looping occurs have been the subject of much speculation and experimental work [52,53]. The direction of looping or lateralization seems to be triggered by a signaling system that affects visceral and cardiac positioning. Failure of effective lateralization is thought to result in the congenital heterotaxy syndromes, asplenia and polysplenia, which have a profound impact on visceral, pulmonary, and cardiac organ systems. Congenitally corrected transposition or isolated ventricular inversion may arise as a result of abnormal segmental differentiation.

Studies have shown the asymmetric presence of various morphogens responsible for left-to-right differentiation in chick embryos. Sonic hedgehog (Shh)

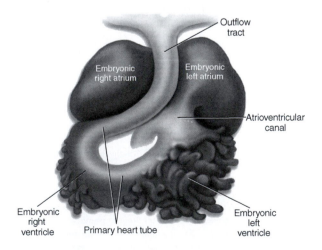

Fig. 4. Lateralization and looping. The primitive heart tube undergoes differential growth and begins to bend, first ventrally and then with the convexity of a curve to the right. Looping positions the atrioventricular canal over the developing left and right ventricles. (*From* Streeter GL. In: O'Rahilly R, Muller F, editors. Developmental stages in human embryos. Washington, DC: Carnegie Institute of Washington; 1987; with permission.)

leads to the expression of Nodal and lefty, members of the TGFβ family in the left lateral mesoderm [54]. Through a series of intermediary signaling molecules, the transcription factor Ptx2 is then expressed on the left side. This protein binds to DNA and regulates expression of mRNA, establishing left-to-right asymmetry of the heart, lungs, and gut. Murine models of left-to-right defects demonstrate absent, bilaterally symmetric, or reversed Nodal and Ptx2 expression, most often resulting in failure of cardiac looping abnormalities and embryonic death [55]. In human beings, mutations in the ACVR2B gene, which codes for human activin receptor IIB, have been associated with left-to-right axis malformations [56].

Wedging

After cardiac looping, individual cardiac chambers become evident. The atrioventricular canal relocates over the right and left ventricles (Fig. 5). The bulbus cordis position is brought toward the future atrioventricular sulcus and

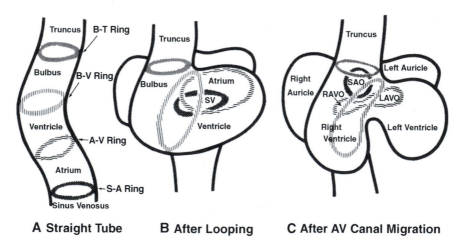

A Straight Tube   B After Looping   C After AV Canal Migration

Fig. 5. (A–B) Wedging. The outflow areas consisting of the bulbus cordis and truncus arteriosus are moving to the embryo's left to provide an outflow for the developing left ventricle. Four specialized tissue or rings, sinoatrial (S-A), atrioventricular (A-V), bulboventricular (B-V) and bulbotruncal (B-T), delimit the segments of the heart tube and are brought into approximation, or "wedged." The outflow areas nestle anterior to the atria, sitting astride the developing interventricular septum. The ventricular septum is eventually closed superiorly with endocardial tissue from the atrioventricular canal, the outlet septum, and fibrous tissue from the perimembranous area. (C) The bulbotruncal ring approximates or "wedges" into the A-V valve ring dividing it into the right-sided atrioventricular orifice (RAVO) and the left-sided atrioventricular orifice (LAVO). The RAVO gives rise to the tricuspid valve ring, and the LAVO is destined to become the mitral valve ring. SAO, sinoatrial orifice; SV, sinus venosus. (Modified from Anderson RH, Becker AE, Wenink ACG, et al. The development of the cardiac specialized tissue. In: Wellens HJJ, Lie K, Janse MJ, editors. The conduction system of the heart. Philadelphia: Lea & Febiger; 1976; with permission.)

positions itself between the mitral and tricuspid valves, a process known as "wedging" [69]. The ventricles grow outward, each with distinctive anatomic muscle patterning. Some of the most severe forms of congenital heart disease are forms of right or left ventricular hypoplasia and are known to have an increased familial frequency. In murine models, the related basic helix-loop-helix (bHLH) transcription factors dHAND/HAND2 and eHAND/HAND1 are expressed predominantly in the primitive right and left ventricular segments, respectively [57,58]. Deletion of dHAND in mice results in right heart hypoplasia. eHAND and Nkx2-5 have been implicated in left heart hypoplasia [59,60]. In the zebrafish, which has a single ventricle, only one HAND gene (dHAND) has been identified, the mutation of which abolishes the ventricular segment of the heart [61]. Neuregulin growth factors from the endocardium and their myocardial receptors, erbB2 and erbB4, are required for the development of ventricular trabeculae. It also seems that the retinoid X receptor-a (RXRa) gene is involved in ventricular chamber development and delineation of the atrioventricular border between the atria and ventricles [62]. This may be implicated in familial forms of Ebstein's malformation, in which downward displacement and atrialization of the right ventricle occur. Vascular endothelial growth factor (VEGF) and angiopoietin-1 are also required for normal trabeculation and proliferation of cardiomyocytes.

Septation of the atria

Normal atrial development consists of fusion of the pulmonary venous anlage to the left atrium in conjunction with growth of the septum secundum and fusion with the primum or atrioventricular septum (Fig. 6). The brachioce-

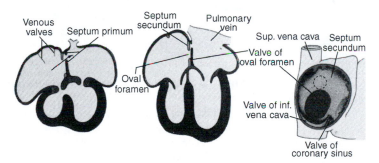

Fig. 6. Atrial septation. Sinus venosus tissue from the atrial back wall fuses with the developing septum primum, which grows caudally to join with cushion tissue from the developing atrioventricular canal. The septum secundum arises to the right of the septum primum and also grows in a crescentic fashion toward the caudal atrioventricular canal. A deficiency in the floor of the septum secundum (fossae ovalis) and the flap of the septum primum serve as the fetal communication known as the foramen ovale. Inf, inferior; Sup, superior (*Modified from* Colvin EV. Cardiac embryology. In: Garson A, Bricker JT, McNamara DG, editors. The science and practice of pediatric cardiology. Philadelphia: Lea & Febiger; 1990. p. 86; with permission.)

phalic vein (innominate vein) transfers blood from the left-sided cardinal vein to the right cardinal vein (superior vena cava). The ductus venosus persists as a connection between the umbilical vein and the right vitelline vein (suprarenal inferior vena cava). The influences controlling regression and persistence of these segments of the embryonic venous structures are largely unknown. Various congenital abnormalities of venous channels are known to occur, including anomalous pulmonary venous drainage channels, various septal defects, interruption of the inferior vena cava, and persistence of a left-sided vena cava. Holt-Oram syndrome, an inheritable form of secundum atrial septal defects associated with radial limb deformities, has been mapped to chromosome 12q2 and has been identified as associated with the TBX gene [63]. In animal models, a nuclear receptor, COUP-TFII, is found in atrial precursors and is required for atrial growth [64].

Development of the atrioventricular valves

Septation of the primary heart tube into distinct chambers is achieved through regional swellings of the extracellular matrix, known as cardiac cushions, that form the anlage of atrioventricular and ventriculoarterial valves. When the cushions first form, they are relatively acellular, but endothelial cells seem to migrate into the cushions and become more spindle shaped [65]. Signaling between the endocardium and myocardial cell layers, mediated in part by TGFβ, induces the transformation of endocardial cells to mesenchymal cells [66]. This transformation does not occur in the absence of myocardiocytes, suggesting that endothelial differentiation is dependent on a signaling chemical trigger. The cell adhesion molecule, N-CAM, is expressed throughout the endocardium before cushion formation, but its expression is downregulated as the endothelial cells migrate into the cardiac jelly. At this point, the endocardial cells begin to express the substrate adhesion molecule (SAM), tenascin. Tenascin has been shown to disrupt cell-substrate adhesion, allowing cells to migrate more freely through the matrix [19]. The common atrioventricular canal differentiates into right- and left-sided valve orifices. This process is often halted in trisomy 21 (Down syndrome), which is typically associated with a common atrioventricular valve. Gene targeting in mice has revealed important roles for the neurofibromatosis (NF)-ATc and Smad6 transcription factors in the formation of the cardiac valves. NF-ATc is a mediator of the calcium-dependent protein phosphatase calcineurin, suggesting a role for calcineurin in transduction of signals for valvulogenesis [67,68]. Additional regulatory molecules include BMP-4 and msx-2 (a member of the homeobox gene family), which have restricted expression within the myocardium of the atrioventricular canal. The differentiation of the cushion mesenchymal cells into valvuloseptal fibroblasts correlates with the expression of fibrillin and fibulin, two microfibrillar proteins thought to serve as a frame for cell adhesion as differentiation occurs.

Conotruncus and development of the aortic and pulmonary arteries

The ventriculoarterial cushions of the conotruncus are histologically similar to the endocardial cushions of the atrioventricular canal. It is generally accepted that there are two pairs of ridges that fuse to form a spiral septum separating the aortic and pulmonary outflow tracts (Fig. 7). The ridges fuse first at the distal outlet septum and then migrate proximally in the outlet conus, fusing with the superior rim of the ventricular septum. Essentially the same type of transformation occurs for the conal cushions, except for the invasion of the cushions by myocardial cells, because there is no muscular component to the terminally differentiated semilunar valves. Neural crest cells originating from the hindbrain region at the level of rhombomeres 6, 7, and 8 migrate to the caudal three pharyngeal arches and become condensed in the mesenchyme, known as the aorticopulmonary septation complex [69]. Thus, neural crest cells in the outlet septum underlie the endothelium that migrates into the pulmonary outflow tract to fuse with the ventricular septum. Many examples of conotruncal anomalies, including truncus arteriosus, tetralogy of Fallot, and double-outlet right ventricle, can be reliably produced in chick embryos by removal of the caudal neural crest at the level of the otic placode to somite 3 (rhombomeres 6, 7, and 8) before neural crest cell migration [70,71].

Deficient contributions from the cranial neural crest are thought to contribute to the congenital diseases DiGeorge syndrome and velocardiofacial syndrome (see the article in this issue on DiGeorge syndrome by Goldmuntz) [72]. The most common features of these syndromes include an interrupted aortic arch, outflow tract malformation, hypoplastic thymus, and hypoparathyroidism [73]. DiGeorge syndrome and velocardiofacial syndrome carry microdeletions in the q11.2 region of chromosome 22. Several critical regions in the area of 22q11 that contribute to the neural crest and multiple candidate genes suspected to play a role in conotruncal septation have now been identified, including cHIRA and Pax3 [25] as well as UFD1 and TBX1 [1]. Functional attenuation of cHIRA in the chick cardiac neural crest results in a significantly increased incidence of truncus arteriosus but does not affect the repatterning of aortic arch arteries, the ventricular function, or the alignment of the outflow tract [25]. Mutations of the TGFβ2 gene result in a failure of the muscular component of the outflow arteries to form, and various abnormalities in the retinoic acid (RA) signal transduction pathway cause several types of outflow tract defects. Mutation of the NF-1 gene in mice causes a double-outlet right ventricle, and ET-1 and dPax-3 mutations are known to cause persistent truncus arteriosus or abnormalities in the aortic arch artery. The diverse group of conotruncal disorders (DiGeorge syndrome, velocardiofacial syndrome, and conotruncal facial syndrome) collectively termed CATCH 22 (cardiac anomalies, abnormal facies, thymic hypoplasia, cleft palate, and hypocalcemia) result from a deletion of the subband in 22q11, which may be detected by fluorescent in situ hybridization (FISH). There is a DiGeorge critical region on chromosome 22 containing several genes, although none has yet been confirmed as functionally involved in cardiogenesis [74–76]. It is possible that

A

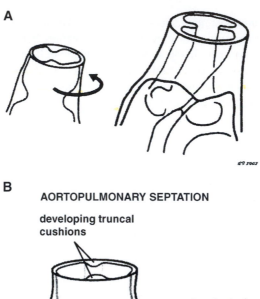

B

AORTOPULMONARY SEPTATION

developing truncal
cushions

counter clockwise
rotation

developing infundibular
cushions

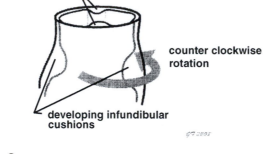

C

AORTOPULMONARY SEPTATION

developing
Ao outflow

developing pulmonary
valve

left AV valve

infundibulum

ventricular septal
defect

right AV valve

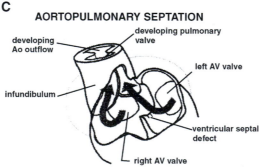

Fig. 7. Development of the aortic and pulmonary valves. (*A*) Frontal view. The single orifice of the truncus arteriosus is initially divided by the anterior and posterior truncal swellings, which grow together to form the initial aorticopulmonary septum. (*B*) At the same time, there is counterclockwise rotation of the entire root, such that the normal aorta moves into a posterior position relative to the pulmonary artery. (*C*) At the same time, the infundibulum or bulbus conus is developing beneath the normal pulmonary valve but regressing beneath the normal aortic valve, resulting in a downward movement of the aortic annulus and valve and a superior leftward movement of the pulmonary valve. This results in the normal relation of a superior leftward pulmonary valve and inferior slightly rightward aortic valve. Ao, aortic; AV, atrioventricular. (*From* Collins-Nakai R, McLaughlin P. How congenital heart disease originates in fetal life. Cardiol Clin 2002;20:377; with permission.)

genes on other chromosomes, specifically 4 and 10, may also play a role in neurogenic cell migration and activity. Because babies born with conotruncal abnormalities may have clinically significant immune deficiency and hypocalcemia, FISH probe assessment should be performed early in all patients with conotruncal anomalies, including truncus arteriosus, aortic arch interruption, right aortic arch, and tetralogy of Fallot.

Aortic arch and its branches

The aortic arch and brachiocephalic vessels arise from components of the branchial cleft vessels that join the ventral aorta sac with the paired dorsal aortae (Fig. 8). Four numbered brachial arteries are apparent in mammals, although as many as six arches are present in other species. Selective regression or persistence of these segments gives rise to the normal aortic arch branching pattern and various anomalies of the aortic arch. Although neural crest migration is not required for the initial formation of the aortic arch arteries, it is required for the maintenance of these vessels [77]. Neural crest components are related to segmentation of the hindbrain and neural crest, which is controlled by homeobox or hox genes. Consequently, the hox proteins expressed by the neural crest control

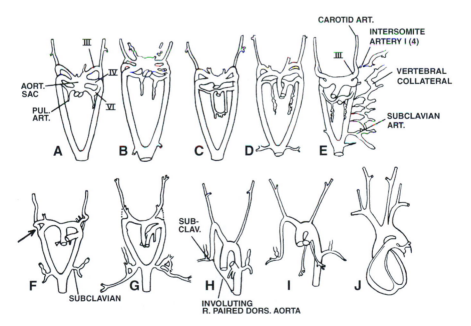

Fig. 8. (*A–J*) Aortic arch and its branches. Development stages in the transformation of the branchial arch system to an asymmetric left aortic arch. The ventral aortic sac connects through a series of six branchial arterial arches to the paired dorsal aortae. AORT, aortic; ART, artery; DORS, dorsal; R, right. (*Modified from* Congdon ED. In: Goor DA, Lillehei CW, editors. Congenital malformations of the heart. New York: Grune and Stratton; 1975. p. 80; with permission.)

the patterning of the aortic arches via migrating neural crest cells. These hox genes do not seem to participate in the outflow tract septation of the heart [78]. Char syndrome, an autosomal dominant trait characterized by patent ductus arteriosus, hand anomalies, and facial dysmorphism, reveals dominant-negative mutations in the transcription factor TFAP2B, which is expressed in the neural crest [79]. Patterning of the pharyngeal arches and outflow regions can be affected not only by neural crest ablation but by the degree of embryonic cervical flexure, direct manipulation of the outflow tract, and teratogens, such as RA. Many of the anomalies that affect the neural crest–derived outflow tract also cause disturbances of aortic arches, suggesting that similar gene patterning is involved. Because failure of neural crest migration seems to be involved in a number of clinically relevant abnormalities (specifically those of the cardiac outflow and aortic arch, with additional involvement of the laryngopharyngeal pouch derivatives, thymus, and parathyroid glands), genetic studies should be considered in this population.

Teratology in cardiovascular development

The period of known cardiac development begins with gastrulation at 15 days of gestation and is morphologically complete by 12 weeks of gestation. Additional disturbances as well as toxicologic, infectious, and as yet unknown influences during this interval may contribute to the development of cardiac malformations.

Known risk factors for congenital heart disease include diabetes mellitus, exposure to rubella, and the use of certain anticonvulsant medications or isotretinoin [25,80] There is a greater than a nine-fold increased risk of transposition of the great arteries for retinol intakes of 10,000 IU or more, as reported by Botto and colleagues [81] using data from the Baltimore-Washington Infant Study.

The presence of maternal fever increased the risk of congenital heart defects by 1.8 times [82]. It has been postulated that there is a threshold (38.9°C) for teratogenesis in human beings [83]. Whether this relates to fever or the infectious agent is unknown.

Recently, it has been suggested that trichloroethylene, a common organic solvent constituent, is also a selective cardiac teratogen inhibiting the development of embryonic heart valve precursors, most commonly resulting in atrial and ventricular septal defects and pulmonary or aortic valvular stenosis. Advanced maternal age was also seen as a contributing risk factor in this study [84]. Maternal age seems to have an influence in association with other teratogens, such as alcohol [85], in addition to being an independent risk factor in adverse birth outcomes, particularly chromosomal abnormalities [86]. The reason for an increased risk in this population is not clear.

Heavy metals (eg, lead, mercury), ethylene oxide, alcohol, and ionizing radiation are confirmed environmental teratogens contributing to pregnancy loss.

Caffeine, cigarette smoking, and hyperthermia are suspected teratogens, and the teratogenic impact of pesticides remains unknown.

In addition to factors causally related to congenital heart disease, the association of several environmental factors, including such diverse influences as air travel, video display terminals, food additives, cosmetics, and pesticides, on fetal loss has been recently reviewed [87]. Before definitive conclusions can be reached regarding the teratogenicity of environmental factors, the following issues need to be considered:

- Gestational age at the time of exposure
- Amount of toxin reaching the conceptus
- Duration of exposure
- Impact of other factors or agents to which the mother or the conceptus is simultaneously exposed
- Physiologic status of mother and conceptus: genetic differences
- Interrelation between frequency of exposures, frequency of effect, and recognizability of adverse outcome

Identification of environmental causal influences of congenital cardiac abnormalities is significantly limited by the relatively low incidence of congenital heart disease and requirement for large numbers of patients for study. There are relatively few toxic chemical levels that can be accurately measured postnatally. The retrospective nature of epidemiologic studies and questionnaires is adversely affected by recall bias. Improvements in databasing, universal coding of all congenital defects, and prospects for potential multicenter trials hold the best prospect for progress in this area.

Summary

Congenital heart disease remains a significant cause of morbidity and mortality. In recent years, significant advances in molecular genetics, improved understanding of morphogenesis, recognition of specific patterning of abnormalities within and between species, and the impact of the Human Genome Project have accounted for these advances. Continued rapid developments in genomics and proteomics are anticipated. Epidemiologic investigations continue to be necessary to assess the influence of the environment on genetics. It is exciting to know that we are on the threshold of influencing the occurrence of congenital heart diseases.

Acknowledgments

Appreciation extended to Kathryn Elizabeth Pelech for editing assistance.

References

[1] Dobell ARC, Van Praagh R. The Holmes heart: historic associations and pathologic anatomy. Am Heart J 1996;132(2):437–45.

[2] Abbott ME. Unique case of malformation of the heart? Defect of the interventricular septum; rudimentary right ventricle; patent foramen ovale; great dilatation of right auricle and right auricular appendix. Montreal Med J 1901;30:522–32.

[3] Abbott ME. Congenital cardiac disease. In: Osler W, McCrae T, editors. Modern medicine. 2nd edition. Philadelphia: Lea & Febiger; 1915. p. 323–448.

[4] Abbott ME. Atlas of congenital cardiac disease. New York: American Heart Association; 1936.

[5] Roland CG. Maude Abbott, MD, "Madonna of the Heart." Med Pediatr Oncol 2000;35:64–5.

[6] von Haller A. Sur la Formation du Coeur [On the formation of the heart]. Lausanne, Switzerland: M.M. Bousquet Publishing Company; 1758 [in French].

[7] Waterston D. The development of the heart in man. Trans R Soc Edinburgh 1918;52:257–302.

[8] Born G. Beitrage zur Entwicklungsgeschichte des Saugetierherzens [History of the development of the sucking animal heart.]. Arch Mikroskop Anat 1889;33:284–378 [in German].

[9] Davis CL. Description of a human embryo having twenty paired somites. Contrib Embryol 1923;15:1–51.

[10] Streeter GL. Developmental horizons in human embryos: description of age group xi, 13–20 somites, and age group xii, 21 to 29 somites. Contrib Embryol 1942;30:211–45.

[11] Streeter GL. Developmental horizons in human embryos: description of age group xiii, embryos about 4 or 5 millimeters long, and age group xiv, period of indention of the lens vesicle. Contrib Embryol 1945;31:27–63.

[12] Streeter GL. Developmental horizons in human embryos: description of age groups xv, xvi, xvii, and xviii, being the third issue of a survey of the Carnegie collection. Contrib Embryol 1948; 32:133–203.

[13] Sissman MJ. Development landmarks and cardiac morphogenesis: comparative chronology. Am J Cardiol 1970;25:141–8.

[14] Shimada Y, Ho E. Scanning electron microscopy of the embryonic chick heart: formation of the epicardium and surface structure of the four heterotypic cells that constitute the embryonic heart. In: Van Praagh R, Takao A, editors. Etiology and morphogenesis of congential heart disease. Mount Kisco, NY: Futura; 1979.

[15] de la Cruz MV, Gomez CS, Arteaga MM, et al. Experimental study of the development of the truncus and the conus in the chick embryo. J Anat 1977;123:661–86.

[16] Ruckman RN, Cassling RJ, Clark EB, et al. Cardiac function in the embryonic chick. In: Pexieder T, editor. Perspectives in cardiovascular research, vol. 5. Mechanisms of cardiac morphogenesis and teratogenesis. New York: Raven Press; 1981.

[17] Paschoud N, Pexieder T. Patterns of proliferation during the organogenetic phase of heart development. In: Pexieder T, editor. Perspectives in cardiovascular research, vol. 5. Mechanisms of cardiac morphogenesis and teratogenesis. New York: Raven Press; 1981.

[18] Arguello C, Servin M. The importance of extracellular matrix components in development of the embryonic chick heart. In: Pexieder T, editor. Perspectives in cardiovascular research, vol. 5. Mechanisms of cardiac morphogenesis and teratogenesis. New York: Raven Press; 1981.

[19] Foroud T. Introduction to genetic linkage analysis. Can Invest 1977;15:548–52.

[20] Savill J. Science, medicine, and the future: molecular genetic approaches to understanding disease. BMJ 1997;314:126–9.

[21] Aerssens J, Armstrong M, Gilissen R, et al. The human genome: an introduction. Oncologist 2001;6:100–9.

[22] Beland MJ, Franklin RC, Jacobs JP, et al. Update from the International Working Group for Mapping and Coding of Nomenclatures for Paediatric and Congenital Heart Disease. Cardiol Young 2004;14(2):225–9.

[23] Hanson-Morris K, Pelech AN. The Wisconsin Pediatric Cardiac Registry: a mechanism for exploring etiologies of congenital heart defects. Wis Med J, in press.

[24] Rasmussen SA, Lammer EJ, Shaw GM, et al. Integration of DNA sample collection into a multi-site birth defects case control study. Teratology 2002;66(4):177–84.

[25] Ferencz C, Correa-Villasenor A, Loffredo CA, et al. Genetics and environmental risk factors of major cardiovascular malformations: the Baltimore-Washington Infant Study: 1981–1989. In: Anderson RH, editor. Perspectives in pediatric cardiology, vol. 5. Armonk (NY): Futura Publishing; 1997. p. 59–102.

[26] Garg V, Kathiriya IS, Barnes R, et al. GATA4 mutations cause human congenital heart defects and reveal an interaction with TBX5. Nature 2003;424(6947):443–7.

[27] McBride KL, Pignatelli RL, Ho T, et al. Inheritance analysis of congenital left ventricular outflow tract obstruction malformations: segregation, multiplex relative risk, and heritability. Am J Med Genet A 2005;134(2):180–6.

[28] Risch N, Merikangas K. The future of genetic studies of complex human diseases. Science 1996;273:1516–7.

[29] Spielman RS, McGinnis RE, Ewens WJ. Transmission test for linkage disequilibrium: the insulin gene region and insulin-dependent diabetes mellitus (IDDM). Am J Hum Genet 1993;52(3):506–16.

[30] Pritchard JK, Rosenberg NA. Use of unlinked genetic markers to detect population stratification in association studies. Am J Hum Genet 1999;65(1):220–8.

[31] Pritchard JK, Stephens M, Donnelly P. Inference of population structure using multilocus genotype data. Genetics 2000;155(2):945–59.

[32] Pritchard JK, Stephens M, Rosenberg NA, et al. Association mapping in structured populations. Am J Hum Genet 2000;67(1):170–81.

[33] Matsuzaki H, Dong S, Loi H, et al. Genotyping over 100,000 SNPs on a pair of oligonucleotide arrays. Nat Methods 2004;1(2):109–11.

[34] Edwards AO, Ritter III R, Abel KJ, et al. Complement factor H polymorphism and age-related macular degeneration. Science 2005;308(5720):421–4.

[35] Klein RJ, Zeiss C, Chew EY, et al. Complement factor H polymorphism in age-related macular degeneration. Science 2005;308(5720):385–9.

[36] Collins-Nakai R, McLaughlin P. How congenital heart disease originates in fetal life. Cardiol Clin 2002;20(3):367–83.

[37] Srivastava D, Olson E. A genetic blueprint for cardiac development. Nature 2000;407:221–6.

[38] Rosenquist GC. Migration of precardiac cells from their origin in epiblast until they form the definitive heart in the chick embryo. In: Ferrans VA, Rosenquist GC, Weinstein C, editors. Cardiac morphogenesis. New York: Elsevier; 1985. p. 44–54.

[39] Stalsberg H, DeHaan R. The precardiac areas and formation of the tubular heart in the chick embryo. Dev Biol 1969;19:128–59.

[40] Rosenquist GC, DeHaan RL. Migration of precardiac cells in the chick embryo: a radioautographic study. Contrib Embryol 1966;38:111–21.

[41] Schultheis TM, Zydas S, Lassar AB. Induction of avian cardiac myogenesis by anterior endoderm. Development 1995;121:4203–14.

[42] Fu Y, Yan W, Mohun TJ, et al. Vertebrate tinman homologues XNkx2–3 and XNkx2–5 are required for heart formation in a functionally redundant manner. Development 1998;125:4439–49.

[43] Grow MW, Kreig PA. Tinman function is essential for vertebrate heart development: elimination of cardiac differentiation by dominant inhibitory mutants of the tinman-related genes, XNkx2–3 and XNkx2–5. Dev Biol 1998;204:187–96.

[44] Heikinheimo M, Scandrett JM, Wilson DB. Localization of transcription factor GATA-4 to regions of the mouse embryo involved in cardiac development. Dev Biol 1994;164:361–73.

[45] Lackie JM. Cell movement and cell behaviour. London: Allen & Unwin; 1986.

[46] McQuinn TC, Takao A. Experimental embryology and teratology. In: Garson A, Bricker JT, McNamara DG, editors. The science and practice of pediatric cardiology. Philadelphia: Lea & Febiger; 1990. p. 152–70.

[47] Ruoslahti E, Pierschbacher MD. Arg-Gly-Asp: a versatile cell recognition signal. Cell 1986;44:517–8.

[48] Naidet C, Sémériva M, Yamada KM, et al. Peptides containing the cell-attachment recognition signal Arg-Gly-Asp prevent gastrulation in Drosophila embryos [letter]. Nature 1987;325: 348–50.

[49] Davis CL. Description of a human embryo having twenty paired somites. Contrib Embryol 1923; 15:1–51.

[50] Stalsberg H, DeHaan R. The precardiac areas and formation of the tubular heart in the chick embryo. Dev Biol 1969;19:128–59.

[51] Pexieder T. Development of the outflow tract of the embryonic heart. In: Rosenquist GC, Bergsma D, editors. Morphogenesis and malformation of the cardiovascular system. (Birth defects: original article series, vol. 14.) New York: Alan R. Liss; 1978. p. 29–68.

[52] Manasek FJ. Determinants of heart shape in early embryos. Fed Proc 1981;40:2011–6.

[53] Icardo JM, Ojeda JL. Effects of colchicine on the formation and looping of the tubular heart of the embryonic chick. Acta Anat (Basel) 1984;119:1–9.

[54] Stalsberg H, DeHaan R. The precardiac areas and formation of the tubular heart in the chick embryo. Dev Biol 1969;19:128–59.

[55] Capdevila J, Vogan KJ, Tabin CJ, et al. Mechanisms of left-right determination in vertebrates. Cell 2000;101:9–21.

[56] Kosaki R, Gebbia M, Kosaki K, et al. Left-right axis malformations associated with mutations in ACVR2B, the gene for human activin receptor type IIB. Am J Genet 1999;82(1):70–6.

[57] Srivastava D, Cserjesi P, Olson EN. New subclass of bHLH proteins required for cardiac morphogenesis. Science 1995;270:1995–9.

[58] Srivastava D, Thomas T, Lin Q, et al. Regulation of cardiac mesodermal and neural crest development by the bHLH transcription factor, dHAND. Nat Genet 1997;16:154–60.

[59] Firulli AB, McFadden DG, Lin Q, et al. Heart and extra embryonic mesodermal defects in mouse embryos lacking the bHLH transcription factor Hand1. Nat Genet 1998;8:266–70.

[60] Riley P, Anson-Cartwright L, Cross JC. The Hand1 bHLH transcription factor is essential for placentation and cardiac morphogenesis. Nat Genet 1998;18:271–5.

[61] Yelon D, Ticho B, Halpern ME, et al. Parallel roles for the bHLH transcription factor HAND2 in zebrafish and pectoral fin development. Development 2000;127:2573–82.

[62] Dyson E, Sucor HM, Kubalak SW, et al. Atrial-like phenotype is associated with embryonic ventricular failure in retinoid X receptor alpha−/− mice. Proc Natl Acad Sci USA 1995;92: 7386–90.

[63] Li QY, Newbury-Ecob RA, Terrett JA, et al. Holt-Oram syndrome is caused by mutations in TBX5, a member of the Brachyury (T) gene family. Nat Genet 1997;15:21–9.

[64] Pereira FA, Qui Y, Zhou G, et al. The orphan nuclear receptor COUP-TFII is required for angiogenesis and heart development. Gene Dev 1999;13:1037–49.

[65] Markwald RR, Fitzharris TP, Bolender DL, et al. Structural analysis of cell matrix association during the morphogenesis of atrioventricular cushion tissue. Dev Biol 1979;69:634–54.

[66] Brown CB, Boyer AS, Runyan RB, et al. Requirement of type III TGF beta receptor for endocardial cell transformation in the heart. Science 1999;283:2080–2.

[67] Ranger AM, Grusby MJ, Hodge MR, et al. The transcription factor NF-Atc is essential for cardiac valve formation. Nature 1998;392:186–90.

[68] De la Pompa JL, Timmerman LA, Takimoto H, et al. Role of the NF-Atc transcription factor in morphogenesis of cardiac valves and septum. Nature 1998;392:182–6.

[69] Kirby ML, Waldo KL. Neural crest and cardiovascular patterning. Circ Res 1995;77:211–5.

[70] Nishibatake M, Kirby ML, van Mierop LH. Pathogenesis of persistent truncus arteriosus and dextroposed aorta in the chick embryo after neural crest ablation. Circulation 1987;75: 255–64.

[71] Kirby ML, Waldo KL. Neural crest and cardiovascular patterning. Circ Res 1995;77:211–5.

[72] Goldmuntz E, Emanuel BS. Genetic disorders of cardiac morphogenesis: the DiGeorge and velocardiofacial syndromes. Circ Res 1997;80:437–43.

[73] Wilson DI, Burn J, Scambler P, et al. DiGeorge syndrome: part of CATCH 22. J Med Genet 1993;30:852–6.

[74] Epstein JA, Buck CA. Transcriptional regulation of cardiac development: implications for congenital heart disease and DiGeorge syndrome. Pediatr Res 2000;48(6):717–24.

[75] Jerome AL, Papaiuannou V. DiGeorge syndrome phenotype in mice mutant for the T-box gene, Tbx1. Nat Genet 2001;27:286–91.

[76] Kim MS, Basson CT. Wrapping up DiGeorge syndrome in a T-box? Pediatr Res 2001;50(3): 307–8.

[77] Suvov HM. Molecular insights into cardiac development. Annu Rev Physiol 1998;60:287–308.

[78] Leaatherbury L. Embryology and genetics. In: Collins-Nakai RL, editor. Pediatric and adult congential cardiac self-assessment program. Bethesda (MD): American College of Cardiology; 1998.

[79] Srivastava D, Olson E. A genetic blueprint for cardiac development. Nature 2000;407:221–6.

[80] Lammer EJ, Chen DT, Hoar RM, et al. Retinoic acid embryopathy. N Engl J Med 1985;313(14): 837–41.

[81] Botto LD, Loffredo C, Scanlon KS, et al. Vitamin A and cardiac outflow tract defects. Epidemiology 2001;12(5):491–6.

[82] Botto LD, Lynberg MC, Erickson JD. Congenital heart defects, maternal febrile illness, and multivitamin use: a population-based study. Epidemiology 2001;12(5):485–90.

[83] Graham Jr JM, Edwards MJ, Edwards MJ. Teratogen update: gestational effects of maternal hyperthermia due to febrile illnesses and resultant patterns of defects in humans. Teratology 1998;58(5):209–21.

[84] Yauck JS, Malloy ME, Blair K, et al. Proximity of residence to trichloroethylene-emitting sites and increased risk of offspring congenital heart defects among older women. Birth defects research (part A). Clinical and Molecular Teratology 2004;70:808–14.

[85] Jacobsen JL, Jacobson SW, Sokol RJ, et al. Relation of maternal age and pattern of pregnancy drinking to functionally significant cognitive deficit in infancy. Alcohol Clin Exp Res 1998; 22:345–51.

[86] Pradat P, Francannet C, Harris JA, et al. The epidemiology of cardiovascular defects, I. part, a study based on data from three large registries of congenital malformations. Pediatr Cardiol 2003;24:195–221.

[87] Gardella JR, Hill JA. Environmental toxins associated with recurrent pregnancy loss. Semin Reprod Med 2000;18(4):407–24.

ELSEVIER
SAUNDERS

CLINICS IN
PERINATOLOGY

Clin Perinatol 32 (2005) 845–855

Cardiac Development: New concepts

Peter J. Gruber, MD, PhD[a,b,*]

^a*Cardiac Center, The Children's Hospital of Philadelphia,*
University of Pennsylvania School of Medicine, Suite 8527, 34th Street and Civic Center Boulevard,
Philadelphia, PA 19104, USA
^b*The Molecular Cardiology Research Center, University of Pennsylvania School of Medicine,*
Suite 8527, 34th Street and Civic Center Boulevard, Philadelphia, PA 19104, USA

Congenital heart disease (CHD) is a devastating complex of diseases resulting from defects of development. It affects more than 1 of every 100 live births and is responsible for most prenatal losses [1,2]. Additionally, 3 per 1000 live births require an intervention (catheter based or surgical) during the first year of life. Despite its prevalence and severity, the causes of CHD are largely unknown. A clear molecular mechanism has been identified in only a small number of instances. In most of these situations, there is a vast gap between identifying the causative gene and understanding the mechanism by which structural or functional defects occur. Indeed, the ability to identify potential disease targets now far outstrips the capacity to test these hypotheses and define their mechanisms. What are the obstacles to unraveling the molecular controls of heart morphogenesis, and are there real-time solutions?

Presently, there is an acceleration of significant discovery that should reshape our understanding of congenital cardiac disorders. These advances include the description of an increasing number of gene-targeted mouse models of human cardiac disease; the availability of nearly complete genome sequence information for multiple organisms, including human beings; and increasingly sophisticated bioinformatics tools with which to use these data. The manipulation of gene expression is now possible not only in mouse models, where homologous recombination can be used to inactivate or modify a gene, but in organisms like zebrafish and Xenopus (frogs), where newer techniques can be used to analyze gene expression rapidly and efficiently. Increasingly, investigators are using

---

* The Cardiac Center, Children's Hospital of Philadelphia, University of Pennsylvania School of Medicine, Suite 8527, 34th Street and Civic Center Boulevard, Philadelphia, PA 19104.
E-mail address: pgruber@mail.med.upenn.edu

0095-5108/05/$ – see front matter © 2005 Elsevier Inc. All rights reserved.
doi:10.1016/j.clp.2005.09.003

multiple organisms to model human disease because each provides distinct advantages. This review highlights the most recent and promising avenues of current research in cardiac development in terms of emerging molecular data and model systems.

Approaches to congenital heart disease

How does one experimentally identify genetic associations with disease? Traditionally, these fall into two broad categories: forward or reverse genetic approaches. Historically, primitive model organisms, such as *Drosophila mela-nogaster* (fruit fly) or *Caenorhabditid elegans* (worm), were used in a classic forward genetic approach. In forward genetics, a genetic screen is used to identify mutants that produce a phenotype. Mutant organisms are isolated, and genes are identified by association of a genetic marker (a physical location on a chromosome) with a phenotype. The limiting factor in this type of study has been the ability to associate, or map, a gene to the mutant location (locus), a function of the density of the markers or locators on the DNA strand. In human beings, a similar approach is taken in which patients with a disease are examined for the presence of markers that cosegregate with the disease. In contrast to induced mutations in flies, a group of patients with a disease (natural mutants) are linked to genetic markers. With a close set of physical markers (usually single nucleotide polymorphisms [SNPs]), one can map the disease location to a fine resolution, such that candidate genes can be identified. Because most interesting cardiac morphologic abnormalities rare, informative CHD data sets are usually small, making this process difficult. In contrast, investigators studying oncogenesis frequently study patient data sets that number in the thousands [3]. This process, known as linkage analysis, was a formidable task, because markers were scarce. To overcome this problem, an increasingly dense physical map was required. Practically, with near completion of the Human Genome Project in the last 5 years, this hurdle of marker density has now become much easier. Now, it is often easier to find genes in human beings than it is in more primitive model organisms simply on the basis of sequence availability. The Haplotype Mapping (HapMap) project is a new initiative that should improve the speed and accuracy of these forward genetic approaches even further. The HapMap project endeavors to use haplotypes, or groups of SNPs that behave similarly, simultaneously to reduce the complexity of the number of markers as well as increase the power of genetic associations [4]. Certainly, classic forward genetic methods of gene identification are more powerful than ever before and ripe for further harvest.

A second method of gene identification is a reverse genetic approach. Instead of starting with a disease and finding the gene, one begins with a hypothesis in which a candidate gene is mutated in an animal model to produce a phenotype. This method is direct in that it not only associates a mutation with a phenotype but often provides powerful insights into its mechanism of action. Subsequently, human populations that mimic the animal model are examined for mutations in

the candidate gene. But how does one start? Which genes should one test? Increasingly, new technologies are making this approach less expensive in terms of time and money. Increasingly, techniques, such as conditional gene targeting, that incorporate temporal and spatial specificity to gene manipulation experiments are now routine. Forward and reverse approaches have been successful in identifying causative disease genes, although the most powerful studies use animal models to provide the mechanism and human genetics to validate animal hypotheses.

Yet an even more powerful (and considerably less expensive) way to improve the resolution of forward genetic experiments is to expand data sets through collaboration. Making rare samples available to multiple investigators should become a priority, using Comprehensive Cancer Center tissue banks as a paradigm for resource sharing. In 1992, the Department of Energy (DOE) and National Institutes of Health (NIH) published a series of guidelines on data sharing entitled *DOE-NIH Guidelines Policy for Sharing Data and Resources* [5]. Although these guidelines were intended to enforce timely sharing of resources generated by the Human Genome Project, the precedent was set for a broader application. Indeed, since 2002, 50% of program announcements (PAs) and 60% of requests for applications (RFAs) now require a data-sharing policy. Recent recommendations by the National Academy of Sciences denoted UPSIDE (uniform principle for sharing integral data expeditiously) [6,7] to emphasize the advantages of collaborative approaches. As further emphasis, over the past 3 years, the NIH has become explicit in its policy toward sharing of published publicly funded resources, with 50% of PAs and 60% of RFAs now requiring an explicit data-sharing policy; recent reports now suggest that this figure is becoming 100%. Considerable bioinformatic, logistic, and financial hurdles need to be addressed to ensure the wide adaptation of these principles, but political impediments should be abandoned. I next discuss examples of recent animal models that fulfill these criteria and phenocopy human disease. The critical next step is the difficult task of filling in the signaling details that should eventually allow one to manipulate the system to identify the actual mechanisms by which these diseases occur.

TBX1

DiGeorge syndrome is a complex of abnormalities that can be caused by a deletion in chromosome 22q11.2 and by a mutation in the gene *TBX1* (see the article on DiGeorge syndrome by Goldmuntz in this issue). It consists of thymic and parathyroid hypoplasia, resulting in hypocalcemia as well as defects in the outflow tract of the heart. These defects are all attributable to disturbances in the migration of neural crest cells into pharyngeal arches and pouches. The neural crest is a multipotential group of cells that migrate into the heart and are critical to the development of septae and outflow tract structures. An increasing number of genes affecting neural crest migration and function (eg, Pax3, semaphorins,

Notch) have been shown to produce cardiac defects when mutated [8–11]. DiGeorge syndrome may present as a number of overlapping phenotypes, including velocardiofacial syndrome (VCFS), conotruncal anomaly face syndrome, or isolated defects of cardiac outflow tract development [12]. *TBX1* itself is a gene that maps to the center of the DiGeorge chromosomal region of 22q11.2 and is a member of a set of phylogenetically conserved genes that share a common DNA binding domain, the T-box [13]. Although there are other conserved protein domains, they are considerably more divergent. At the current time, there are at least 20 distinct members, of which a number (*Tbx1*, *Tbx2*, *Tbx3*, *Tbx5*, *Tbx18*, and *Tbx20*) are expressed in regions that portend their clinical phenotype [14].

The identification of the role of *TBX1* in the formation of DiGeorge syndrome is an excellent example of the confluence of forward and reverse genetic techniques required to investigate complex phenotypes. As a first step, using classic forward genetic approaches, a 3-megabase critical chromosomal microdeletion of approximately 20 genes was associated with the clinical phenotype of DiGeorge syndrome. Subsequent mapping of the syndrome to an individual gene was confounded by the fact that the severity of the phenotype was not related to the size of the deletion, however. Further obscuring mapping attempts, several distinct nonoverlapping chromosomal microdeletions result in similar clinical pictures. By testing individual genes in the region identified through human forward genetic mapping approaches, patients with clinical phenotypes consistent with DiGeorge syndrome but lacking chromosomal deletions were examined for evidence of mutations. Despite considerable efforts, no convincing evidence of a single gene mutation was found [15]. Alternative approaches were required, and the focus shifted toward animal models.

Mice are similar to human beings in genetic and physical structure. Despite some differences, they are an excellent model to study cardiac development. One such difference is that the location of the DiGeorge region of human chromosome 22q11 is on mouse chromosome 16. Importantly, the relative genetic structure (composition and order of the genes) of the area is nearly identical, such that alterations of this region of mouse chromosome 16 should predict those of human chromosome 22 [16,17]. In a seminal experiment, mice engineered with deletion deficient for this homologous region displayed abnormalities similar to those of DiGeorge syndrome. Importantly, reintroducing individual genes located in this region corrected the cardiac defects, thus providing strong evidence for the direct involvement of these genes in the pathogenesis of DiGeorge syndrome [18]. Further microdeletions engineered in other laboratories narrowed down this region in a fashion identical to the original performed in human beings. These experiments showed that only abnormalities in *Tbx1* phenocopy the cardiac abnormalities seen in DiGeorge syndrome [19–21]. Importantly, further investigations using specific *Tbx1* gene-targeted mice conclusively demonstrated that an altered *Tbx1* dosage recapitulates the full spectrum of DiGeorge syndrome and VCFS defects [22]. Further mechanistic insight came from the zebrafish animal model, in which there is a mutation called *van gogh*. This mutant was originally identified in a screen for jaw mutations in fish. During this mutational screen, a mutant was identified whose most prominent external feature was a small ear. Subsequently, the gene associated with this defect was found to disrupt the gene *tbx1*, and the corresponding embryos were further found to have defective development of pharyngeal neural crest derivatives [23]. Finally, moving back to human beings, mutations in *TBX1* were screened in 13 patients from 10 families that had clinical features of DiGeorge syndrome but harbored no microdeletions. Two mutations were found in 2 unrelated patients, and a third mutation was found in 3 patients in a family with the closely related VCFS [24]. With three animal systems (fish, mouse, and human) all supporting the hypothesis, *tbx1* (*Tbx1*, *TBX1*) can now be confidently described as the critical (although not only) gene involved in the pathogenesis of DiGeorge syndrome.

Regardless of the identification of *Tbx1* as the gene responsible for the cardiac defects of DiGeorge syndrome and closely related 22q11 syndromes, the mechanism responsible for the clinical phenotype remains obscure. How does a mutation in a single protein result in morphologic limb and cardiac defects? In fact, *Tbx1* alone cannot entirely account for the defects of DiGeorge syndrome, and other genes are likely to be important. It is largely through studies in mice and lower organisms that these few molecular insights have come. As mentioned previously, *Tbx1* is expressed in certain regions of the heart but also in areas surrounding the neural crest. With what proteins does *Tbx1* interact, and what genes does it regulate? Using genetic studies in fish, flies, and rodents, *Tbx1* has been found to regulate expression of fibroblast growth factors (Fgfs) 8 and 10, and deletion of *Fgf* "downstream genes" in the region of expression of *Tbx1* reproduces the defects seen in DiGeorge syndrome [25]. Other genes, such as *Vegf* and members of the *Forkhead* family, are now adding yet one more layer of details into the mechanism of these defects [26]. Importantly, none of the advances detailed here would have been possible without the cross-fertilization of human molecular genetics, genetic engineering of mice, large-scale genetic screens of lower organisms, and bioinformatics, and, increasingly, the pace of these changes is accelerating because of just this confluence of technologies.

GATA4

In contrast to *Tbx1*, where a classic forward genetic approach was the first clue toward identification of the molecular basis of DiGeorge syndrome, *GATA4* is a disease gene that was first examined in pure reverse genetics and then amplified in understanding with human studies. The *GATA* genes are a small family of evolutionarily ancient proteins that share a common DNA recognition core sequence (the nucleotides G-A-T-A) on DNA promoters and regulatory regions to which they bind and act as transcriptional regulators [27–29]. The proteins have two zinc-finger DNA binding motifs that mediate DNA-protein interactions as well as protein-protein interactions. First discovered in the early 1980s, there are two primary families, *GATA 1*, *2*, and *3*, which are important in various aspects of hematopoiesis, and *GATA 4, 5*, and *6*, which are important for the development of mesodermal derivatives, including the gut, heart, liver, and gonads. Decades of experiments in tissue culture, rodents, chicks, and frogs all demonstrated that *Gata4* is important for cardiac differentiation, although the precise role of the protein in cardiac morphogenesis is not clear. Nearly 10 years later, chromosomal deletions in the region of 8p23.1 (where the human *GATA4* locus resides) were confirmed in patients with CHD, with a wide variety of CHD diagnoses (eg, atrial and ventricular septal defects, double-outlet right ventricle, complete common atrioventricular canal, pulmonary stenosis, hypoplastic left heart syndrome) suggesting that haploinsufficiency of *GATA4* may contribute to the formation of human CHD [30]. Further studies in nonsyndromic human beings expanded these findings, with the identification of *GATA4* point mutations in nonchromosomal patients [31]. Using a forward genetic approach with a large kindred spanning five generations, a whole-genome linkage analysis was performed, localizing the associated mutation to 8p22. By direct sequencing of *GATA4*, a single-base DNA change was identified that led to a single amino acid change in the GATA4 protein. In itself, this was a significant finding, although it was the pursuit of the mechanism that made this work more remarkable. Moving back again to in vitro model systems, identical mutant GATA4 was engineered and examined in tissue culture cells for its ability to activate genes important in cardiac development. Mimic mutations did indeed reduce the transcriptional activity of the GATA4. By what molecular mechanism does this take place, however?

GATA4 interacts with TBX-5 and NKX2-5, two molecules critical for cardiac morphogenesis. Did the identified human mutation alter the ability of GATA4 to interact functionally with these proteins or others important for cardiac development? Experiments in tissue culture cells using engineered proteins demonstrated that this was the case and additionally demonstrated a new interaction between GATA4 and TBX5. Additionally, *TBX5* mutations linked to similar cardiac abnormalities were examined and found to interrupt the GATA 4 interaction motif, providing reciprocal evidence for this important interaction. This combination of human genetics and biochemical analyses built on a molecular and bioinformatics background using multiple animal models demonstrates the power of current technology and also points toward a profound understanding of the mechanisms that produce CHD.

Cofactors and epigenetics

Traditional approaches identifying transcription factor mutations and analysis have largely been mined. We can estimate that this is the case because of the redundancy we now see in mouse mutants: phenotypes now fall into a predictable set of subclasses, only a small fraction of which actually resemble clinical CHD. Rather than identifying new primary effectors, new insights are now coming from adaptor molecules or cofactors (connector molecules that transduce or amplify signals). Myocardin is a member of the SAP family of transcription factors that associate with serum response factor (SRF), which is itself a widely expressed transcription factor that regulates the expression of many cardiac genes. Although the dynamics and signaling pathways of SRF function have been extensively probed in many animal model systems, new insights are being discovered by its interactions with other proteins, such as myocardin. Subsequently, other partners of myocardin named myocardin related transcription factor (MRTF)s have been uncovered. These demonstrate yet a third layer of complexity in this transcription factor network, and some mutants of these genes produce CHD in rodents [32–35]. Undoubtedly, this provided the heart with more ways to adapt to physiologic perturbations and provided a means for developmental and/or evolutionary complexity and robustness [36]. Comparison between primitive and complex developmental models may provide clues as to how these layers contribute to the above-mentioned attributes. The cross-talk between signaling systems is the next level that should reveal relations that can be harvested for basic biologic understanding as well as therapy.

A second example of these is the recent discovery of the profound effect of epigenetic modulators in development and disease [37]. Global regulators of transcriptional processes conceptually allow the simultaneous modulation of genetic loci. Sequence-specific DNA binding proteins recruit epigenetic modulators, such as histone deactylases (HDACs), histone acetyl transferase (HAT), and DNA methyl transferases (DNMT). These, in turn, alter the conformation of the DNA strand and thus the activity of the genes contained in that location. HDACs are global regulators of transcriptional activity that have been identified to have profound effects on cardiac development and disease. The family of HDACs is composed of at least 11 family members with unique expression patterns. Seminal insights by Olson and others [36] have led to a generalizable model in which the recruitment of HDACs to a chromosomal locus results in the deactylation and, in general, deactivation of transcriptional units. The critical role of class II HDACs, such as HDAC9, in the modulation of cardiac hypertrophy was elegantly demonstrated by overexpression and gene deletion studies in rodents [38]. Importantly, the activity of many of these proteins can be inhibited by small molecules and may be used to modulate cardiac function in a clinically relevant manner.

Again, to consider intervening in the process of CHD, understanding the mechanism—not just the gene responsible—is the key. Molecules that are critical to the initiation of cardiac morphogenesis have been studied in great detail (*Nkx2–5*, *Gata*, and *Tbx* family members), but only in rare cases has a partial mechanism for the defects been elucidated. This is an important point for cross-fertilization between the clinician and the scientist. For the most part, the molecular data to date are interesting to biologists and geneticists but not yet suitable for clinical consumption. From a human genetic perspective, despite advances in technology, it is not yet financially feasible (or scientifically plausible) to examine all patients with CHD for defects in candidate genes. We simply do not yet know enough about the molecular pathogenesis of these diseases to provide useful information for families or physicians. From the developmental biologic perspective, knowledge of GATA4 interactions with a small number of other transcription factors does not yet tell us with sufficient depth why patients have holes in their heart, thickened leaflets, or altered conal muscular orientations. What is the mechanism by which the ventricular septal crest, atrial septum, and endocardial cushions are guided, meet, join, and differentiate into mature cardiac structures? Are these relatively late morphogenic events dictated directly by these same molecules, or are entirely different combinatorial sets of molecules still waiting to be discovered? How can these questions be approached?

It is a confluence of techniques, animal systems, and increasingly, a systems biologic approach that must be used to tackle complexity directly. It is likely that the further away from an early nodal point of cardiac differentiation one examines, the greater is the complexity of the interactions. The use of microarrays, or chips, especially those that evaluate global genomic information in terms of RNA production (expression arrays), location (BAC arrays), or function (chromatin immunoprecipitation on chips), is likely to be critical to generate large-scale simultaneous information. Importantly, these increasingly large data sets need to be processed, housed, and made available in such a format that they (the data sets) can all talk to each other. Through these naive-based approaches, novel hypotheses can then be generated to test in animal model systems. Three additional steps also have to be filled with respect to these ends. First, funding bodies have to recognize the value of the generation of these data sets outside the traditional paradigm of narrow hypothesis-driven investigation— what we are looking for is new hypotheses. Second, we need to evaluate these hypotheses rapidly, something for which lower animal systems, such as zebrafish, may be ideally suited. The ability to use knockdown (rather than the more precise but cumbersome knockout) technologies, such as RNA interference (RNAi), in a time-sensitive manner is providing a method to cull the pathways of interest, such that only the most promising need to be tested in expensive time-consuming mouse genetic models. Third, precise clinical phenotypes (in rodents and human beings) need to be integrated with molecular data. It is no longer appropriate for an article in the basic scientific literature to report a ventricular septal defect without specifying its specific subtype (eg, conoventricular, muscular, conoseptal). Similarly, an atrial septal defect must be identified by the specific location in the atrial septum and differentiated from a patent foramen ovale.

New approaches

What systems provide the best hope for future progress? Despite the great success that organisms like worms, flies, and zebrafish have, mice have at least three distinct advantages. First, they are mammals and, despite some differences as outlined previously, provide an excellent animal model of cardiac development. Second, more than 99% of mouse genes have homologues in human beings, and, third, the mouse genome supports targeted mutagenesis, allowing genes to be altered efficiently and precisely. These facts have catalyzed efforts to create large-scale mutation resources. Several large-scale mouse genetics programs are now fully operational. One such program, the N-ethyl-N-nitrosourea (ENU) Mouse Mutagenesis Program, uses genetic approaches to model human genetic disease and identify some key pathways [39]. The research program was aimed at generating large numbers of new mouse phenotypes, many of which are planned to carry disorders that model human genetic disease. Characterization of selected phenotypes using a positional candidate cloning approach should identify the underlying genes causing the phenotypes and yield information about the genetic pathways involved. Approximately 500 novel mouse phenotypes were identified from the mutagenesis screen in phase I, although screening for cardiac defects has not been a focus because morphologic defects are often lethal and therefore more cumbersome to study. The International Gene Trap Consortium has established banks of mutated embryonic stem (ES) cells with sequence-verified gene traps; however, to date, only approximately 10% of all genes have been deleted [40]. The Knockout Mouse project and the European Conditional Mouse Mutagenesis Program are now coordinating efforts in many areas to provide a complete catalog of gene mutations [41,42]. A promising new mode of gene interference is posttranscriptional gene silencing by RNAi. Introduction of RNA duplexes is an additional tool that can be used to reduce expression of a specific gene [43,44]. Indeed, RNAi technologies may provide many advantages over conventional gene targeting and should certainly complement classic gene deletion techniques. Largely unmined are the potentials of proteomics and epigenomics as well as epiproteomics. There is some evidence that protein modifications, such as sumolyation, glycosylation, and lipid modifications, such as myristilasation and farnesylisation, can profoundly influence later protein activity, with developmental and pathophysiologic ramifications [45–47]. These and other new approaches will lead to better research, diagnosis, and treatment of children with congenital heart disease.

References

[1] Hoffman JI. Incidence of congenital heart disease: I. Postnatal incidence. Pediatr Cardiol 1995;16:103–13.

[2] Hoffman JI, Kaplan S. The incidence of congenital heart disease. J Am Coll Cardiol 2002; 39:1890–900.

[3] Poynter JN, Gruber SB, Higgins PD, et al. Statins and the risk of colorectal cancer. N Engl J Med 2005;352:2184–92.

[4] Foster MW, Sharp RR. Beyond race: towards a whole-genome perspective on human populations and genetic variation. Nat Rev Genet 2004;5:790–6.

[5] Department of Energy/National Institutes of Health. DOE-NIH guidelines for sharing data and resources policy. Human Genome News 1992;4:4.

[6] Czech T. Sharing publication-related and materials: responsibilities of authorship in the life sciences. Washington, DC: The National Academy Press. p. 1–16.

[7] Cozzarelli NR. UPSIDE: uniform principle for sharing integral data and materials expeditiously. Proc Natl Acad Sci USA 2004;101:3721–2.

[8] Brown CB, Feiner L, Lu MM, et al. PlexinA2 and semaphorin signaling during cardiac neural crest development. Development 2001;128:3071–80.

[9] Feiner L, Webber AL, Brown CB, et al. Targeted disruption of semaphorin 3C leads to persistent truncus arteriosus and aortic arch interruption. Development 2001;128:3061–70.

[10] Jarriault S, Brou C, Logeat F, et al. Signalling downstream of activated mammalian Notch. Nature 1995;377:355–8.

[11] Li L, Krantz ID, Deng Y, et al. Alagille syndrome is caused by mutations in human Jagged1, which encodes a ligand for Notch1. Nat Genet 1997;16:243–51.

[12] McKusick V. DiGeorge syndrome. In: Online Mendelian inheritance in man. 2004. Available at: http://www.ncbi.nlm.nih.gov/entrez/dispomim.cgi?id=188400.

[13] Tiller G, McKusick V. T-box 1. Online Mendelian inheritance in man. 2005. Available at: http://www.ncbi.nlm.nih.gov/entrez/dispomim.cgi?id=602054.

[14] Plageman Jr TF, Yutzey KE. T-box genes and heart development: putting the "T" in heart. Dev Dyn 2005;232:11–20.

[15] Epstein JA. Developing models of DiGeorge syndrome. Trends Genet 2001;17(Suppl):S13–7.

[16] Galili N, Baldwin HS, Lund J, et al. A region of mouse chromosome 16 is syntenic to the DiGeorge, velocardiofacial syndrome minimal critical region. Genome Res 1997;7:399.

[17] Lund J, Roe B, Chen F, et al. Sequence-ready physical map of the mouse chromosome 16 region with conserved synteny to the human velocardiofacial syndrome region on 22q11.2. Mamm Genome 1999;10:438–43.

[18] Lindsay EA, Botta A, Jurecic V, et al. Congenital heart disease in mice deficient for the DiGeorge syndrome region. Nature 1999;401:379–83.

[19] Jerome LA, Papaioannou VE. DiGeorge syndrome phenotype in mice mutant for the T-box gene, Tbx1. Nat Genet 2001;27:286–91.

[20] Lindsay EA, Vitelli F, Su H, et al. Tbx1 haploinsufficiency in the DiGeorge syndrome region causes aortic arch defects in mice. Nature 2001;410:97–101.

[21] Merscher S, Funke B, Epstein JA, et al. TBX1 is responsible for cardiovascular defects in velo-cardio-facial/DiGeorge syndrome. Cell 2001;104:619–29.

[22] Liao J, Kochilas L, Nowotschin S, et al. Full spectrum of malformations in velo-cardio-facial syndrome/DiGeorge syndrome mouse models by altering Tbx1 dosage. Hum Mol Genet 2004; 13:1577–85.

[23] Piotrowski T, Ahn DG, Schilling TF, et al. The zebrafish van gogh mutation disrupts tbx1, which is involved in the DiGeorge deletion syndrome in humans. Development 2003;130:5043–52.

[24] Yagi H, Furutani Y, Hamada H, et al. Role of TBX1 in human del22q11.2 syndrome. Lancet 2003;362:1366–73.

[25] Brown CB, Wenning JM, Lu MM, et al. Cre-mediated excision of Fgf8 in the Tbx1 expression domain reveals a critical role for Fgf8 in cardiovascular development in the mouse. Dev Biol 2004;267:190–202.

[26] Hu T, Yamagishi H, Maeda J, et al. Tbx1 regulates fibroblast growth factors in the anterior heart field through a reinforcing autoregulatory loop involving forkhead transcription factors. Development 2004;131:5491–502.

[27] Burch JB. Regulation of GATA gene expression during vertebrate development. Semin Cell Dev Biol 2005;16:71–81.

[28] Peterkin T, Gibson A, Loose M, et al. The roles of GATA-4, -5 and -6 in vertebrate heart development. Semin Cell Dev Biol 2005;16:83–94.

[29] Shimizu R, Yamamoto M. Gene expression regulation and domain function of hematopoietic GATA factors. Semin Cell Dev Biol 2005;16:129–36.

[30] Pehlivan T, Pober BR, Brueckner M, et al. GATA4 haploinsufficiency in patients with interstitial deletion of chromosome region 8p23.1 and congenital heart disease. Am J Med Genet 1999; 83:201–6.

[31] Garg V, Kathiriya IS, Barnes R, et al. GATA4 mutations cause human congenital heart defects and reveal an interaction with TBX5. Nature 2003;424:443–7.

[32] Wang D, Chang PS, Wang Z, et al. Activation of cardiac gene expression by myocardin, a transcriptional cofactor for serum response factor. Cell 2001;105:851–62.

[33] Wang DZ, Li S, Hockemeyer D, et al. Potentiation of serum response factor activity by a family of myocardin-related transcription factors. Proc Natl Acad Sci USA 2002;99:14855–60.

[34] Li J, Zhu X, Chen M, et al. Myocardin-related transcription factor B is required in cardiac neural crest for smooth muscle differentiation and cardiovascular development. Proc Natl Acad Sci USA 2005;102:8916–21.

[35] Niu Z, Yu W, Zhang SX, et al. Conditional mutagenesis of the murine serum response factor gene blocks cardiogenesis and the transcription of downstream gene targets. J Biol Chem 2005; 280:32531–8.

[36] Wang DZ, Olson EN. Control of smooth muscle development by the myocardin family of transcriptional coactivators. Curr Opin Genet Dev 2004;14:558–66.

[37] McKinsey TA, Olson EN. Toward transcriptional therapies for the failing heart: chemical screens to modulate genes. J Clin Invest 2005;115:538–46.

[38] McKinsey TA, Zhang CL, Olson EN. Control of muscle development by dueling HATs and HDACs. Curr Opin Genet Dev 2001;11:497–504.

[39] Nolan PM, Peters J, Strivens M, et al. A systematic, genome-wide, phenotype-driven muta-genesis programme for gene function studies in the mouse. Nat Genet 2000;25:440–3.

[40] Skarnes WC, von Melchner H, Wurst W, et al. A public gene trap resource for mouse func-tional genomics. Nat Genet 2004;36:543–4.

[41] Austin CP, Battey JF, Bradley A, et al. The knockout mouse project. Nat Genet 2004;36:921–4.

[42] Auwerx J, Avner P, Baldock R, et al. The European dimension for the mouse genome muta-genesis program. Nat Genet 2004;36:925–7.

[43] Gura T. A silence that speaks volumes. Nature 2000;404:804–8.

[44] Hammond SM, Caudy AA, Hannon GJ. Post-transcriptional gene silencing by double-stranded RNA. Nat Rev Genet 2001;2:110–9.

[45] Haltiwanger RS, Lowe JB. Role of glycosylation in development. Annu Rev Biochem 2004; 73:491–537.

[46] Wells L, Hart GW. O-GlcNAc turns twenty: functional implications for post-translational modification of nuclear and cytosolic proteins with a sugar. FEBS Lett 2003;546:154–8.

[47] Takada Y, Khuri FR, Aggarwal BB. Protein farnesyltransferase inhibitor (SCH 66336) abolishes NF-kappaB activation induced by various carcinogens and inflammatory stimuli leading to suppression of NF-kappaB-regulated gene expression and up-regulation of apoptosis. J Biol Chem 2004;279:26287–99.

CLINICS IN
PERINATOLOGY

Clin Perinatol 32 (2005) 857–875

Current Concepts in Fetal Cardiovascular Disease

Anita Szwast, MD[a,b], Jack Rychik, MD[b,c,*]

[a]*The Children's Hospital of Philadelphia, 34th Street and Civic Center Boulevard,
Philadelphia, PA 19104, USA*
[b]*University of Pennsylvania School of Medicine, Philadelphia, PA 19104, USA*
[c]*Fetal Heart Program, Cardiac Center, The Children's Hospital of Philadelphia,
34th Street and Civic Center Boulevard, Philadelphia, PA 19104, USA*

Fetal imaging has advanced tremendously over the past 20 years. The developing fetus can be monitored in exquisite detail. Observations pertaining to fetal anatomy and physiology can be made with great reliability. As a result, congenital anomalies previously diagnosed postnatally are now being diagnosed in utero and managed to optimize outcome. Accurate transabdominal cardiovascular imaging can be performed as early as 16 weeks' gestation [1]. Transvaginal imaging may be performed as early as 10 to 12 weeks, although image acquisition in multiple orthogonal planes is limited by space constraints and fetal position [2]. As fetal imaging modalities continue to improve, insight into the physiology and pathophysiology of the fetal cardiovascular system broadens. This article describes the uniqueness of the fetal cardiovascular system and highlights some recent advances in the understanding of fetal cardiovascular medicine, specifically (1) fetal cardiac interventions and (2) the enigmatic process of twin–twin transfusion syndrome.

The uniqueness of the fetal cardiovascular myocardium

The fetal cardiovascular system differs from the mature, adult cardiovascular system in several ways. First, the structural elements of the fetal myocardium

* Corresponding author. Fetal Heart Program, The Children's Hospital of Philadelphia, 34th Street and Civic Center Boulevard, Philadelphia, PA 19104.
E-mail address: rychik@email.chop.edu (J. Rychik).

0095-5108/05/$ – see front matter © 2005 Elsevier Inc. All rights reserved.
doi:10.1016/j.clp.2005.09.012

differ from those of the adult myocardium. Early fetal myocytes may undergo replication, or increase in cell number, leading to hyperplasia. Adult myocytes may only increase cell size, leading to hypertrophy. Fetal myocardium is also much stiffer compared with the adult myocardium. The fetal myocardium is comprised of 60% noncontractile elements compared with only 30% noncontractile elements in the adult myocardium [3]. Furthermore, the rapid removal of calcium from troponin C, the mechanism responsible for myocardial relaxation, is less efficient in the fetus compared with the adult [4]. Consequently, compared with adult myocardium, fetal myocardium demonstrates impaired relaxation properties, evidenced by reversed differences in the Doppler echocardiography-derived flow patterns obtained when sampling across the atrioventricular valve inflow into the fetal ventricle (Fig. 1). In the adult, early diastolic filling predominates with an E wave (early passive filling) to A wave (active atrial contraction) velocity ratio (E:A ratio) exceeding 1. In the fetus, passive early filling is impaired with active atrial contraction accounting for most of ventricular filling [5]. Hence, the E:A ratio in the fetus is usually less than 1. Finally, the fetus has a limited ability to increase stroke volume. Morton and Thornberg [6] demonstrated that stroke volume peaks at an atrial pressure equal to 4 or 5 mm Hg in fetal lambs. Further increases in preload do not result in increases in stroke volume [6]. Many investigators believe that the unique fetal myocardial properties primarily account for the limited preload reserve. Grant and colleagues [7] proposed that the noncompliant tissues surrounding the heart, such as the pericardium, chest wall, and lungs, limit ventricular excursion. At birth, aeration of the lungs and removal of lung fluid enables better filling of the ventricles, leading to increases in ventricular preload and increases in ventricular stroke volumes [8–10].

 The stiffness of the fetal myocardium explains why hydrops is oftentimes the common clinical manifestation of fetal cardiovascular compromise. Any disease process that results in a slight increase in atrial pressure is poorly tolerated, leading to the findings of ascites, peripheral edema, and hydrops.

The fetal cardiovascular circulation

Fetal blood flow patterns are unique, optimized to deliver oxygen and nutrients to vital organs while shunting blood away from less important fetal structures [11]. The placenta serves as the site for oxygenation and nutrient delivery to the fetus. Consequently, the resistance within the placenta is extremely low to promote shunting of blood to the placenta. The iliac arteries give rise to the two umbilical arteries that carry an admixture of deoxygenated arterial blood to the placenta. Within the placenta, oxygen is exchanged for carbon dioxide within the capillary bed. A single umbilical vein leaves the placenta carrying richly oxygenated blood back to the fetus through the umbilical cord. The umbilical vein inserts into the ductus venosus to bypass most of the liver. The ductus venosus, in turn, connects with the inferior vena cava to enter the right atrium.

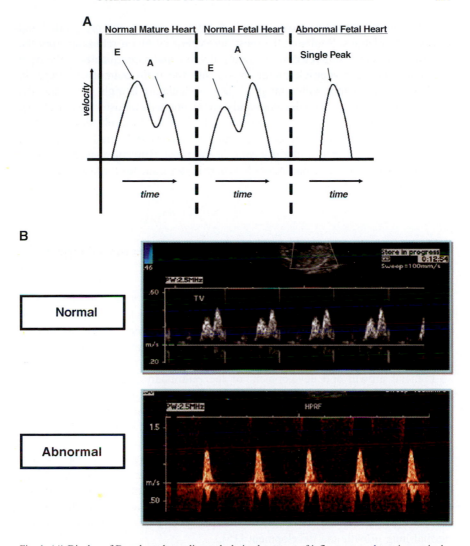

Fig. 1. (*A*) Display of Doppler echocardiograph-derived patterns of inflow across the atrioventricular valve. In the normal mature heart, the early wave (E wave) exceeds the later atrial contraction wave (A wave) in peak velocity. In the fetal heart, because of differences in compliance, the A wave peak velocity is normally higher than the E wave peak velocity. In disorders of fetal compliance and stiffness, such as in the twin–twin transfusion syndrome, the two inflow waves may summate and fuse into a single peak. (*B*) Doppler echocardiography displays normal inflow pattern in the top panel and an abnormal flow pattern in the lower panel.

The angle at which the ductus venosus inserts into the inferior vena cava–right atrium junction directs most of the richly oxygenated blood across the foramen ovale and into the left ventricle. The left ventricle, in turn, perfuses the coronary arteries and the cerebral vasculature. These fetal physiologic adaptations ensure that the most richly oxygenated blood (that returning from the ductus venosus) is delivered to the structures most in need of oxygen, namely the myocardial and cerebral circulations. Similarly, the most deoxygenated blood returning from the superior vena cava is directed to the tricuspid valve and subsequently to the right ventricle. The right ventricle pumps blood into the main pulmonary artery. In the fetus, the resistance within the pulmonary vasculature is high. Consequently, blood is directed away from the lungs and into the ductus arteriosus to return to the descending aorta and ultimately the umbilical arteries. These physiologic adaptations likewise ensure that deoxygenated blood is delivered to the fetal oxygenating organ, that is, the placenta, in the most efficient manner possible. (See the article by Johnson and Ades elsewhere in this issue for further explanation of this topic.)

Patterns of fetal blood flow in congenital heart disease: the pulmonary circulation

The pulmonary circulation is closely intertwined with the developing cardiovascular system during fetal life. Changes within the heart may profoundly influence pulmonary vascular development; hence comprehending the patterns of pulmonary blood flow in the fetus that has and that does not have heart disease is of interest.

Prenatal growth and development of the pulmonary vasculature is closely linked to the development of the bronchial tree. By 16 weeks' gestation, the bronchial tree has formed and the preacinar arteries have formed [12–14]. By 20 weeks' gestation, the preacinar veins have formed. During the canalicular phase of lung development, which occurs between 16 and 28 weeks' gestation, the basic structure of the gas-exchanging portion of the lung is formed and vascularized. In experimental sheep models, ligation of the left pulmonary artery during this late canalicular phase of lung development created pulmonary hypoplasia within the distribution of the ligated pulmonary artery [15]. These results highlight the importance of normal pulmonary arterial flow in ensuring normal lung growth and development [15].

The fetal pulmonary vasculature maintains high pressures and high resistances to promote low pulmonary blood flows [16]. Investigators initially believed that the amount of fetal pulmonary blood flow remained constant throughout gestation, comprising less than 20% of the combined cardiac outputs [17–19]. Recent work by Rasanen et al [20], however, demonstrated that the amount of blood flow delivered to the lungs begins to increase after the second trimester. In human fetuses, 13% of the combined cardiac output is pumped to the lungs at 20 weeks' gestation. Pulmonary blood flow increases to 25% of combined cardiac output at 30 weeks' gestation and remains constant thereafter. Rasanen and colleagues [21] further demonstrated that the pulmonary vascular bed exhibits dynamic vasoreactivity in response to supplemental oxygen after 31 weeks' gestation. By administering 60% oxygen to mothers of normal fetuses, they demonstrated that the Doppler ultrasound-derived "pulsatility index" (PI) in the pulmonary vascular bed decreased [21]. The PI may be thought of as a surrogate for pulmonary vascular resistance. With decreasing pulmonary vascular resistance with maternal oxygen administration, pulmonary blood flow increases during maternal hyperoxygenation, but only after 31 weeks' gestation. This development of pulmonary vascular reactivity to changes in oxygen tension may be explained by a marked increase in the number of small resistive arteries within the pulmonary vascular bed as gestation proceeds [22]. The walls of these small vessels have smooth muscle, which serve to maintain a vasoconstricted state in settings of low oxygen tension [16,22]. With increasing oxygen tension, the pulmonary arterial bed vasodilates, leading to increased pulmonary blood flow [23,24]. Broth et al [25] used the hyperoxygenation test for pulmonary artery reactivity to predict which fetuses would be at risk for lethal pulmonary hypoplasia. In their study of 29 fetuses with congenital anomalies that may cause pulmonary hypoplasia, a reactive hyperoxygenation test, defined as a decrease in 20% in the PI of either branch pulmonary artery, predicted 92% survival. A nonreactive test predicted 79% of deaths caused by pulmonary hypoplasia [25].

There is a complex interactive dependency between the developing heart and pulmonary vasculature. Differences in cardiac structure such as are found in various forms of congenital heart disease may variably impact on the developing pulmonary vascular tree. Haworth and Reid [26,27] first described postnatal anatomic lung abnormalities associated with altered fetal pulmonary blood flow patterns in patients who have different types of congenital heart disease. In fetuses that have hypoplastic left heart syndrome (HLHS) and a restrictive atrial communication, there is significant obstruction to pulmonary venous return, which results in increased pressures within the pulmonary vascular bed. The pulmonary veins compensate by becoming more muscularized [28,29]. As a result, pulmonary vascular resistance increases and pulmonary blood flow decreases, leading to significant changes in the pulmonary vasculature that have important prognostic implications. Fetuses that have HLHS and an open atrial communication typically have survival rates in excess of 90%. Unfortunately, survival rates in fetuses that have HLHS and a restrictive atrial communication decrease to 52% secondary to pulmonary vascular hypoplasia and maldevelopment [30]. Identifying and, potentially, intervening in fetuses that have a restrictive atrial communication may alter the natural history of this disorder. Preliminary work at the Children's Hospital of Philadelphia suggests that fetuses that have HLHS and an unobstructed atrial communication have a normal response to maternal hyperoxygenation. In other words, these fetuses have a decrease in the PI in the pulmonary arteries and an increase in pulmonary blood flow in response to maternal oxygen administration similar to normal fetuses. Further defining the response to maternal hyperoxygenation, in particular in the fetus that has a restrictive interatrial communication, may lead to better understanding of the uniqueness of the developing pulmonary vasculature in the fetus that has HLHS. This work may lead to pharmacologic or intervention therapies that would allow for prenatal remodeling of the pulmonary vasculature.

Fetal cardiovascular interventions: at the dawn of a promising era

With the increasing application of fetal echocardiography and the ability to peer into the womb, it has become apparent that some forms of congenital heart disease undergo structural developmental change during the second and third trimesters of gestation [31]. Lesions that initially present as a simple anomaly at early gestational time point A may progress to a more serious and complex anomaly at later gestational time point B, or at birth. Identification of this phenomenon has led to great interest in fetal intervention to halt the progression of the disease. Successful fetal intervention may alleviate some of the morbidity and mortality seen at birth. Knowing when to intervene to achieve a successful outcome remains problematic. Recent interest has focused on whether fetal echocardiography may be able to identify fetuses that may benefit from prenatal intervention.

In general, fetal intervention is indicated when either (1) the fetus is at risk for demise, or (2) the intervention can substantially alter the postnatal course of the disease. Performing fetal cardiac intervention is controversial, as prenatal demise in utero because of the cardiac anomaly at hand is a rare phenomenon. In addition, there are currently excellent postnatal surgical results for nearly all forms of congenital heart disease. Fetal intervention must also be considered within the context of potential risk to the mother. Any fetal cardiac intervention performed has the potential risk for "200% morbidity or mortality," as both mother and fetus may be deleteriously affected. Fetal cardiac intervention is therefore directed at changing the fundamental make-up of the disease, theoretically lessening its severity, in the hopes of improving postnatal morbidity, while at all times minimizing potential risks to the mother (see Table 1).

Table 1
Forms of structural prenatal heart disease currently under consideration for potential fetal intervention

Candidate anomaly	Outcome without fetal intervention	Fetal intervention	Anticipated outcome with fetal intervention
Aortic stenosis progressing to hypoplastic left heart syndrome (HLHS)	HLHS with reconstructive surgery consisting of 3 operations leading to single ventricle and Fontan circulation	Balloon valvuloplasty of aortic valve	Two-ventricle heart with aortic valve disease
Pulmonic stenosis progressing to hypoplastic right heart	Hypoplasia of the right ventricle leading to single ventricle and Fontan circulation	Balloon valvuloplasty of pulmonic valve	Two-ventricle heart with pulmonic valve disease
HLHS and intact atrial septum	HLHS with high mortality	Atrial septoplasty	HLHS with low mortality
TGA with intact atrial septum	TGA with high mortality	Atrial septoplasty	TGA with low mortality

Abbreviations: LV, left ventricle; RV, right ventricle; TGA, transposition of the great arteries.

Critical aortic stenosis

Some fetuses that have aortic stenosis have been observed to progress and acquire left ventricular hypoplasia, and in the extreme develop into HLHS. The hypothesized explanation for this phenomenon is that impediment to a normal complement of forward blood flow through the left ventricle caused by aortic stenosis can in some circumstances result in impaired ventricular growth. The principle motivating intervention in the fetus is that prenatal opening of the aortic valve may allow for improved flow through the left ventricle, thereby promoting growth and preventing development of left ventricular hypoplasia.

Treatment of HLHS after birth involves three operations resulting in a staged surgical reconstruction in which the right ventricle performs the task of providing for the systemic circulation. Whereas surgical survival currently exceeds 90%, there are several long-term complications that plague many of these children. Despite dramatic improvements in surgical survival, children who have HLHS exist under the unique physiologic constraints of a single ventricle palliation. These patients have their single, well formed right ventricle assigned to perfuse the systemic circulation, while pulmonary blood flow is achieved by way of passive filling of the pulmonary vascular bed following surgical connection of the systemic veins directly to the pulmonary arteries (the Fontan operation). Under this construct, the pulmonary and systemic circulations are separated; however, a normal cardiovascular system is not achieved because there is still absence of a pulmonary ventricle. The possibility of diverting the cardiovascular system of a fetus developing left ventricular hypoplasia from a single ventricle pathway into a two-ventricle system would be a great achievement and is of great interest.

In critical aortic stenosis, various criteria have been proposed to determine the indications for fetal intervention. Left-to-right shunting at the atrial level and retrograde flow in the aortic arch have been proposed as possible predictors of development of left ventricular hypoplasia. Successful fetal intervention for aortic stenosis has been technically achieved. Tworetzky et al [32] selected candidates for fetal intervention based on the echocardiographic evidence of severe aortic stenosis defined as a gradient up to 2m/s across the aortic valve in association with left ventricular dysfunction. In their series, the left ventricular length at time of intervention was not less than 2 SD below the mean. Some fetuses had dilated left ventricles with evidence of endocardial brightening, whereas others had mitral regurgitation [32]. Allen et al [33] described successful balloon dilation of a fetus that had critical aortic stenosis. Their patient had a thickened, doming aortic valve and a dilated, poorly contractile left ventricle. The peak gradient across the aortic valve was 2 m/s. The mitral valve papillary muscles appeared "echobright." There was reversal of flow from left to right across the atrial communication [33]. McCaffrey and Sherman [34] documented evolution of critical aortic stenosis to HLHS in five of nine fetuses followed serially from the second gestation to term. In their series, fetuses that have critical aortic stenosis likely to progress to HLHS had limited aortic annulus growth, limited left ventricle (LV) short axis growth, and limited LV volume growth [34]. Unfortunately, the small number of patients included in the study precluded formal statistical analysis.

Clear-cut predictive criteria for development of HLHS in the fetus that has second trimester aortic stenosis are lacking. Current results of fetal intervention for aortic stenosis are equivocal in "preventing" left ventricular hypoplasia. Sufficiently determining those at risk and hence identifying appropriate candidates at the outset are important factors that will influence the validity of a resulting two-ventricle outcome for the fetus undergoing intervention. Nevertheless, excitement has been generated by the preliminary data, which suggests that aortic valvuloplasty in the fetus is technically feasible.

Critical pulmonic stenosis/pulmonary atresia with intact ventricular septum

Similar to the fetus that has aortic stenosis, one that has pulmonary stenosis or atresia is at risk for development of right ventricular hypoplasia. The intention of fetal intervention is to open the pulmonary outflow tract and theoretically promote growth of the right ventricle, thereby allowing for a two-ventricle treatment strategy after birth.

Critical pulmonic stenosis (PS) or pulmonary atresia with intact ventricular septum (PA/IVS) is generally well-tolerated in fetal life. Allen et al [35] reported a 9% in utero mortality rate for all fetuses that have PA/IVS or severe PS in the absence of significant tricuspid regurgitation [35]. Selection criteria for fetal intervention are not yet well established. Tulzer et al [36] recently reported their experience with two fetuses, one diagnosed as having PA/IVS the other as having critical PS at 28 weeks' and 30 weeks' gestation, respectively. Both fetuses had evidence of impending hydrops, defined as abnormal venous Doppler waveforms, impaired ventricular filling caused by severe tricuspid regurgitation extending into diastole, and a pericardial effusion. Both fetuses underwent successful balloon dilation of the pulmonary valve with resultant pulmonary insufficiency and right ventricle (RV) growth. The investigators considered very hypertrophied ventricles as poor candidates for fetal intervention [36]. Maeno et al [37] described a series of 20 patients with prenatal diagnoses of critical PS or PA/IVS. In their series, fetuses that had PA/IVS and were treated with a single ventricle type of management had more severe tricuspid annular hypoplasia and main pulmonary artery hypoplasia, with Z scores less than 2 SD below the mean [37].

Determining candidacy for fetal intervention by reliably predicting those that will progress to ventricular hypoplasia may be more difficult in right-sided disease than in left-sided disease. The threshold for ventricular inadequacy may be different for the right ventricle than for the left ventricle. A much smaller right ventricle may be tolerated for perfusing the pulmonary circulation than would be a small left ventricle for perfusing the systemic circulation. Identifying reliable criteria for potential right ventricle inadequacy in the fetus is another important challenge facing investigators.

Restrictive atrial communication and hypoplastic left heart syndrome

In HLHS, restrictive atrial communication occurs in 6% to 22% of patients [28,38,39]. Unfortunately, in this group of patients, neonatal mortality rates are as high as 48% despite urgent neonatal balloon atrial septostomy [30]. Impediment to left atrial egress, as occurs in the fetus that has left atrioventricular valve atresia and an intact atrial septum, leads to marked left atrial and pulmonary venous hypertension (Fig. 2). Histopathologic changes consisting of "arterialization" of the pulmonary veins have been found on postnatal necropsy analysis of the lung vasculature in the newborn who has HLHS and intact atrial septum (Fig. 3) [28].

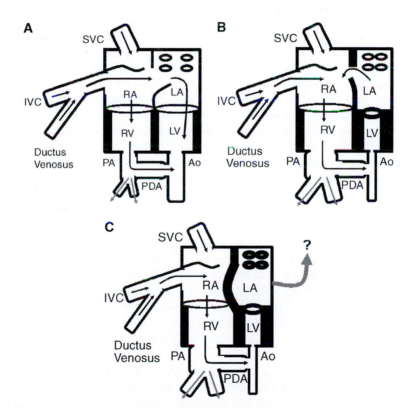

Fig. 2. Normal fetal circulation (*A*) and the circulatory changes in the fetus with HLHS (*B*) and HLHS with intact atrial septum (*C*). In the fetus that has HLHS and a patent foramen ovale, pulmonary venous return can drain across the atrial septum and mix with systemic venous return in the right atrium in an unobstructed manner. In the fetus with HLHS and an intact atrial septum, pulmonary venous return has no exit from the left atrium, resulting in left atrial hypertension and pulmonary venous congestion. This condition may negatively impact on pulmonary vascular development. Despite a timely and successful opening of the atrial septum after birth, such patients have significant pulmonary disease and persistent marked cyanosis.

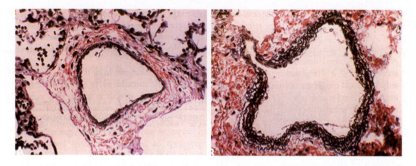

Fig. 3. Histopathology of the pulmonary veins in a neonate with HLHS and an open atrial septum (*left panel*) and a neonate with HLHS and intact atrial septum (*right panel*). Note the thickened wall and increased number of internal elastic laminae, suggesting an "arterialization" of the pulmonary veins in the patient who has HLHS and intact atrial septum.

Impediment to left atrial egress alters fetal pulmonary vascular development during gestation, resulting in a damaged lung at birth. This finding may explain the poor outcome in these newborns despite early diagnosis and aggressive treatment attempts at opening the septum.

Consequently, fetal techniques for balloon atrial septostomy have emerged. Marshall et al [40] selected fetal candidates for balloon atrial septostomy based on the echocardiographic appearance of prominent flow reversal in dilated pulmonary veins. Huhta et al [41] selected candidates for atrial septal defect creation using a laser with a nonreactive fetal pulmonary vasoreactivity study. Doppler echocardiographic identification of reversal of flow in the pulmonary veins is a strong predictor of this disease (Fig. 4). Hence HLHS with intact atrial septum is an ideal anomaly for fetal intervention in that the selection criteria are predictive of the disease, and the outcome using conventional strategies is poor. By performing an opening of the atrial septum in utero, the hope is to allow for normal drainage of the pulmonary vasculature and normal development of the lung. The most effective gestational timing of such a procedure is unknown.

Restrictive atrial communication and transposition of the great arteries

In d-transposition of the great arteries (d-TGA), preoperative mortality rates secondary to inadequate mixing at the atrial or ductal level approach 4%. Maeno et al [42] studied 16 fetuses that had a prenatal diagnosis of d-TGA with an intact or small ventricular septal defect. Their series identified two fetuses that had both a restrictive foramen ovale (defined as a fixed, flat, or redundant septum) and a restrictive ductus arteriosus (defined as narrowing at the pulmonary artery end and a diameter Z score less than −2 on prenatal scans). Both of these fetuses died immediately after birth [42]. Jouannic et al [43] studied 130 fetuses that had d-TGA over 5.5 years. Prenatally, 23 fetuses had restrictive foramen ovale, 5 had a restrictive ductus arteriosus, and 4 had abnormalities of both. At birth, 7 of

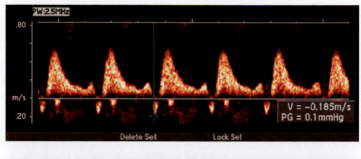

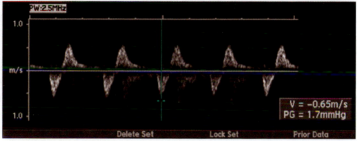

Fig. 4. Doppler echocacardiography sample from a fetus that has HLHS and an open atrial septum (*top panel*) and a fetus that has HLHS and intact atrial septum (*bottom panel*). The cross-hair marker in each is placed onto the wave corresponding to atrial contraction. The fetus that has HLHS and intact atrial septum has a different Doppler flow pattern with a much greater "reversal" of flow with atrial contraction, and much less forward flow in general relative to the fetus that has HLHS and an open atrial septum. This pattern is distinctive and predictive of a fetus that will have difficulties at birth.

24 neonates who had a prenatally detected abnormality of the foramen ovale or ductus arteriosus were critically ill and hypoxemic at birth. In contrast, of 95 fetuses deemed to have a normal foramen ovale and ductus arteriosus on prenatal scanning, only six were critically ill at birth. If an abnormality of either the foramen ovale or ductus arteriosus was seen on the prenatal scan, the specificity and sensitivity for predicting an emergency neonatal intervention was 84% and 54%, respectively. If abnormalities of both foramen ovale and ductus arteriosus were seen, then the specificity rose to 100%, while the sensitivity fell to 31% [43]. Opening of the atrial septum in such fetuses may impact positively by allowing for mixing and a more favorable physiology once the fetus is separated from the placental circulation.

There is much yet to be learned about the structural and physiologic changes that take place during gestational development in the human fetus. Identifying predictors for progression of disease is essential if appropriate candidates are to be chosen for fetal intervention. A large-scale multicenter study looking at the natural history of progression of congenital heart anomalies is necessary. Such an investigation will provide for better identification of candidates who will benefit from fetal intervention.

Twin–twin transfusion syndrome

The twin–twin transfusion syndrome (TTTS) is an enigmatic disease with a fascinating pathophysiology. Understanding this disease process may help in elucidating one of the mechanisms for development of cardiac structural abnormalities in the fetus. TTTS complicates 10% to 15% of all monochorionic, diamniotic twin pregnancies [44]. The pathophysiology of the disorder remains poorly understood, but has traditionally been attributed to a net transfusion of blood by way of vascular anastomoses within the placenta from the donor twin to the recipient twin. This situation leads to hypervolemia and polycthemia with consequent polyhydramnios in the recipient twin and to hypovolemia, anemia, and oligohydramnios in the donor twin (Fig. 5). Recent work by Bajora et al [45] identified unilateral vascular anastomoses deep within the placenta of monochorionic multiple gestations. Moreover, superficial bidirectional arterio–arterial connections, which may be protective in maintaining a net zero transfusion balance between donor and recipient, are absent in TTTS [45,46]. TTTS remains a challenging therapeutic problem in fetal medicine. If left untreated, mortality rates approach 100% [47,48]. The introduction of techniques such as serial amnioreduction or laser ablation of placental vascular anastomoses has improved survival rates to as high as 60% to 70% [49–53]. Unfortunately, many survivors suffer long-term adverse neurologic outcomes [54,55]. The incidence of cerebral palsy or global developmental delay ranges from 4% to 26% in TTTS survivors [56–61]. Serious neurologic morbidity was even higher (50%) in surviving twins whose co-twins had died in utero [61]. Recent studies have suggested that neurologic outcome may be improved with selective fetoscopic laser photocoagulation [60].

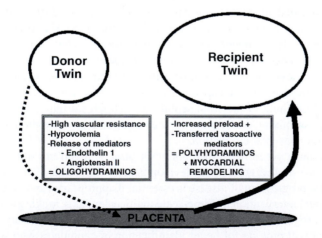

Fig. 5. Physiologic explanation for differences between the twins in twin–twin transfusion syndrome.

Over the past decade, knowledge of the cardiovascular manifestations of TTTS has increased tremendously. In donor twins, as a consequence of the hypovolemia, there is nephrosclerosis. Invasive studies have documented elevated levels of angiotensin II in donor twins, suggesting stimulation of the renin-angiotensin system to compensate for hypovolemia [62]. Such stimulation of the renin-angiotensin system can lead to serious pathologic changes in the fetus. Robillard et al [63] demonstrated that infusion of angiotensin II in fetal sheep led to increased collagen synthesis, smooth muscle hypertrophy, and vascular medial hypertrophy. Physiologic adaptations to elevated angiotensin levels in utero may explain why donor survivors of TTTS manifest increased vascular stiffness as children [64]. The question arises as to whether vascular maldevelopment in utero may lead to lifelong problems of vascular compliance, a risk factor for atherosclerosis and coronary artery disease in the adult. Intriguingly, Gardiner [65] demonstrated that midgestation intervention with laser photocoagulation prevented these reductions in vascular distensibility. Control twins and survivors of TTTS treated with laser photocoagulation had normal vascular distensibility at birth, but twins treated with serial amnioreduction manifested abnormal patterns of vascular distensibility at birth [65].

Cardiovascular abnormalities in the donor twin are not as common as in the recipient twin. Donor twins, however, do experience increased afterload. Doppler sampling within the umbilical arteries reveals elevated PIs, reflecting increased total vascular resistance with diminished diastolic flow. Donor twins do not, however, develop atrioventricular valvular regurgitation or cardiomyopathy. Karatza et al [66] reported normal combined cardiac performance indices for donor twins, although a recent study in our laboratory at The Children's Hospital of Philadelphia (unpublished data) demonstrates that donor twins have lower combined cardiac output indices relative to their recipient twins and to normal controls. Ventricular performance is preserved in donor twins, as evidenced by normal left ventricular shortening fractions and normal LV and RV myocardial performance indices [67]. The myocardial performance index, or Tei index, is a load-independent measure of systolic and diastolic ventricular performance measured by performing Doppler echocardiography. It is defined as the combined isovolumic contraction time plus isovolumic relaxation time, divided by the ejection time. Raboisson et al [67] proposed differentiating twins who have TTTS from twins who have discordant growth secondary to intrauterine growth retardation (IUGR) by determining differences in myocardial performance indices. Twins who have IUGR should theoretically demonstrate no differences in myocardial performance, whereas twin sets that have TTTS should manifest such differences. Comparing the smaller twin to the larger twin, a change in the LV myocardial performance index greater than or equal to 0.09 combined with a change in the RV myocardial performance index greater than or equal to 0.05 identified TTTS with a sensitivity of 75% and a false positive rate of 9% [67]. TTTS is clearly a cardiovascular disease process, and it can be identified by the presence of intertwin differences in sensitive measures of myocardial dysfunction.

Cardiovascular abnormalities are common in recipient twins (Table 2). Recipient twins have significant volume loading of the heart, which leads to progressive ventricular dilation and hypertrophy. Atrioventricular valvular regurgitation is common and may be severe. Right ventricular pressures by tricuspid regurgitant jets may be 2 to 3 times normal. Progressive right ventricular hypertrophy may develop in conjunction with pulmonary infundibular stenosis, leading to acquired "congenital" PS or even pulmonic atresia [68,69]. Mediators produced by the donor twin to counteract hypovolemia, such as angiotensin II, may cross the placenta and stimulate myocardial hypertrophy in the recipient twin. In a fetal sheep model, Segar et al [70] demonstrated a direct hormonal effect of angiotensin II in stimulating myocardial hypertrophy, independent of increases in systemic afterload. Other investigators have demonstrated that concentrations of endothelin-1, another potent vasoconstrictor, are 2.5 times higher in recipient twins compared with their donor co-twins [71]. These two vasoconstrictors may act in conjunction in recipient twins to cause myocardial hypertrophy and dysfunction. In the extreme case, hypertrophic obstructive cardiomyopathy may develop. As a consequence of the hypertrophy, recipient twins have diastolic dysfunction, as evidenced by elevated myocardial performance indices [67]. Systolic performance, as evidenced by lower shortening fractions compared with

Table 2
Progressive changes in the cardiovascular system of fetuses that have the twin-twin transfusion syndrome

Changes	Area affected	Recipient	Donor
Early/mild	Right side of heart	RV cavity dilation	Normal RV cavity
		RV myocardial hypertrophy	Normal RV myocardial thickness
		Tricuspid regurgitation (>mild)	Tricuspid regurgitation (<mild)
		Diminution in diastolic flow velocity of the ductus venosus	Normal ductus venosus flow
	Left side of heart	LV cavity dilation	Normal LV cavity
		LV myocardial hypertrophy	Normal LV myocardial thickness
		Mitral regurgitation (>mild)	Mitral regurgitation (<mild)
	Umbilical cord	Umbilical venous pulsations	No evidence for umbilical venous pulsations
Late/severe		Umbilical artery initially normal, then increased resistance when in premorbid state	Umbilical artery uniformly demonstrates increased resistance early, then progresses to absent or reversed diastolic flow

donor cotwins, may also be impaired [67]. Ultimately, ventricular performance may become so dysfunctional that hydrops fetalis ensues.

Treatment options for TTTS have included serial amnioreduction, amniotic septostomy, laser ablation of placental vessels, and selective fetocide. A recent study by Senat et al [72] compared outcomes of severely affected TTTS fetuses randomly assigned to serial amnioreduction versus laser therapy combined with a single amnioreduction procedure. Laser therapy was associated with improved perinatal and improved six-month survival. Moreover, there was a lower incidence of periventricular leukomalacia [72]. In milder forms of TTTS, however, serial amnioreduction may be the treatment of choice [73].

Of great interest is the variability in outcome of recipient TTTS fetuses that have severe findings (Fig. 6). One subset of recipient fetuses undergoes the process of change described in the earlier discussion and ultimately succumbs with progressive myocardial dysfunction, hydrops, and fetal demise. Another subset seems to adapt to the cardiovascular changes, and continues forward within the pregnancy. These recipient twins exist in a form of "chronic" cardiomyopathy, with a thickened, dysfunctional heart with atrioventricular regurgitation. Perhaps treatment impacts on the outcome in this group, or natural changes alone within the placenta alter the primary stimulative process, such that further progression is halted and these fetuses survive. Most interesting is the third group of recipient fetuses, in which the progressive cardiomyopathic changes of RV dilation, hypertrophy, and dysfunction lead to development of RV outflow tract obstruction, PS, and even pulmonary atresia. The authors, and others, have directly observed a remarkable process of change in these recipient fetuses. What starts out to be a normal-size right ventricle with a normal pulmonary valve develops marked RV hypertrophy and obstruction to RV outflow and ultimately evolves into the form of congenital heart disease known as PA/IVS [74]. A serious form of congenital heart disease is observed to develop in a normal heart under direct observation. TTTS demonstrates the plasticity of the fetal heart, even

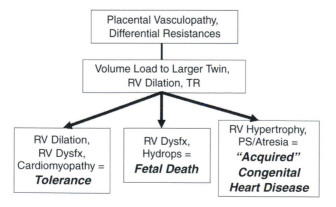

Fig. 6. Outcome model for the recipient twin with severe findings in twin–twin transfusion syndrome.

late in gestation. Further understanding of the phenomenon of TTTS may offer clues as to the overall development of congenital heart disease.

Summary

   With the technical capability and ubiquity of obstetrical ultrasound has come an increasing focus on fetal health and a shift in timing of diagnosis of major congenital anomalies from after birth to before birth. Fetal echocardiography allows the probing of the developing human fetus and the observation of fascinating phenomena, heretofore not seen. Several interesting, challenging, and somewhat novel disease processes may afflict the fetal cardiovascular system. In the new arena of "prenatal cardiology," investigational efforts are now focused on improving diagnostic understanding of the fetus and ways to effect change by interventional techniques. These factors contribute to a continuing change in the approach to cardiovascular disease in the developing human.

References

[1] Haak MC, van Vugt JM. Echocardiography in early pregnancy. J Ultrasound Med 2003;21: 490–3.
[2] Johnson P, Sharland G, Maxwell D, et al. The role of transvaginal sonography in the early detection of congenital heart disease. Ultrasound Obstet Gynecol 1994;4:248–51.
[3] Friedman WF. The intrinsic physiologic properties of the developing heart. Prog Cardiovasc Dis 1972;15:87–111.
[4] Mahoney L. Calcium homeostasis and control of contractility in the developing heart. Semin Perinatol 1996;20:510–9.
[5] Reed KL, Meijboom EK, Sahn DJ, et al. Cardiac Doppler flow velocities in human fetuses. Circulation 1986;73:41–6.
[6] Thornburg KL, Morton MJ. Filling and arterial pressures as determinants of left ventricular stroke volume in unanesthetized fetal lambs. Am J Physiol 1986;251:H961–8.
[7] Grant DA. Ventricular constraint in the fetus and newborn. Can J Cardiol 1992;15:95–104.
[8] Grant DA, Kondo CS, Maloney JR, et al. Changes in pericardial pressure during the perinatal period. Circulation 1992;86:1615–21.
[9] Grant DA, Maloney JE, Tyberg JV, et al. Effects of external constraint on the fetal left ventricular function curve. Am Heart J 1992;123:1601–9.
[10] Grant DA, Walker AM. Pleural pressures limit fetal right ventricular output. Circulation 1996;94:555–61.
[11] Rudolph AM. Distribution and regulation of blood flow in the fetal and neonatal lamb. Circ Res 1985;57:811–21.
[12] Inselman LS, Mellins RB. Growth and development of the lung. J Pediatr 1981;98:1–15.
[13] Pringle KC. Human fetal lung development and related animal models. Clin Obstet Gynecol 1986;29:502–13.
[14] Laudy JAM, Wladimiroff JW. The fetal lung 1: developmental aspects. Ultrasound Obstet Gynecol 2000;16:284–90.
[15] Wallen LD, Perry SF, Alston JT, et al. Morphometric study of the role of pulmonary arterial flow in fetal lung growth in sheep. Pediatr Res 1990;27:122–7.
[16] Emerson DS, Cartier MS. The fetal pulmonary circulation. In: Copel JA, Reed KL, editors. Doppler ultrasound in obstetrics and gynecology. New York: Raven Press, Ltd.; 1995. p. 307–23.

[17] St John Sutton M, Groves A, MacNeill A, et al. Assessment of changes in blood flow through the lungs and foramen ovale in the normal human fetus with gestational age: a prospective Doppler echocardiographic study. Br Heart J 1994;71:232–7.

[18] Rudolph AM, Heymann MA. Circulatory changes during growth in the fetal lamb. Circ Res 1970;26:289–99.

[19] Morin III FC, Egan EA, Ferguson W, et al. Development of pulmonary vascular response to oxygen. Am J Physiol 1988;254:H542–6.

[20] Rasanen J, Wood DC, Weiner S, et al. Role of the pulmonary circulation in the distribution of human fetal cardiac output during the second half of pregnancy. Circulation 1996;94: 1068–73.

[21] Rasanen J, Wood DC, Debbs RH, et al. Reactivity of the human fetal pulmonary circulation to maternal hyperoxygenation increases during the second half of pregnancy. Circulation 1998;97:257–62.

[22] Levin DL, Rudolph AM, Heymann MA, et al. Morphological development of the pulmonary vascular bed in fetal lambs. Circulation 1976;53:144–51.

[23] Morin FC, Egan EA. Pulmonary hemodynamics in fetal lambs during development at normal and increased oxygen tension. J Appl Physiol 1992;73(1):213–8.

[24] Lewis AB, Heymann MA, Rudolph AM. Gestational changes in pulmonary vascular responses in fetal lambs in utero. Circ Res 1976;39:536–41.

[25] Broth RE, Wood DC, Rasanen J, et al. Prenatal prediction of lethal pulmonary hypoplasia: the hyperoxygenation test for pulmonary artery reactivity. Am J Obstet Gynecol 2002;187: 940–5.

[26] Haworth SG, Reid L. Quantitative structural study of pulmonary circulation in the newborn with aortic atresia, stenosis, or coarctation. Thorax 1977;32:121–8.

[27] Haworth SG, Reid L. Quantitative structural study of pulmonary circulation in the newborn with pulmonary atresia. Thorax 1977;32:129–33.

[28] Rychik J, Rome JJ, Collins MH, et al. The hypoplastic left heart syndrome with intact atrial septum: atrial morphology, pulmonary vascular histopathology, and outcome. J Am Coll Cardiol 1999;34:554–60.

[29] Graziano JN, Heidelberger KP, Ensing GJ, et al. The influence of a restrictive atrial septal defect on pulmonary vascular morphology in patients with hypoplastic left heart syndrome. Pediatr Cardiol 2002;23:146–51.

[30] Vlahos AP, Lock JE, McElhinney DB, et al. Hypoplastic left heart syndrome with intact or highly restrictive atrial septum: outcome after neonatal transcatheter atrial septostomy. Circulation 2004;109:2326–30.

[31] Trines J, Hornberger LK. Evolution of heart disease in utero. Pediatr Cardiol 2004;25: 287–98.

[32] Tworetzky W, Wilkins-Haug L, Jennings RW, et al. Balloon dilation of severe aortic stenosis in the fetus: potential for prevention of hypoplastic left heart syndrome: candidate selection, technique, and results of successful intervention. Circulation 2004;110:2125–31.

[33] Allan LD, Maxwell DJ, Carminati M, et al. Survival after fetal aortic balloon valvoplasty. Ultrasound Obstet Gynecol 1995;5:90–1.

[34] McCaffrey FM, Sherman FS. Prenatal diagnosis of severe aortic stenosis. Pediatr Cardiol 1997;18:276–81.

[35] Allen LD, Crawford DC, Tynan MJ. Pulmonary atresia in prenatal life. J Am Coll Cardiol 1986;8:1131–6.

[36] Tulzer G, Arzt W, Franklin RCG, et al. Fetal pulmonary valvuloplasty for critical pulmonary stenosis or atresia with intact septum. Lancet 2002;360:1567–8.

[37] Maeno YV, Boutin C, Hornberger LK, et al. Prenatal diagnosis of right ventricular outflow tract obstruction with intact ventricular septum, and detection of ventriculocoronary connections. Heart 1999;81:661–8.

[38] Forbess JM, Cook N, Roth SJ, et al. Ten-year institutional experience with palliative surgery for hypoplastic left heart syndrome: risk factors related to stage I mortality. Circulation 1995;92(Suppl II):II262–6.

[39] Aiello VD, Ho SY, Anderson RH, et al. Morphologic features of the hypoplastic left heart syndrome: a reappraisal. Pediatr Pathol 1990;10:931–43.

[40] Marshall AC, van der Velde ME, Tworetzky W, et al. Creation of an atrial septal defect in utero for fetuses with hypoplastic left heart syndrome and intact or highly restrictive atrial septum. Circulation 2004;110(3):253–8.

[41] Huhta J, Quintero RA, Suh E, et al. Advances in fetal cardiac intervention. Curr Opin Pediatr 2004;16(5):487–93.

[42] Maeno YV, Kamenir SA, Sinclair B, et al. Prenatal features of ductus arteriosus constriction and restrictive foramen ovale in d-transposition of the great arteries. Circulation 1999;99: 1209–14.

[43] Jouannic J-M, Gavard L, Fermont L, et al. Sensitivity and specificity of prenatal features of physiologic shunts to predict neonatal clinical status in transposition of the great arteries. Circulation 2004;110:1743–6.

[44] Sebire NJ, Snijders RJM, Hughes K, et al. The hidden mortality of monochorionic twin pregnancies. Br J Obstet Gynaecol 1997;104:1203–7.

[45] Bajora R, Wigglesworth J, Fisk NM. Angioarchitecture of monochorionic placentas in relation to the twin-twin transfusion syndrome. Am J Obstet Gynecol 1995;172:856–63.

[46] Machin G, Stikk K, Lalani T. Correlations of placental vascular anatomy and clinical outcomes in 69 monochorionic twin pregnancies. Am J Med Genet 1996;61:229–36.

[47] Weir PE, Ratten GH, Beischer NA. Acute polyhydramnios—a complication of monozygous twin pregnancy. Br J Obstet Gynaecol 1979;86:849–53.

[48] Gonsoulin W, Moise K, Kirshon B, et al. Outcome of twin-twin transfusion diagnosed before 28 weeks of gestation. Obstet Gynecol 1990;75:214–6.

[49] Quintero RA, Dickinson JE, Morales WJ, et al. Stage-based treatment of twin-twin transfusion syndome. Am J Obstet Gynecol 2003;188:1333–40.

[50] Hecher K, Diehl W, Zikulnig L, et al. Endoscopic laser coagulation of placental anastomoses in 200 pregnancies with severe mid-trimester twin-to-twin transfusion syndrome. Eur J Obstet Gynecol Reprod Biol 2000;92:135–9.

[51] Hecher K, Plath H, Bregenzer T, et al. Endoscopic laser surgery versus serial amniocentesis in the treatment of severe twin-twin transfusion syndrome. Am J Obstet Gynecol 1999;180: 717–24.

[52] Mari G, Roberts A, Detti L, et al. Perinatal morbidity and mortality rates in severe twin-twin transfusion syndrome: results of the International Amnioreduction Registry. Am J Obstet Gynecol 2001;185:708–15.

[53] Dickinson JE, Evans SF. Obstetric and perinatal outcomes from the Australian and New Zealand twin-twin transfusion syndrome registry. Am J Obstet Gynecol 2000;182:706–12.

[54] Banek CS, Hecker K, Hackeloer BJ, et al. Long-term neurodevelopmental outcome after intrauterine laser treatment for severe twin-twin transfusion syndrome. Am J Obstet Gynecol 2003;188:876–80.

[55] Wee LY, Fisk NM. The twin-twin transfusion syndrome. Sem Neonatol 2002;7:187–202.

[56] Mari G, Detti L, Oz U, et al. Long-term outcome in twin-twin transfusion syndrome treated with serial aggressive amnioreduction. Am J Obstet Gynecol 2000;183:211–7.

[57] Seng YC, Rajadurai VS. Twin-twin transfusion syndrome: a five-year review. Arch Dis Child 2000;83:F168–70.

[58] Cincotta RB, Gray PH, Phythian G, et al. Long term outcome of twin-twin transfusion syndrome. Arch Dis Child 2000;83:F171–6.

[59] Haverkamp F, Lex C, Hanisch C, et al. Neurodevelopmental risks in twin-to-twin transfusion syndrome: preliminary findings. Eur J Pediatr Neurol 2001;5:21–7.

[60] Sutcliffe AG, Sebire NJ, Pigott AJ, et al. Outcome for children born after in utero laser ablation therapy for severe twin-to-twin transfusion syndrome. Br J Obstet Gynaecol 2001;108: 1246–50.

[61] Lopriore E, Nagel HTC, Vandenbussche FPHA, et al. Long-term neurodevelopmental outcome in twin-to-twin transfusion syndrome. Am J Obstet Gynecol 2003;189:1314–9.

[62] Mahiey-Caputo D, Muller F, Joly D, et al. Pathogenesis of twin-twin transfusion syndrome: the renin-angiotensin system hypothesis. Fetal Diagn Ther 2001;16:241–4.

[63] Robillard JE, Gomez RA, Meernik JG, et al. Role of angiotensin II on the adrenal and vascular responses to hemorrhage during development in fetal lambs. Circ Res 1982;50:645–50.

[64] Cheung YF, Taylor MJ, Fisk NM, et al. Fetal origins of reduced arterial distensibility in the donor twin in twin-twin transfusion syndrome. Lancet 2000;355:1157–8.

[65] Gardiner HM, Taylor MJO, Karatza A, et al. Twin-twin transfusion syndrome: the influence of intrauterine laser photocoagulation on arterial distensibility in childhood. Circulation 2003; 107:1906–11.

[66] Karatza AA, Wolfenden JL, Taylor MJO, et al. Influence of twin-twin transfusion syndrome on fetal cardiovascular structure and function: prospective case-control study of 136 monochorionic twin pregnancies. Heart 2002;88:271–7.

[67] Raboisson MJ, Fouron JC, Lamoureux J, et al. Early intertwin differences in myocardial performance during the twin-to-twin transfusion syndrome. Circulation 2004;110:3043–8.

[68] Lougheed J, Sinclair BG, Funk KFK, et al. Acquired right ventricular outflow tract obstruction in the recipient twin in twin-twin transfusion syndrome. J Am Coll Cardiol 2001;38:1533–8.

[69] Zosmer N, Bajoria R, Weiner E, et al. Clinical and echographic features of in utero cardiac dysfunction in the recipient twin in twin-twin transfusion syndrome. Br Heart J 1994;72(1): 74–9.

[70] Segar JL, Dalshaug GB, Bedell KA, et al. Angiotensin II in cardiac pressure-overload hypertrophy in fetal sheep. Am J Physiol Regul Integr Comp Physiol 2001;281:R2037–47.

[71] Bajoria R, Sullivan M, Fisk NM. Endothelin concentrations in monochorionic twins with severe twin-twin transfusion syndrome. Hum Reprod 1999;14(6):1614–8.

[72] Senat M-V, Deprest J, Boulvain M, et al. Endoscopic laser surgery versus serial amnioreduction for severe twin-to-twin transfusion syndrome. N Engl J Med 2004;351:136–44.

[73] van Gemert MJ, Umur A, Tijssen JG, et al. Twin-twin transfusion syndrome: etiology, severity, and rational management. Curr Opin Obstet Gynecol 2001;13(2):193–206.

[74] Lougheed J, Sinclair BG, Fung Kee Fung K, et al. Acquired right ventricular outflow tract obstruction in the recipient twin in twin-twin transfusion syndrome. J Am Coll Cardiol 2001; 38:1533–8.

CLINICS IN
PERINATOLOGY

Clin Perinatol 32 (2005) 877–890

Does Fetal Diagnosis Make a Difference?

Meryl S. Cohen, MD[a],*, Michele A. Frommelt, MD[b]

[a]Division of Cardiology, The Children's Hospital of Philadelphia, 34th Street and
Civic Center Boulevard, Philadelphia, PA 19104, USA
[b]Division of Cardiology, Children's Hospital of Wisconsin, 9000 West Wisconsin Avenue,
Milwaukee, WI 53201, USA

Fetal echocardiography has made substantial differences in the world of pediatric cardiology today. It has taught us much about the natural history of congenital heart disease in utero, particularly that certain lesions are progressive and undergo significant change throughout gestation. Fetal echocardiography has guided us in identifying candidates for prenatal cardiac intervention and has aided us to perform these procedures technically with success. It has enabled us to diagnose, monitor, and treat arrhythmias and, in some cases, to observe rapid conversion to a normal sinus rhythm with prompt resolution of ventricular dysfunction and fetal hydrops. With prenatal identification, we are able to counsel families about their child's cardiac disease and the anticipated course after birth. Recognition of congenital heart disease in utero often affects the location and timing of delivery and often avoids hemodynamic compromise, especially with ductal-dependent lesions. Fetal echocardiography has extended the care of children with congenital heart disease to include the fetus and has opened a new frontier within pediatric cardiology.

Indications for fetal echocardiography

Recent advances in two-dimensional and Doppler echocardiography have allowed more accurate and earlier detection of congenital cardiac abnormalities. Because most cases of congenital heart disease occur in pregnancies with no known risk factors, routine obstetric screening of the fetal heart becomes

* Corresponding author.
  E-mail address: cohenm@email.chop.edu (M.S. Cohen).

0095-5108/05/$ – see front matter © 2005 Elsevier Inc. All rights reserved.
doi:10.1016/j.clp.2005.09.007   *perinatology.theclinics.com*

imperative. Unfortunately, many defects continue to be missed in the low-risk population, because only a four-chamber view of the heart is obtained, typically at approximately 18 weeks of gestation. Many studies have demonstrated that this does not suffice as a prenatal screening test for congenital heart disease, because the more common congenital heart abnormalities go undetected if outflow tracts are not included or the abnormality may progress throughout gestation [1–3]. Although the American College of Obstetrics and Gynecology recommends

---

Box 1. Indications for fetal echocardiography

Fetal
    Extracardiac anomalies, including
        Omphalocele
        Diaphragmatic hernia
        Duodenal atresia
        Transesophageal fistula
        Horseshoe kidney
        Renal agenesis
        Single umbilical artery
        Velocardiofacial syndrome
        Trisomy 13, 18, or 21
    Nonimmune hydrops
    Sustained arrhythmias
    Abnormal four-chamber view
    Abnormal outflow tract view
    Increased first-trimester nuchal translucency measurement
Maternal
    Maternal congenital heart defect
    Metabolic disorder
        Diabetes mellitus
        Collagen vascular disease
        Phenylketonuria
    Teratogen exposure
        Alcohol
        Lithium
        Anticonvulsants
Familial
    Previous child with congenital heart disease
    Mendelian syndrome
        Tuberous sclerosis
        Noonan
        Marfan
        Hypertrophic cardiomyopathy

obtaining only a four-chamber view of the heart on a low-risk ultrasound scan, we advocate the addition of outflow tract imaging. The addition of outflow tract imaging to screening ultrasound has been shown to improve the effectiveness of routine prenatal screening for major congenital heart defects [4,5]. It improves identification of conotruncal abnormalities, such as transposition of the great arteries, tetralogy of Fallot, a double-outlet right ventricle, and truncus arteriosus. Although these lesions are typically quiescent throughout gestation, transition to the neonatal circulation can be problematic in some patients, leading to the need for prompt resuscitation and/or intervention at a tertiary care facility. Importantly, many of these lesions are surgically amenable to complete repair with an excellent long-term outcome.

The indications for a high-risk fetal echocardiogram, including multiple anatomic views and Doppler analysis of the heart, are traditionally divided into three categories: fetal, maternal, and familial (Box 1). The likelihood of a positive yield varies with each indication, so much so that one might consider some indications unnecessary and others absolutely essential. For example, it is well known that isolated extrasystoles in the fetus are common and rarely associated with structural heart disease [6]. The biggest risk, albeit low, seems to be the development of a sustained tachyarrhythmia, which would be best monitored locally by the obstetrician and the mother carrying the fetus. Contrast that to the fetal indication of an abnormal four-chamber view, where the yield is extremely high, somewhere in the range of 50%. The structural lesions identified are often complex, necessitating close prenatal follow-up, parental counseling, and, possibly, delivery at a tertiary care facility.

Abnormal nuchal fold thickening in early gestation (10–14 weeks) is one of the newly recognized risk factors for major congenital heart disease [7,8]. Hyett and colleagues [7] reviewed a total of 29,000 chromosomally normal fetuses undergoing nuchal fold measurements. More than 50% of fetuses with major cardiac malformations had abnormal nuchal fold measurements in early gestation. Also, as nuchal fold thickening increased, there was an increased prevalence of cardiac defects. The reason for this association remains unclear. Other indications yielding a high incidence of congenital heart disease include the presence of extracardiac or chromosomal abnormalities in the fetus, nonimmune fetal hydrops, and maternal metabolic disorders, such as diabetes mellitus and collagen vascular disease [9–12].

Natural history of congenital heart disease

The development and use of fetal echocardiography has given pediatric cardiologists a unique opportunity to observe and follow the natural history of congenital heart disease in utero. Our understanding of many aspects of cardiac development and cardiovascular physiology has been significantly enhanced by these antenatal observations and has led to the development of fetal cardiac intervention as a new and innovative field within pediatric cardiology. It has become clear that congenital heart disease is not a static but rather a dynamic process that evolves over the course of gestation. Furthermore, progression of fetal heart disease is often affected by the timing of the insult during gestation, with earlier injury more likely to lead to more significant progression. Although some cardiac defects, such as obstructive or regurgitant valvular disease, change rapidly during gestation, others, such as transposition of the great arteries, are relatively quiescent during fetal life but have profound hemodynamic abnormalities at birth. In addition to structural congenital heart disease, sustained fetal arrhythmias may have a significant impact on the function of the fetal heart and the well-being of the fetus over the course of gestation. Arrhythmias can be diagnosed and monitored with the use of m-mode and Doppler fetal echocardiography, and the initiation and effects of medical therapy can be guided by the observations on serial studies. We now know that fetal hydrops related to sustained tachyarrhythmias can resolve with appropriate medical therapy. Fetal bradyarrhythmias are historically more difficult to manage; however, successful fetal pacing is certainly on the horizon.

Altered flow theory

One of the most important hypotheses substantiated from observations in fetal echocardiography is the altered flow theory. The fetal circulation is a unique system with parallel systemic and pulmonary circuits; communication between the two circulations is provided by the patent foramen ovale and patent ductus arteriosus. This physiology allows for blood flow to shift from one circuit to the other, especially if there is increased resistance to flow in one pathway. Diminished forward flow into a chamber or great vessel resulting in abnormal growth of fetal cardiac structures has been observed by fetal echocardiography, especially in fetuses with early obstructive or regurgitant lesions. Many examples exist to validate this theory.

After birth, the normal left ventricle receives blood almost exclusively from the pulmonary veins. In contrast, the fetal left ventricle is predominantly filled by oxygenated blood that returns from the placenta and traverses the foramen ovale [13]. If a hemodynamic disturbance results in diminished flow across the foramen ovale, the combined cardiac output is diverted to the right ventricle and pulmonary artery, resulting in less impetus for normal growth of the left-sided structures. Although adequate blood flow is provided to the pulmonary bed and the systemic bed via the patent foramen ovale and ductus arteriosus, there is now the potential for evolution of hypoplastic left heart syndrome.

Several mechanisms may cause diminished flow across the foramen ovale, including restrictive foramen ovale size [14], structural left-sided disease (eg, mitral stenosis, aortic stenosis) [15], extrinsic compression of the heart (eg, left congenital diaphragmatic hernia) [16], or an intrinsic abnormality of the myocardium. Because aortic valve disease is relatively common, many fetal studies have focused on and serially followed this abnormality throughout gestation. We now know that a bicuspid aortic valve and mild aortic stenosis are often well tolerated during fetal life. With more significant aortic stenosis, however, alterations in left ventricular compliance may occur secondary to the development of left ventricular hypertrophy or to the development of left ventricular dilatation and dysfunction with endocardial fibroelastosis. Endocardial fibroelastosis is a poorly understood phenomenon in which the endocardial lining of the left ventricle becomes fibrotic. If the disease state persists, flow across the foramen ovale (normally right to left in utero) reverses and flows from the left atrium to the right atrium. This reversal of foramen ovale flow, detectable by pulsed and color Doppler ultrasound, heralds severe left heart obstruction, the result of which may be the cessation of left ventricular growth [17] (Fig. 1). A

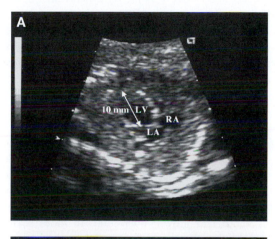

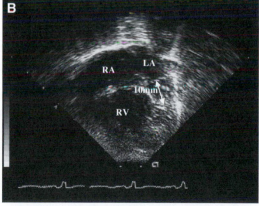

Fig. 1. (A) Fetal four-chamber view demonstrating a dilated but well-developed left ventricular chamber with areas of endocardial fibroelastosis in an 18-week-old fetus with critical aortic stenosis. The arrow indicates a left ventricular internal dimension of 10 mm. (B) Apical four-chamber view in the same patient at birth demonstrating marked hypoplasia of the left ventricle consistent with hypoplastic left heart syndrome. The arrow indicates a left ventricular internal dimension of 10 mm, unchanged since 18 weeks of gestation. LA, left atrium; LV, left ventricle; RA, right atrium; RV, right ventricle.

dilated and poorly functioning left ventricle of adequate size at midgestation may ultimately become a hypoplastic and akinetic left ventricular chamber at birth [18–21]. Hornberger and coworkers [21] followed 21 fetuses with left heart obstruction using serial echocardiography. Although the left ventricular measurements were normal at the midtrimester examination, left heart hypoplasia developed by the time of birth. A small mitral valve and ascending aorta at midgestation predicted a smaller left ventricle at term. Less severe forms of left heart obstruction may also progress. Babies born with coarctation of the aorta often have progressive hypoplasia of the transverse arch and isthmus of the aorta during middle to late gestation [22,23].

Similar to left heart obstructive lesions, right heart obstruction may result in cessation of growth of distal structures. Diminished growth of the pulmonary arteries has been observed in tetralogy of Fallot, where severe subpulmonary obstruction leads to diversion of blood in the right ventricle across the ventricular septal defect directly into the aorta [24,25]. This abnormal flow pattern promotes the development of a dilated aortic root, one of the earliest reported fetal echocardiographic markers of tetralogy of Fallot. In tricuspid atresia, pulmonary artery size is often related to the size of the ventricular septal defect that provides flow to the pulmonary vascular bed exclusively; a large ventricular septal defect provides unobstructed flow to the branch pulmonary arteries, which are usually well developed, whereas a small ventricular septal defect is typically associated with pulmonary outflow obstruction. Severe pulmonary stenosis has also been observed to become pulmonary atresia before birth [26]. Altered right ventricular compliance may lead to augmented right-to-left atrial level shunting, causing cessation of right ventricular growth over time. In more severe forms of the disease, fistulae develop between the right ventricle and coronary arteries so that the blood entering the right ventricle fills the coronaries in a retrograde manner [27,28]. Because this type of pulmonary atresia carries a significantly worse prognosis than other less severe forms of the disease, early fetal intervention for a severely stenotic pulmonary valve seems attractive.

Forward flow can also be impeded when there is significant valvular regurgitation. In Ebstein's anomaly with severe tricuspid regurgitation, forward flow to the pulmonary arteries is diminished. Although antegrade pulmonary blood flow may have been relatively normal early in gestation, it is not uncommon to see the development of severe pulmonary stenosis and even pulmonary atresia by the time of delivery [29,30].

In addition to the unique parallel circulation of the fetal cardiovascular system, there are several features of fetal myocardium that differ from the adult myocardium. Fetal myocardial cells have more noncontractile elements and different relaxation properties than adult cardiac cells, resulting in a less compliant myocardium [31]. This is reflected in the fetal Doppler inflow pattern of the atrioventricular valves, which exhibit a prominent A wave (atrial contraction) with less passive early filling. Some investigators advocate that it is not the intrinsic properties but rather the extrinsic compression of the fetal heart that causes diminished compliance [32]. In any case, a demand for increased cardiac output is poorly tolerated in the fetus, because stroke volume cannot be significantly augmented by increased preload [33]. Instead, atrial pressure begins to increase and hydrops fetalis may develop. These factors make the fetal myocardium particularly vulnerable to lesions that increase preload. Several disease states can cause fetal heart failure, including arteriovenous malformations, sacrococcygeal teratoma, congenital cystic adenomatoid malformation of the lung, anemia, sustained arrhythmias (bradycardia or tachycardia), and significant atrioventricular valve regurgitation.

Fetal heart failure is manifested as increasing heart size, diminished ventricular shortening, atrioventricular valve regurgitation, development of hydrops fetalis, and, eventually, abnormal umbilical and ductus venosus Doppler patterns (Fig. 2) [34]. The development of umbilical venous pulsations and reversal of flow in the umbilical artery are poor prognostic signs and predict fetal demise. Fetal heart failure is often difficult to treat unless the disease process causing the hemodynamic abnormality is reversed. For example, fetal surgical intervention to remove sacrococcygeal teratoma in fetuses with hydrops has resulted in reversal of the hydrops and improved survival in some cases [35].

The severity of structural and acquired heart defects may evolve over time, with full manifestation of disease only in late gestation, thus serial fetal echocardiographic studies continue to be a critically important part of our work. Collaboration with other centers should add to our ever-expanding knowledge base and provide valuable information on the constantly changing fetal

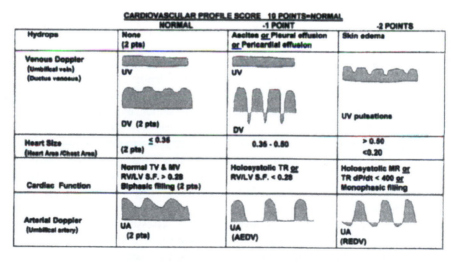

Fig. 2. The heart failure score is 10 if there are no abnormal signs and reflects 2 points for each of five categories: hydrops, venous Doppler, heart size, cardiac function, and arterial Doppler. AEDV, absent end-diastolic velocity; *dP/dt*, change in pressure over time of TR jet; DV, ductus venosus; LV, left ventricle; MR, mitral valve regurgitation; MV, mitral valve; pts, points; SF, ventricular shortening fraction; TR, tricuspid valve regurgitation; TV, tricuspid valve; REDV, reversed end-diastolic velocity; RV, right ventricle; UV, umbilical vein. (*From* Huhta JC. Guidelines for the evaluation of heart failure in the fetus with or without hydrops. Pediatr Cardiol 2004;25:276; with permission.)

cardiovascular system. Serial studies are also important to monitor for the development of progressive obstruction or ventricular dysfunction and to assess the growth rate of structures that may be affected by abnormal forward flow. The data obtained should also help to guide us as to the timing and need for fetal cardiac intervention, whether it be medical or "surgical." It should also provide us with information about the best candidates for fetal cardiac intervention.

Finally, we have also learned that some fetal cardiac hemodynamics do not always worsen by the time of birth. Subtle cardiac abnormalities, such as pericardial effusion and some forms of cardiomyopathy, may improve by the end of gestation, such that there is no demonstrable disease at birth. Moreover, true structural defects, such as ventricular septal defects, may be more prevalent than previously thought. Paladini and colleagues [36] reported that approximately one third of ventricular septal defects close before birth and that the likelihood of closure is determined by the size and location of the defect, with muscular defects being the most common to close spontaneously. Fetal arrhythmias may also improve over the course of gestation. Some forms of atrial arrhythmias convert to normal rhythm spontaneously. If the rhythm converts spontaneously or with medical intervention, the hydrops (if present) may improve.

Outcome for prenatal diagnosis of congenital heart disease

During the past 25 years, neonatal cardiac surgery has grown and developed into a tremendously successful and innovative field. The surgical outcomes for many cardiac defects have improved significantly over this period, such that there are few lesions that cannot be palliated or corrected in the current era. Recently, other measures of success have become relevant, including surgical reoperation rate, frequency of hospitalization, and exercise tolerance. Neurodevelopmental issues in our patients are now being recognized, including poor school performance, psychiatric disorders, and attention deficit hyperactivity disorder. With our patients now surviving into adulthood, quality of life becomes critical. How many adults with congenital heart disease are going to marry and be able to have children, maintain employment, and live long lives? These questions are only beginning to be answered. Also, with surgical and intensive care innovation as well as the broad application of accurate prenatal diagnosis, patients operated on in 2005 are likely to have a better long-term outcome than those who had surgery 25 years ago. Recent studies that have assessed the impact of prenatal diagnosis on outcome have typically addressed only surgical survival; the answers to many of the other long-term questions are yet to come but remain essential.

Surgical mortality and morbidity

Although a fetus with severe congenital heart disease is generally quite stable in the antenatal environment, transition to the neonatal period often results in hemodynamic compromise; this is particularly true for patients with ductal-dependent circulation. In right heart obstructive lesions, ductal closure results in severe hypoxemia from diminished pulmonary blood flow. In contrast, ductal closure in left heart obstructive lesions causes markedly diminished systemic blood flow and end-organ shock, resulting in severe metabolic acidosis and eventual death. Thus, identification of such lesions in utero provides caregivers the ability to maintain ductal patency and hemodynamic stability with prostaglandin E_1 therapy.

Despite the prompt administration of prostaglandin E_1 to prenatally diagnosed patients, many studies have not shown a significant improvement in surgical survival for these patients when compared with those diagnosed postnatally [37–42]. Fountain-Dommer and coworkers [42] recently reported their experience with prenatal diagnosis of patients undergoing the Norwood procedure. Of the prenatally diagnosed patients who underwent surgery, 83% survived compared with 79% of the postnatally diagnosed group. In fact, no differences were found between the groups with regard to preoperative stability or postoperative morbidity. In contrast, there are a few published reports that have demonstrated improved survival for patients with prenatal diagnosis [43,44]. Tworetzky and colleagues [43] reported that patients with a prenatal diagnosis of hypoplastic left heart syndrome had 100% survival (n = 14) after the Norwood procedure compared with 66% survival (n = 38) in those diagnosed after birth. Improved early survival in this study was attributed to better preoperative clinical condition. Similar results have been reported for coarctation of the aorta [44]. Transposition of the great arteries, a cardiac lesion that may not be ductal dependent but can present with severe cyanosis, has also arguably been influenced by prenatal diagnosis. Bonnet and coworkers [45] reported that the prenatal diagnosis of transposition improved preoperative as well as postoperative mortality compared with those cases diagnosed postnatally. In contrast, Kumar and colleagues [38] did not find a significant difference in surgical mortality between prenatally and postnatally diagnosed patients with transposition of the great arteries.

So many factors other than early recognition of disease have an impact on surgical survival for congenital heart disease (eg, cardiopulmonary bypass time, circulatory arrest, surgical procedure, cardiac anesthesia, postoperative intensive care), therefore it is not surprising that controversy exists about the impact of prenatal diagnosis on outcome. In addition, some would argue that patients with a prenatal diagnosis have more severe disease than those diagnosed postnatally, which may contribute to morbidity and mortality. For example, patients with heterotaxy syndrome are more likely to be identified in utero if complete heart block is also seen. Complete heart block presents as fetal bradycardia, which alerts the obstetrician to evaluate the fetus for cardiac abnormalities. Complete heart block in association with heterotaxy syndrome is almost uniformly fatal no matter the timing or type of intervention [46]. Other lesions may be easier to identify prenatally when the presentation is more severe. A fetus with a small left ventricle may not be recognized on level II ultrasound, but the same fetus with severe tricuspid regurgitation is more likely to be identified and referred to a pediatric cardiologist. Severe tricuspid regurgitation is a significant risk factor for poor outcome in patients with hypoplastic left heart syndrome [47,48]. In addition, patients with extracardiac anomalies or chromosomal abnormalities who have associated congenital heart disease are likely to be identified before birth; these anomalies are also significant risk factors for poor outcome of neonatal cardiac surgery [49].

Although hospital mortality may not be significantly improved by prenatal diagnosis, morbidity is positively affected by early identification of disease in many studies. Verheijen and colleagues [41,50] reported that infants with a prenatal diagnosis of congenital heart disease were more likely to have better pH, higher base excess, and lower lactate levels than those with a postnatal diagnosis; this was particularly true for those patients with ductal-dependent physiology. For hypoplastic left heart syndrome, prenatal diagnosis has been associated with less metabolic acidosis, improved ventricular function, and less severe tricuspid valve regurgitation [40,43]. Prenatal diagnosis has also been shown to reduce delay in hospital admission and subsequent surgical intervention [39,40,44,45,51]. With regard to neurodevelopmental outcome, there are few reports in the literature. Mahle and coworkers [40] reported that prenatal diagnosis of hypoplastic left heart syndrome had a favorable impact on short-term neurologic outcome. In this cohort, fewer patients diagnosed prenatally had neurologic events after the Norwood procedure compared with those diagnosed after birth. In contrast, prenatal identification of transposition of the great arteries does not seem to influence short-term neurodevelopmental outcome. Bartlett and colleagues [52] performed the Psychomotor Development Index and Mental Development Index on 1-year-old infants with transposition of the great arteries and found no differences in the scores if a prenatal diagnosis was made. This study was limited by the fact that the prenatal group contained a small number of patients; therefore, subtle differences would not have been identified. Although these studies do suggest that prenatal diagnosis improves short-term morbidity, the long-term impact of prenatal diagnosis remains to be seen.

Family planning

Perhaps the most important but somewhat immeasurable impacts of fetal echocardiography and prenatal diagnosis are those that affect the family. It is well known that the spectrum of heart disease diagnosed prenatally is quite different than that seen by the general pediatric cardiologist. Complex disease is over-represented with the present practice of four-chamber view imaging, and the heart disease is often associated with other extracardiac abnormalities. Unless prenatal ultrasound is completely abandoned, these complex patients should continue to appear and may increase in number as low-risk scanning techniques improve. How are these families best served?

When congenital heart disease is suspected prenatally, a multidisciplinary approach is needed to evaluate and support the mother, fetus, and family. No one specialist has sufficient knowledge or training to work alone in this setting. Many centers have developed specialized fetal cardiology programs, where pediatric cardiologists, perinatologists, neonatologists, cardiac surgeons, geneticists, social workers, and even psychologists work together to provide complete care for the fetus and family.

Accuracy of the prenatal diagnosis is critical for parental counseling and for further management of the pregnancy and delivery. Many recent studies have demonstrated that the addition of a pediatric cardiologist in the multidisciplinary group leads to improved accuracy of detected congenital heart disease [53,54]. In a recent study by Cuneo and colleagues [53], the integration of a pediatric cardiologist into the perinatal team led to an increased rate of detection of critical congenital heart disease as well as improved diagnostic accuracy (97% positive predictive value with integration versus 75% without). In an earlier study by Berghella and coworkers [54], maternal fetal medicine specialists and pediatric cardiologists were equally able to detect congenital heart disease; however, the pediatric cardiologist was more accurate in identifying the exact diagnosis.

Once the diagnosis of congenital heart disease is confirmed, a complete anatomic survey of the fetus is also performed. With the recent collaboration of the pediatric cardiologist, and perinatologist, studies can be performed together so that a timely and complete diagnosis can be made. Genetic counseling should be immediately available, especially in the setting of a suspected abnormal karyotype. Also, it has been well documented that prenatally detected congenital anomalies of any sort can result in great stress to affected families. Social services and psychologic support may be necessary for the family, including the mother, father, and siblings.

Before discharging the family from the clinic, follow-up should be carefully arranged. In many cases, serial ultrasound is important to monitor the growth and well-being of the fetus as well as to evaluate any important changes in the fetal cardiac structure or function. Arrangements for delivery should be discussed, because many of the lesions diagnosed prenatally require prompt resuscitation or intervention. Delivery at a tertiary care facility can avoid transport-related morbidity and is likely to improve overall mortality. Also, delivery at a tertiary care facility allows the parents to be close to their newborn as the mother recovers from the birth and allows the family to have access to the medical and surgical team caring for their baby. These factors certainly improve the already stressful experience that parents face when delivering a newborn with critical congenital heart disease.

Future

During the next 20 years, there should be continued improvements in screening for congenital heart disease, with improved diagnostic accuracy, even in the low-risk population. Advances in ultrasound technology and image resolution may lead to earlier diagnosis, and possibly earlier intervention. Three-dimensional echocardiography may provide additional information and improve accuracy by rapid uniform data acquisition. Collaborative studies should add to our present knowledge of fetal cardiac development and physiology and should guide us in our therapies. Fetal cardiac intervention has already had some success in the setting of critical aortic stenosis and is likely to continue to expand and improve.

Recently, the impact of prenatal diagnosis on the overall incidence of congenital heart disease has been brought into question. Many factors play a role in parental decision making, including the severity of the cardiac anomaly, the addition of extracardiac anomalies, and even the availability of postnatal treatment in some countries. In an earlier study by Allan and coworkers [55], a significant decrease in the overall incidence of hypoplastic left heart syndrome over time was reported, because the rate of pregnancy termination was quite high. In a more recent study by Daubeney and colleagues [56], a termination rate of 60% was reported when the diagnosis of pulmonary atresia with intact ventricular septum was made; this resulted in a significant decrease in the incidence of this disease over a 5-year period. This information is more difficult to collect in the United States, but there are presently no documented reports of a change in the incidence of critical congenital heart disease.

Summary

Fetal echocardiography has clearly made a difference in the world of pediatric cardiology today. It has taught us much about the natural history of fetal cardiac disease, and with ongoing collaborative studies, it should continue to enhance our knowledge base. Fetal echocardiography has enabled us to identify potential candidates for fetal cardiac intervention and has promoted the development of an exciting new discipline within pediatric cardiology. We hope that the recognition of critical congenital heart disease in utero improves the long-term outcome of our patients, including neurodevelopmental outcome and quality of life.

References

[1] Allan LD, Crawford DC, Chita SK, et al. Prenatal screening for congenital heart disease. BMJ 1986;292:1717–9.
[2] Achiron R, Glaser J, Gelernter I, et al. Extended fetal echocardiographic examination for detecting cardiac malformations in low risk pregnancies. BMJ 1992;304:671–4.
[3] Bromley B, Estroff JA, Sanders SP, et al. Fetal echocardiography: accuracy and limitations in a population at high and low risk for heart defects. Am J Obstet Gynecol 1992;166:1473–81.
[4] Carvalho JS, Mavrides E, Shinebourne EA, et al. Improving the effectiveness of routine prenatal screening for major congenital heart defects. Heart 2002;88:387–91.
[5] Kirk JS, Riggs TW, Comstock CH, et al. Prenatal screening for cardiac anomalies: the value of routine addition of the aortic root to the four-chamber view. Obstet Gynecol 1994;84:427–31.
[6] Kleinman CS, Copel JA. Fetal cardiac arrhythmias: diagnosis and therapy. In: Resnick R, Creasy R, editors. Maternal fetal medicine. Philadelphia: WB Saunders; 1994. p. 326–41.

[7] Hyett JA, Perdu M, Gurleen S, et al. Using fetal nuchal translucency to screen for major congenital cardiac defects at 10–14 weeks of gestation: population-based cohort study. BMJ 1999;318:81–5.

[8] Galindo A, Comas C, Martinez JM, et al. Cardiac defects in chromosomally normal fetuses with increased nuchal translucency at 10–14 weeks of gestation. J Matern Fetal Neonatal Med 2003;13:163–70.

[9] Copel JA, Pilu G, Kleinman CS. Extracardiac anomalies and congenital heart disease. Semin Perinatol 1993;17:89–105.

[10] Becerra JE, Khoury MJ, Cordero JF, et al. Diabetes mellitus during pregnancy and the risks for specific birth defects: a population-based case-control study. Pediatrics 1990;85:1–9.

[11] Buyon JP, Hiebert R, Copel J, et al. Autoimmune-associated congenital heart block: demographics, mortality, morbidity and recurrence rates obtained from a national neonatal lupus registry. J Am Coll Cardiol 1998;31:1658–66.

[12] Jones DC. Non-immune hydrops fetalis. Semin Perinatol 1995;19:447–61.

[13] Atkins DL, Clark EB, Marvin WJ. Foramen ovale/atrial septum ratio: a marker of transatrial blood flow. Circulation 1982;66:281–3.

[14] Chabot V, Hornberger LK, Hagen-Ansert S, et al. Prenatal detection of restrictive foramen ovale. J Am Soc Echocardiogr 1990;3:15–9.

[15] McCaffrey FM, Sherman FS. Prenatal diagnosis of severe aortic stenosis. Pediatr Cardiol 1997; 18:276–81.

[16] Baumgart S, Paul JJ, Huhta JC, et al. Cardiac malposition, redistribution of fetal cardiac output and left heart hypoplasia reduce survival in neonates with congenital diaphragmatic hernia requiring extracorporeal membrane oxygenation. J Pediatr 1998;133:57–62.

[17] Berning RA, Silverman NH, Villegas M, et al. Reversed shunting across the ductus arteriosus or atrial septum in utero heralds severe congenital heart disease. J Am Coll Cardiol 1996;27:481–6.

[18] Allan LD, Sharland GK, Tynan MJ. The natural history of hypoplastic left heart syndrome. Int J Cardiol 1989;25:341–3.

[19] Sharland GK, Chila SK, Fagg NLK, et al. Left ventricular dysfunction in the fetus: relation to aortic valve anomalies and endocardial fibroelastosis. Br Heart J 1991;66:419–24.

[20] Danford DA, Cronican P. Hypoplastic left heart syndrome: progression of left ventricular dilation and dysfunction to left ventricular hypoplasia in utero. Am Heart J 1992;123:1712–3.

[21] Hornberger LK, Sanders SP, Rein AJ, et al. Left heart obstructive lesions and left ventricular growth in the midtrimester fetus: a longitudinal study. Circulation 1995;92:1531–8.

[22] Allan LD, Chita SK, Anderson RH, et al. Coarctation of the aorta in prenatal life: an echocardiographic, anatomical, and functional study. Br Heart J 1988;59:356–60.

[23] Hornberger LK, Sahn DJ, Kleinman CS, et al. Antenatal diagnosis of coarctation of the aorta: a multicenter experience. J Am Coll Cardiol 1994;23:417–23.

[24] Allan LD, Sharland GK. Prognosis in fetal tetralogy of Fallot. Pediatr Cardiol 1992;13:1–4.

[25] Hornberger LK, Sanders SP, Sahn DJ, et al. In utero pulmonary artery and aortic growth and potential for progression of pulmonary outflow tract obstruction in tetralogy of Fallot. J Am Coll Cardiol 1995;23:739–45.

[26] Rice MJ, McDonald RW, Reller MD. Progressive pulmonary obstruction in the fetus: two case reports. Am J Perinatol 1993;10:424–7.

[27] Maeno YV, Boutin C, Hornberger LK, et al. Prenatal diagnosis of right ventricular outflow tract obstruction with intact ventricular septum, and detection of ventriculocoronary connections. Heart 1999;81:661–8.

[28] Sandor GG, Cook AC, Sharland GK, et al. Coronary arterial abnormalities in pulmonary atresia with intact ventricular septum diagnosed during fetal life. Cardiol Young 2002;12:436–44.

[29] Hornberger LK, Sahn DK, Kleinman CS, et al. Tricuspid valve disease with significant tricuspid insufficiency in the fetus: diagnosis and outcome. J Am Coll Cardiol 1991;17:167–73.

[30] Sharland GK, Chita SK, Allan LD. Tricuspid valve dysplasia or displacement in intrauterine life. J Am Coll Cardiol 1991;17:944–9.

[31] Friedman WF. The intrinsic physiologic properties of the developing heart. Prog Cardiovasc Dis 1972;15:87–111.

[32] Grant DA. Ventricular constraint in the fetus and newborn. Can J Cardiol 1999;15:95–104.

[33] Rychik J. Fetal cardiovascular physiology. Pediatr Cardiol 2004;25:201–9.

[34] Huhta JC. Guidelines for the evaluation of heart failure in the fetus with or without hydrops. Pediatr Cardiol 2004;25:274–86.

[35] Hedrick HL, Flake AW, Crombleholme TM, et al. Sacrococcygeal teratoma: prenatal assessment, fetal intervention, and outcome. J Pediatr Surg 2004;39:430–8.

[36] Paladini D, Palmieri S, Lamberti A, et al. Characterization and natural history of ventricular septal defects in the fetus. Ultrasound Obstet Gynecol 2000;16:118–22.

[37] Copel JA, Tan AS, Kleinman CS. Does a prenatal diagnosis of congenital heart disease alter short-term outcome? Ultrasound Obstet Gynecol 1997;10:237–41.

[38] Kumar RK, Newburger JW, Gauvreau K, et al. Comparison of outcome when hypoplastic left heart syndrome and transposition of the great arteries are diagnosed prenatally versus when diagnosis of these two conditions is made only postnatally. Am J Cardiol 1999;83:1649–53.

[39] Eapen RS, Rowland DG, Franklin WH. Effect of prenatal diagnosis of critical left heart obstruction on perinatal morbidity and mortality. Am J Perinatol 1998;15:237–42.

[40] Mahle WT, Clancy RR, McGaurn SP, et al. Impact of prenatal diagnosis on survival and early neurologic morbidity in neonates with the hypoplastic left heart syndrome. Pediatrics 2001;107:1277–82.

[41] Verheijen PM, Lisowski LA, Stoutenbeek P, et al. Prenatal diagnosis of congenital heart disease affects preoperative acidosis of the newborn patient. J Thorac Cardiovasc Surg 2001;121:798–803.

[42] Fountain-Dommer RR, Bradley SM, Stroud MR, et al. Outcome following, and impact of, pre-natal identification of the candidates for the Norwood procedure. Cardiol Young 2004;14:32–8.

[43] Tworetzky W, McElhinney DB, Reddy VM, et al. Improved surgical outcome after fetal diagnosis of hypoplastic left heart syndrome. Circulation 2001;103:1269–73.

[44] Franklin O, Burch M, Manning N, et al. Prenatal diagnosis of coarctation of the aorta improves survival and reduces morbidity. Heart 2002;87:67–9.

[45] Bonnet D, Coltri A, Butera G, et al. Prenatal diagnosis of transposition of great vessels reduces neonatal morbidity and mortality. Arch Mal Coeur Vaiss 1999;92:637–40.

[46] Cohen MS. Clarifying anatomical complexity: diagnosing heterotaxy syndrome in the fetus. Prog Pediatr Cardiol, in press.

[47] Barber G, Helton JG, Aglira BA, et al. The significance of tricuspid regurgitation in hypoplastic left heart syndrome. Am Heart J 1988;116:1563–7.

[48] Chang AC, Farrell PE, Murdison KA, et al. Hypoplastic left heart syndrome: hemodynamic and angiographic assessment after initial reconstructive surgery and relevance to modified Fontan procedure. J Am Coll Cardiol 1991;17:1143–9.

[49] Gaynor JW, Mahle WT, Cohen MI, et al. Risk factors for mortality after the Norwood procedure. Eur J Cardiothorac Surg 2002;22:82–9.

[50] Verheijen PM, Lisowski LA, Stoutenbeek P, et al. Lactacidosis in the neonate is minimized by prenatal detection of congenital heart disease. Ultrasound Obstet Gynecol 2002;19:552–5.

[51] Chang AC, Huhta JC, Yoon GY, et al. Diagnosis, transport, and outcome in fetuses with left ventricular outflow tract obstruction. J Thorac Cardiovasc Surg 1991;102:841–8.

[52] Bartlett JM, Wypij D, Bellinger DC, et al. Effect of prenatal diagnosis on outcomes in D-transposition of the great arteries. Pediatrics 2004;113:335–40.

[53] Cuneo BF, Curran LF, Davis N, et al. Trends in prenatal diagnosis of critical cardiac defects in an integrated obstetric and pediatric cardiac imaging center. J Perinatol 2004;24:674–8.

[54] Berghella V, Pagotto L, Kaufman M, et al. Accuracy of prenatal diagnosis of congenital heart defects. Fetal Diagn Ther 2001;16:407–12.

[55] Allan LD, Cook A, Sullivan I, et al. Hypoplastic left heart syndrome: effects of fetal echo-cardiography on birth prevalence. Lancet 1991;337:959–61.

[56] Daubeney PE, Sharland GK, Cook AC, et al. Pulmonary atresia with intact ventricular septum: impact of fetal echocardiography on incidence at birth and postnatal outcome. UK and Eire Collaborative Study of Pulmonary Atresia with Intact Ventricular Septum. Circulation 1998;98:562–6.

ELSEVIER
SAUNDERS

CLINICS IN
PERINATOLOGY

Clin Perinatol 32 (2005) 891–912

Prenatal Diagnosis of Fetal Arrhythmias

Janette F. Strasburger, MD[a,b,c,*]

[a]*Medical College of Wisconsin, Milwaukee, WI 53201, USA*
[b]*Children's Hospital of Wisconsin, 9000 West Wisconsin Avenue, MS 713, Milwaukee, WI 53201, USA*
[c]*Children's Hospital of Wisconsin–Fox Valley, 200 Theda Clark Medical Plaza, Suite 480,*
Neenah, WI 54956, USA

Life-threatening fetal arrhythmias are rare and warrant sophisticated specialty prenatal care, often provided by maternal-fetal medicine obstetricians, and pediatric and adult cardiologists. This medical field is in quick transition, and new methods of diagnosis and treatment of the fetus with arrhythmias are emerging. In this article, the mechanisms of arrhythmias are presented in light of recent progress in the new field of fetal electrophysiology. Treatments are reviewed with recommendations based on the small number of series of fetal tachycardia and fetal atrioventricular (AV) block drug treatment strategies published to date. Finally, a summary of areas of potential future research is outlined.

The diagnosis of fetal arrhythmias has undergone a dramatic change within the past decade. Now, in addition to the diagnostic capabilities afforded by echocardiography and Doppler imaging, the new modality of fetal magnetocardiography (FMCG) is defining fetal cardiac conduction and rhythm patterns in a much more precise manner [1–9]. FMCG is capable of providing actual cardiogram signals as opposed to the mechanical motion documented by M-mode, 2-D, and pulsed Doppler; and it provides precise electrophysiologic data, including QRS and QT interval, beat-to-beat heart rate variability, and presence of T-wave alternans (a T-wave pattern associated with sudden death) [6,10]. Tissue Doppler also provides a new means of defining the mechanical relationship of atrial and ventricular wall motion, yielding better prediction of electrophysiologic events [11,12]. This technique measures the motion of the myocardium and allows predictions of diastolic function. Origins of events such as the AV and ventricoatrial (VA) intervals can be predicted (Fig. 1).

---

* Children's Hospital of Wisconsin, 9000 West Wisconsin Avenue, MS 713, Milwaukee, WI 53201.

E-mail address: jstrasbu@mcw.edu

0095-5108/05/$ – see front matter © 2005 Elsevier Inc. All rights reserved.

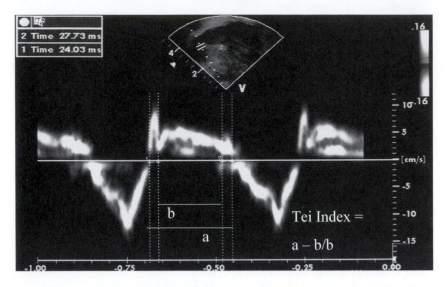

Fig. 1. Tissue Doppler recording: The Tei Index is an index of diastolic function. Shown here is a tracing from the lateral myocardial wall near the AV valve.

It has not been possible to use the fetal electrocardiogram clinically before the onset of labor because of the poor signal-to-noise ratios caused by the insulating effect of the vernix caseo'sa in latter pregnancy and the small signal size [12–15]. Likewise, obstetric fetal heart rhythm assessment has been performed using systems developed for the analysis of heart rate variability within the normal range, but insensitive to the assessment of ectopy (irregular heart beats), or rates well outside of the expected range. Despite limitations in electrophysiologic accuracy in diagnostics over the past three decades, perinatal clinicians have made significant advancements in fetal cardiac drug therapy that are reviewed in this article. There remains a need, however, to tailor the knowledge learned to date by the more accurate diagnostic capabilities that are now available with Doppler, tissue Doppler and FMCG.

Drug therapy has also changed over the past decade, with an increasing awareness of the potential risks of proarrhythmia, with the initiation of new anti-arrhythmic agents into fetal use, with the use of drug combinations in some circumstances, and with the expansion of interventional fetal treatment techniques altering drug delivery. The fetus without hydrops is easily treated with most drugs, is unlikely to die from fetal drug treatment, and, in many cases, does not even warrant medication treatment. The trigger instinct to deliver urgently or to treat the fetus just because of the presence of an arrhythmia, should be eliminated from perinatal medicine and replaced by the more refined assessment of these patients. Less ill fetuses have been included in many published series of fetal tachycardia therapies, thus diluting the mortality incidence and making some drugs appear to have a good therapeutic effect when, in fact, proarrhythmic car-

Table 1
Fetal tachycardia treatment series

	Hansmann, et al [19]	Oudijk, et al [18]	Simpson, et al [17]	Frohn-Mulder, et al [16]	Van Engelen, et al [20]	Allan, et al [21]	Sonneson, et al [22]	Juniak, et al [23]	Strasburger, et al [24]
Year Published	1991	2000	1998	1995	1994	1991	1998	2003	2004
Patients	60	20	110	35	34	14	14	25	24
% HF	35	40	39	37	44	100	57	100	93
SVT (# pts)	54	10	105	35	25	12	14	21	15
% of SVT HF pts cnvt	50	60	66	59	82	100	60	93	93
AFL (# pts)	6	10	22	0	9	2	0	4	9
% HF cnvt AFL		80	0	?	?	85	71	33	33
% Direct therapy	21 (IV)	0?	3 (IV)	?	?	0?	0	0?	86 (IM)
% HF, mortality[a]	T 20%, D 46%	30	T 27%, D 50%	46	13	8	14	12	0
Digoxin (# pts)	14+/45−	0	40+/28−	13+/6−	11+/4−	2	14	9	23−
Verapamil (# pts)	37(+/−?)	0	24+/4−	0	0	0	0	0	0
Flecainide (# pts)	1−	0	20+/5−	7+/4−	9+	14+	0	7+/3−	0
Sotalol (# pts)	0	16+/4−	0	0	0	0	10+/4−	2−	0
Amiodarone (# pts)	1+/1−	0		0	0	0	0	7+/4−	12+/SVT, 3+/6− AF
Multi-drug (# pts)	2+/1−	0	23+/11−	5−	8+/2−	0	0	0	3+SVT
Total	59	20	110	35	34	14	14	25	24

Abbreviations: AFL, atrial flutter; cnvt, converted; D, direct; HF, hydrops fetalis; SUT, supraventricular tachycardia; T, transplacental.
[a] Mortality is expressed only as mortality for the hydropic group.

diac deaths were occurring at an incidence of 8% to 35% in hydropic supraventricular tachycardia (SVT) and atrial flutter fetal groups (Table 1) [16–24]. Recently, amiodarone was shown to have high efficacy alone and in combination with other agents, with no mortality in a large number of hydropic fetuses [23,24].

Tachyarrhythmias

The fetus presenting with a heart rate in excess of 180 beats per minute requires urgent evaluation, and must be triaged into treatment strategies based on severity of disease, gestation at presentation, and maternal or placental factors. Not all fetuses require the initiation of antiarrhythmic therapy, and only fetuses with mature lung development should be considered for delivery [25–27]. One of the leading sources of morbidity in fetal SVT patients remains the injudicious premature delivery of these babies. Studies have shown that care within a tertiary facility by those skilled in the management of these infrequent cases has resulted in lower prematurity rates, cesarean section rates, and morbidity [24,27]. The most important thing for the general obstetrician to know is that rates in excess of 230 beats/min or rates sustained at less than 80 beats/min are almost never fetuses with traditional fetal distress for which delivery is the treatment of choice. Therefore, rather than emergent delivery, emergent maternal–fetal medicine evaluation is the preferred response.

The first challenge is to identify the mechanism of tachycardia. SVT is the most common mechanism, occurring commonly at around 28 to 32 weeks' gestation [27,28]. Hydrops fetalis can rapidly develop in the less mature fetus; it is determined by the duration in hours of the tachycardia and by immature fetal gestation rather than by the rate of the SVT [27]. In a minority of patients, reentrant SVT may be in the rate range of 190 to 220 beats/min, and may be intermittent. Several groups have shown that these patients can be observed closely without treatment because hydrops is rare when SVT rate is less than 220 beats/min [25,29]. After an initial observation period of 4 to 12 hours in the hospital, nonhydropic fetuses with intermittent SVT (<20% to 30% of the time), even at rates greater than 240 beats/min can be observed on an outpatient basis. Mothers can be taught the at-home use of a hand-held Doppler monitoring device that can facilitate recognition of a change in SVT frequency. Usually ultrasounds are obtained at a minimum of one to two times weekly; and in the early phases, daily echocardiograms are optimal. Kannenkeril and colleagues [30] demonstrated that those infants who develop congestive heart failure are more likely to have a left-sided accessory AV pathway, and left-sided accessory connections dominate (90%) in the newborn period. Left-sided activation of the atrium may be more deleterious to the cardiac output because of its effect in restricting the normal right-to-left shunting at the atrial level [31,32]. The distribution of SVT versus atrial flutter in treatment series are shown in Table 1. SVT is usually at rates of 240 to 310 beats/min with 1:1 AV association. It appears extremely regular on heart-rate monitoring. Atrial flutter is characterized by irregular patterns of contraction, high rates of 425 to 500 beats/min in the atrium, and variable AV contraction sequences [17,26,27,33,34].

FMCG has demonstrated that the initiations and terminations of SVT are complex and often involve re-entry [6,35]. Almost all initiations occur with fetal activity. Ectopic beats are extremely frequent, sometimes occurring and initiating SVT several times per minute (Figs. 2 and 3), making short-term therapies for SVT such as adenosine ineffective for long-term management. Unlike the infant, in whom adenosine can effect conversion and reinitiation is uncommon, in the fetus reinitiation almost always occurs. Other mechanisms for initiation include sinus acceleration, re-entry over a second pathway, and antegrade block of Wolfe-Parkinson-White preexcitation [6]. Similarly, patterns of termination are also complex, including dual antegrade AV conduction block, block in the AV node, and block in the accessory connection. These patterns of tachycardia will likely predict efficacy of certain drug classes, although the experience to date is limited using specific drug therapy linked to electrophysiologic mechanism. Fetuses were commonly noted to have preexcitation (about 25%), and multiple accessory pathways are seen in about the same proportion [6]. Loss of preexcitation before delivery is common [36].

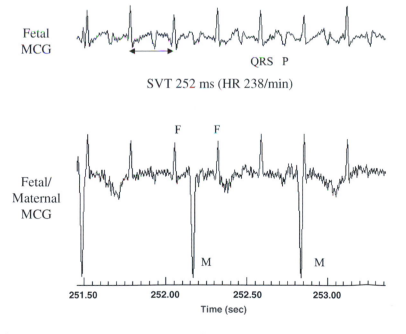

Fig. 2. Fetal (F) and maternal (M) rhythm recordings using magnetocardiography. Note the easily apparent P and QRS waves. The fetal heart rate is 238 beats/min with a VA interval approximately 50% of the RR interval. Figs. 2, 3, 6, 8–10 had cut-off data in supplied file. Please check these corrected figures for accuracy.

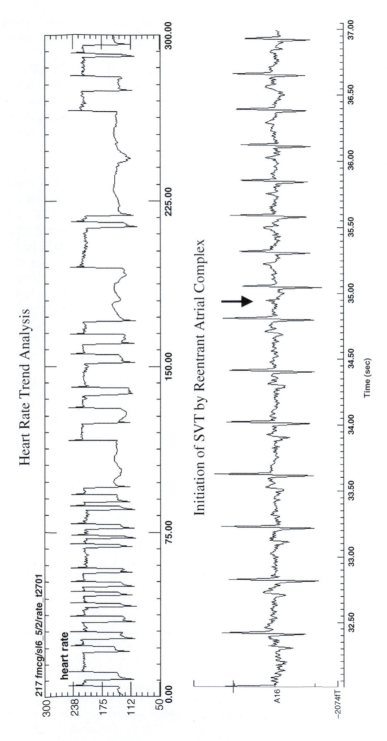

Fig. 3. Top tracing: heart rate trend analysis reveals multiple initiations and terminations of SVT during a 5-minute recording period. The heart rate is approximately 213 beats/min. The sinus rates show good variability and are at about 138 beats/min. Bottom tracing: the first P wave in tachycardia initiates the SVT and has a shorter coupling interval; it is evident on the trend analysis by overshoot on initiation.

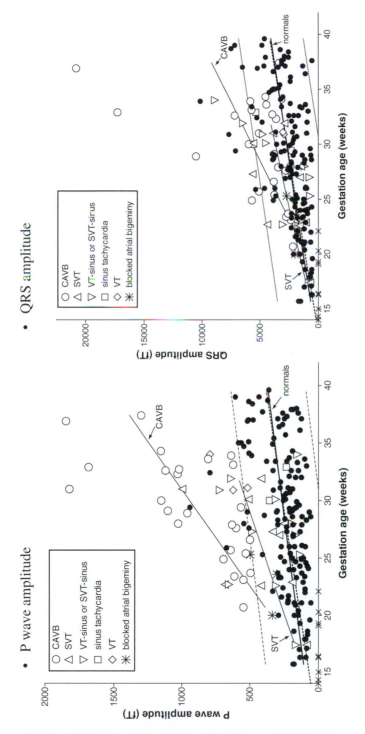

Fig. 4. The amplitudes of the P wave and QRS. The two were measured in normal human fetuses (*black circles*) and fetuses with various arrhythmias (*open symbols*). (*From* Li Z, Strasburger JF, Cuneo BF, et al. Giant fetal magnetocardiogram P-waves in congenital atrioventricular block: a marker of cardiac compensation. Circulation 2004;110:2097–101; with permission).

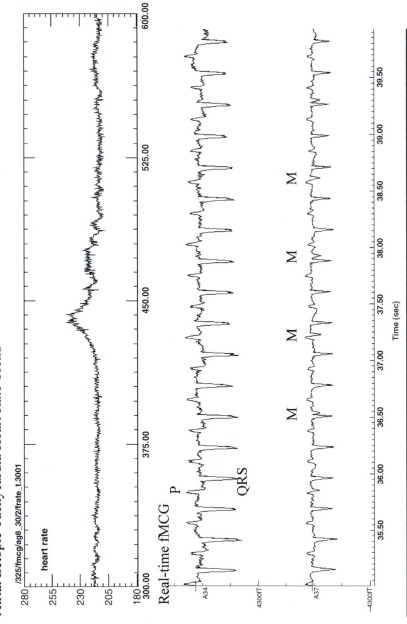

Atrial Ectopic Tachycardia Heart Rate Trend

FMCG has also highlighted the degree of atrial hypertrophy associated with SVT. Compared with complete AV block, it is mild, but in most cases exceeds the normal range (Fig. 4) [37,38].

About 70% to 80% of fetal tachycardia is reentrant SVT, and 20% to 30% is atrial flutter. Almost all SVT involves accessory AV connections, including more than 70% of fetuses with atrial flutter that have a hidden accessory pathway triggering the atrial flutter [27,39]. AV node re-entry is uncommon, although long-RP tachycardia, or the permanent form of junctional reciprocating tachycardia is occasionally encountered [24]. Other rare forms of automatic atrial tachycardias, junctional tachycardias, and ventricular tachycardias (VT) have been observed in isolated reports [25,40–44]. Each has characteristics that help to distinguish it from other forms; however, FMCG is probably the best means of assessing actual mechanism.

There is a strong association between the SVT and atrial flutter. In as many as 70% of fetuses presenting with atrial flutter, underlying reentrant tachycardia is present [27,39,45]. It is more likely to present later in pregnancy and is associated with less hydrops. The combination of atrial flutter and congenital cardiac defects holds a more serious prognosis, and sudden demise has been encountered in this group, which may relate to the underlying potential for proarrhythmia in fetuses with congenital heart disease. Atrial flutter rate is usually 425 to 500 beats/min with variable conduction to the ventricle at rates of about 210 beats/min, and the rhythm is irregular [18,24,27,39,41,45–48].

Atrial ectopic tachycardia (AET), an automatic tachycardia, has been seen alone and in association with rhabdomyomas in one case (B. Cuneo, personal communication, 2004). It varied in rate over time and displayed a "warm-up" phenomenon in which the rate accelerated (Fig. 5). Block in the SVT may be noted at high rates where the atrial rate remains unchanged and only the ventricular response drops. First-degree AV block during atrial tachycardia is common with AET. Permanent junctional reciprocating tachycardia (PJRT) has some similar features with a VA that exceeds the AV interval; however, PJRT is much more incessant and never has AV dissociation during tachycardia because it involves the AV node in the SVT circuit. PJRT has rates of 180 to 260 beats/min, whereas the only two AET cases the author has seen have been between 180 and 250 beats/min. Hydrops can develop with PJRT.

Ventricular and junctional tachycardias are perhaps the most difficult diagnoses to make on the basis of echocardiography alone [7,40,42,49–51]. VT is usually associated with complete heart block, long QT syndrome, or myocarditis; and subtle clues may be present. The ventriculoatrial contraction sequence may be intermittent, or even dissociated. There is usually more ventricular dysfunction at lower heart rates than seen with SVT. When slow enough, there is also fusion

---

Fig. 5. Atrial ectopic tachycardia. Note the period of rate acceleration on the heart rate trend analysis. Also note the large P waves with respect to the QRS amplitude. The tachycardia is incessant.

with underlying rhythm, creating a Doppler pattern that seems to come and go. Significant AV valve regurgitation is often present. The baseline rate, at least in LQTS, is usually bradycardia or with associated second-degree AV block. The combination of tachycardia and bradycardia or AV block in the same patient should always lead to the suspicion of VT The avoidance of QT-prolonging drugs and further attempts to confirm the rhythm using FMCG or tissue Doppler are recommended [24,42,43]. The usual rates of VT are 210 to 260 beats/min. A slow form of VT, known as accelerated ventricular rhythm, is seen with rates just above the sinus rate and competes with sinus rhythm. It rarely exceeds 220 beats/min and is not usually associated with ventricular dysfunction or hydrops.

Excellent reviews detailing the treatment of SVT and other fetal tachyarrhythmias have been previously published [26,33]. Treatment for SVT and atrial flutter are usually similar; however, some differences are worth pointing out. The drug with the highest safety profile in the treatment of either condition is digoxin. After all the studies published in the past 3 decades, digoxin still has the lowest overall mortality rate in association with its isolated use (for the number of patients treated) [33]. It is preferable to administer it to the mother intravenously, because oral digoxin absorption in pregnancy is inconsistent and slow. Most drugs are poorly transferred through the hydropic placenta, and therefore, in the author's experience, intramuscular administration has been effective in rapidly achieving therapeutic fetal effect [52]. For SVT, the preferred second-line treatment in the extremely ill fetus is amiodarone; it can be added within 1 to 2 days [23,24]. There is no published experience to date with maternal intravenous amiodarone administration, but the oral administration of 1200 to 2400 mg/d over 2 to 7 days in combination with 50% lower doses of digoxin, or in a few instances with other medications, has proven effective [24]. The volume of distribution is high and it takes several days to show efficacy, with a gradual slowing of SVT rate in the interim. There are noteworthy side effects of thyroid dysfunction and rare thrombocytopenia and rash. Nonetheless, this regimen has had no associated mortality to date. In severe situations, amiodarone can be initiated along with digoxin on admission, rather than delayed until full loading of digoxin. Amiodarone is not effective for atrial flutter and only seems to slow the rate of the atrial flutter without terminating it.

For the less ill fetus, procainamide, flecainide, and sotalol have also been used as second-line treatments [16–24]. Procainamide is a uterine irritant and can trigger contractions when administered intravenously to the mother. It is relatively safe, but efficacy is only 50% to 60% [4,53,54]. Flecainide is fairly effective, but it has been associated with at least a 7% to 15% mortality rate [16–24]. In at least three case reports, severe conduction disturbances have been noted following flecainide administration, and it does concentrate in the amniotic fluid [55–57]. Sotalol has had a mortality as high as 30% in the hydropic population for SVT, but it seems to be safe and efficacious for atrial flutter in about 80% of cases [18]. It is considered the treatment of choice for refractory atrial flutter. Finally, delivery is an option for the fetus with mature lungs. The neonatal course of the premature infant delivered for SVT and requiring potent

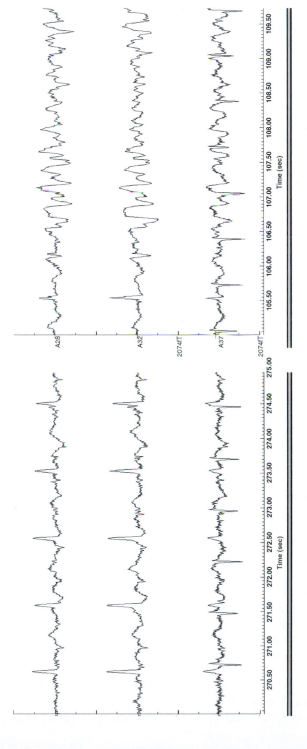

Fig. 6. Congenital long QT syndrome. Tracing on the left shows AV block with a markedly prolonged QT interval. Tracing on the right shows the onset of torsades de pointes ventricular tachycardia.

antiarrhythmic medications to control SVT, is usually typified by significant hyperbilirubinemia caused by drug–bilirubin competition for binding sites, anemia caused by bone marrow suppression from the drugs, and a higher incidence of necrotizing enterocolitis [24]. In utero care is usually the best option until the infant is term. In our experience, cesarean-section rate was 100% for premature infants and about 16% for term infants.

VT and junctional tachycardia are much more complicated to treat [24,26, 42,43]. The author is aware of treatment in labor in one instance, and has previously reported an infant experiencing proarrhythmic torsades de pointes VT from amiodarone at 29 weeks gestation who had congenital long QT syndrome (LQTS) and VT (Fig. 6) [25]. This infant responded to maternal intravenous lidocaine and magnesium administration. The use of beta blocking agents in fetal LQTS in utero is unclear, although they have been used to prevent cardiac arrest in pregnant mothers suffering from LQTS. There is limited transplacental passage to the fetus, and beta blockers have been associated with fetal hypoglycemia [42,51].

Congenital atrioventricular block

Congenital AV block (CAVB) has two predominant presentations. The usual case is that of a fetus with normal cardiac structure, and exposure to maternal SSA or SSB antibodies. The particular subunits most often implicated in severe disease are Anto-Ro52 kd and -60 kd. These fetuses can acquire heart block at any stage of pregnancy, and may also have ventricular dysfunction or transient first-degree AV block [58]. Villain and colleagues [59] found that infants positive for maternal antibody were more likely to require pacing, proceeded to develop cardiomyopathy in up to 30% of cases, and had a more severe form of CAVB than infants who had structurally normal hearts and were antibody negative. This result may relate to apoptosis (myocyte destruction), which is antibody mediated [60]. Most mothers are asymptomatic and are detected only through antibody screening. The risk for a mother with lupus or other collagen vascular disease having a fetus with complete AV block is about 1% to 2%; and risk for recurrence is about 16% to 40%, depending on the series reviewed [61].

Fetuses most often present with second- (incomplete) or third-degree AV block. Although initially there was an attempt to identify at-risk fetuses by echocardiography using a mechanical AV interval at the first-degree AV block stage, it is now believed that this progression is too rapid to recognize as progression; and when mechanical PR prolongation is present, AV mechanical intervals of 150 to 170 ms are usually confirmed as normal when FMCG is used for verification. Regression of first-degree AV block spontaneously has been documented in the human fetus; and what the implications of first-degree AV block are, or whether prophylactic steroid treatment should be instituted in these mothers, is a controversial subject. At Children's Hospital of Wisconsin, it is not done before the onset of either significant ventricular dysfunction, or second-degree AV block. Regular heart rate screening for second-degree AV block is advisable when maternal collagen vascular disease is present. The use of betamethasone, 4 mg/d, a glucocorticoid capable of transplacental transfer in good concentrations, as well as the use of terbutaline, a 2.5- to 5-mg dose given 4 to 6 times daily, to achieve a maternal heart rate of 110 beats/min, has been shown to limit intrauterine and neonatal mortality [61]. Jaeggi recently reported an infant survival rate of 90% at one year, and a permanent pacemaker implant rate in the newborn period of 56% [61]. FMCG has proven effective in defining those who will need to be paced at birth [62]. Ventricular or junctional tachycardia or ectopy are commonly seen in the initial phases of heart block and probably represent an acute inflammatory response [63]. Anecdotally, it seems that betamethasone may suppress this ectopy. The long-term use of betamethasone has unclear benefits, although some have reported regression of endocardial fibroelastosis and improved long-term survival even when third-degree AV block was not reversed [58,61,64]. Betamethasone has been associated with osteoporosis, bone and hip fractures, and other serious side effects in pregnant mothers, and with slow fetal brain development [65]. It should be used with caution, monitored closely, and tapered at the earliest possible point. Significant adrenal suppression can occur in mother and baby, and tapering protocols are necessary when neonatal hypoglycemia is present, suggesting an abnormal adrenocortic axis. Stress doses may need to be administered for major operative procedures in the newborn period.

CAVB associated with congenital heart disease has a poorer prognosis than that associated with collagen vascular disease. Cuneo and colleagues [66] have found that this group will actually respond differently to terbutaline than autoimmune-acquired heart block patients. Usually the heart rate trends are flat, but terbutaline increases the rate by 6 to 15 beats/min and recruits nonstable pacemakers at slightly higher rates, a more dramatic response than is seen in autoimmune CAVB. Intrauterine hydrops and demise are seen in about 7% of fetuses with CAVB. Another 10% to 15% succumb in infancy to severe CHD [67]. The most common defects are atrial isomerism with asplenia or polysplenia, L-transposition of the great arteries with or without single ventricle, and AV septal defect. These patients frequently warrant pacing in the neonate period, because of the increased cardiac output requirements associated with their heart disease [42]. The heart rates in the 2 hours after delivery may be falsely reassuring in both groups in infants who have heart block, and these infants require close observation for the development of occult heart block.

In the biomagnetism laboratory at the University of Wisconsin, 22 fetuses have been evaluated for CAVB with and without CHD. Fig. 7 shows the various clinical stages thus far recognized, and characteristics common to each stage. The fetus must immediately adapt to sudden loss of heart rate with the onset of heart block, and therefore many adaptations facilitating the maintenance of cardiac output occur quickly. The fetus incapable of adapting to low rate develops hydrops or dies suddenly. The features that correlate with more favorable postnatal prognosis include good ventricular heart rate accelerations and atrial vari-

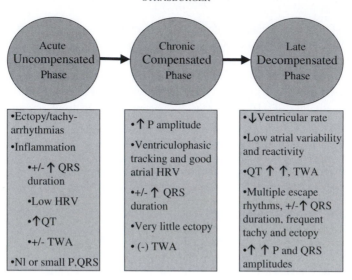

Fig. 7. Schematic of progression of compensation for fetuses with complete AV block. Fetuses can present in any stage. P wave amplitude increases (atrial wall thickening) are difficult to detect using standard echocardiography. FMCG seems to be more sensitive to early findings of compensation. Similarly, brief junctional and ventricular tachycardia events (see Fig. 8) can be undetected during echocardiographic study or fetal heart rate monitoring. *Abbreviations:* HRV, heart rate variability; P, QRS, QT, cardiac intervals; tachy, tachycardia; TWA, T-wave alternans.

ability, absence of structural defects, and a prenatal rate maintaining itself at more than 55 beats/min. Poorer prognosis indicators in this series included low ventricular rates (< 50 beats/min), rapidly decreasing heart rates, poor ventricular function, AV valve regurgitation, or hydrops, presence of T-wave alternans or severely long QTc interval greater than 0.53, and presence of CHD (Figs. 8 and 9). Clearly the sophisticated approach to analyzing these patients using FMCG is likely to allow better assessment of survival and prediction of need for pacing postnatally; and ultimately it may help define which patients would benefit from intrauterine pacing and at what point in their course.

Indications for pacing in the neonate with CAVB have been published as joint scientific statements by the American Heart Association/American College of Cardiology in Circulation and are updated periodically [68]. The delivery room should be equipped adequately for the resuscitation of these bradycardic infants, including temporary external or transvenous pacing capabilities, monitoring devices, and positive chronotropic resuscitation drugs such as isoproterinol or epinephrine. If hydrops is present from any cause, resuscitation may require peritoneal, pericardial, or pleurocentesis.

Fig. 8. Non-sustained junctional tachycardia is noted in this fetus with congenital AV block. This arrhythmia is usually seen in the early uncompensated phase of CAVB and may represent effort to maintain cardiac output before compensatory myocardial hypertrophy. M, maternal; P, QRS, cardiac intervals.

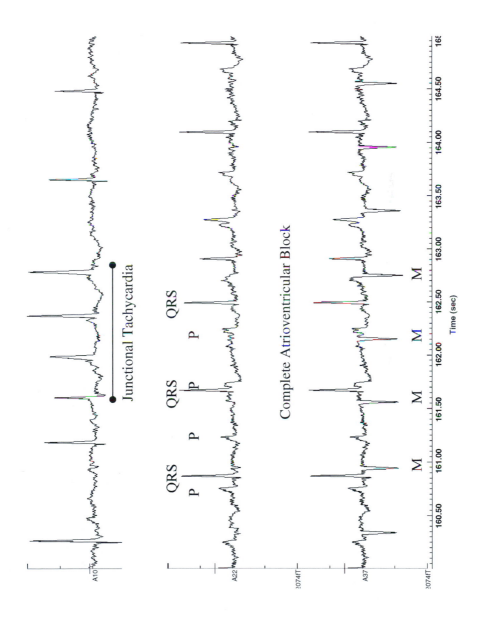

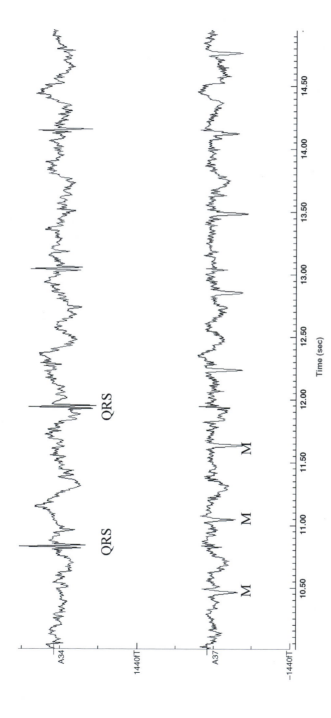

Fig. 9. Fetus with complete AV block. Note the bizarre T waves in the top tracing, which shows macroscopic T-wave alternans. Note the downward T wave in the third complex compared with upward-facing T waves otherwise. The fetal P waves are difficult to observe on this particular recording. Fetal ventricular rate was 54 beats/min. Maternal T waves are visible in association with maternal QRS complexes (M).

Fetal ectopy

Previously, fetal ectopy had been believed to be entirely benign. The occurrence of ectopy in 1% to 3% of all pregnancies makes it a common phenomenon; however, Cuneo [8] found that in 2.5% of fetuses, a prolongation of the PR interval was also seen along with the ectopy, and that this first-degree AV block could predict such abnormalities as LQTS, presence of occult second-degree AV block, risk for atrial flutter, maternal SSA/SSB antibody, and other conditions. All fetuses with ectopy should have a mechanical AV interval recorded with each cardiac scan [8]. In addition, mothers of fetuses that have frequent ectopy should be counseled that they have a risk roughly 40 times that of the general population for developing SVT either prenatally or in the first month after delivery, and that they should look for the signs and symptoms of SVT. When regular and sustained, fetal ectopy can be mistaken for other diagnoses. The most common mistake is suspecting CAVB in a fetus with sustained low rate caused by blocked atrial bigeminy (Fig. 10). These fetuses rarely persist for more than a few days with these low rates, and often have periods of sinus rhythm with frequent ectopy. In summary, although common, fetal ectopy is not always benign and not always easily distinguished from other arrhythmias. For these reasons, having an experienced pediatric cardiologist involved in the evaluation of these patients is important.

Fetal sudden death

The incidence of sudden death in utero beyond the point of fetal viability is about 1:500 in otherwise healthy pregnancies [69–72]. For maternal lupus, diabetes, or hypertension, this incidence increases to as high as 1:33. Much of the sudden death has been attributed to placental problems, growth failure, and cord accidents; however, even with greater autopsy use, 8% to 40% of fetal deaths are entirely unexplained. The possibility that cardiac arrhythmias account for some of these deaths is high. Schwartz [72,73] found that infants at 3 days of age with QT prolongation had a 41-fold higher risk for sudden death than those who had a normal QT interval. Genetic defects in SCN5A were shown to be the cause of recurrent fetal loss in one family [74]. A contradictory finding shows that recurrent fetal loss is uncommon in families with LQTS [75]. These outcomes may relate to these families having less lethal variants of LQTS. FMCG may begin to play a larger role in evaluating the rare mother with multiple unexplained fetal losses.

Research applications

Several areas require additional investigation as developments in fetal electrophysiology unfold. Larger and more detailed multicenter patient treatment

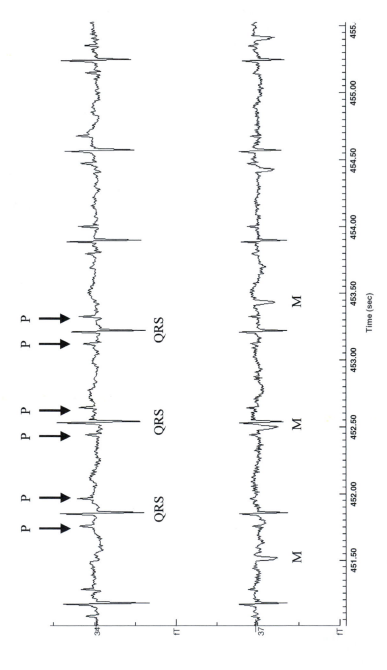

Fig. 10. Blocked atrial bigeminy in the top tracing is characterized by early extra P waves that are not conducted. Although this causes a slower ventricular rate, it is much more benign and self-limiting than atrioventricular block. The functional ventricular rate is only 88 beats/min. M, maternal; P, QRS, cardiac intervals.

strategies in patients with hydrops caused by SVT need to be performed using the various antiarrhythmic agents. There remains a paucity of data on the effects of most antiarrhythmic drugs on the electrocardiogram and general health of the mother. Long-term follow-up of fetuses and mothers treated with amiodarone is indicated to assess for any neurologic or endocrinologic abnormalities. If possible, late neurocognitive studies should be performed on infants treated in utero for any fetal or maternal disease process, to better predict what form of special needs they may require. Whereas major neurologic sequelae are rare, minor speech delay has been observed [24]. More thorough assessment of mechanism-specific treatments needs to occur; however, it is unlikely to be possible until more widespread use of FMCG is available.

For congenital heart block, more serial FMCG evaluation of many fetuses is needed to better evaluate indications and timing for fetal pacing. It is likely that pacing technology will be available within the near future; and the injudicious use of fetal pacing without preoperative analysis of malignant ventricular arrhythmias, QT prolongation, and T-wave alternans—conditions associated with CAVB in the author's experience—is likely to result in fetal death. A large multicenter placebo-controlled study of betamethasone therapy for fetuses with third-degree AV block may be warranted given the risk for long-term betamethasone therapy (but not for second-degree where its use is more established).

Fetal sudden death markers need to be determined in the general fetal population. The author's laboratory has recently identified T-wave alternans as a marker of higher morbidity in fetuses with complete AV block. FMCG may eventually be used as a screening tool and reveal normal fetuses with LQTS, allowing for genetic testing.

Better overall monitoring devices for the fetus are needed. Improvements in microchip technology may afford an implantable or noninvasive monitoring device.

Summary

New methodologies have led to significant progress in fetal electrophyisology. Improvements in monitoring and therapy are likely to lead to greater capacity to treat the fetus in the near future.

References

[1] Menendez T, Achenbach S, Hofbeck M, et al. Prenatal diagnosis of QT prolongation by magnetocardiography. Pacing Clin Electrophysiol 2000;23:1305−7.
[2] Wakai RT, Leuthold A, Wilson AD, et al. Association of fetal junctional rhythm and respiratory arrhythmias detected by magnetocardiography. Pediatr Cardiol 1997;18:201−3.
[3] Wakai RT, Leuthold AC, Martin CB. Atrial and ventricular fetal heart rate patterns in isolated congenital complete heart block detected by magnetocardiography. Am J Obstet Gynecol 1998; 179:258−60.

[4] Wakai RT, Leuthold L, Cripe L, et al. Assessment of fetal rhythm in congenital complete heart block by magnetocardiography. Pacing Clin Electrophysiol, in press.

[5] Van Leeuwen P, Hailer B, Bader W, et al. Magnetocardiography in the diagnosis of fetal arrhythmia. Br J Obstet Gynaecol 1999;11:1200–8.

[6] Wakai RT, Strasburger JF, Li Z, et al. Magnetocardiographic rhythm patterns at initiation and termination of fetal supraventricular tachycardia. Circulation 2003;107:307–12.

[7] Cuneo BF, Ovadia M, Strasburger JF, et al. Prenatal diagnosis and in utero treatment of torsades de pointes associated with congenital long QT syndrome. Am J Cardiol 2003;91:1395–8.

[8] Cuneo BF, Wakai RT, Strasburger JF, et al. Conduction system disease in fetuses with irregular rhythm diagnosed in utero by abnormal mechanical PR interval and confirmed by fetal magnetocardiography. Fetal Diagn Ther 2005, in press.

[9] Stinstra J, Golbach E, van Leeuwen P, et al. Multicentre study of fetal cardiac time intervals using magnetocardiography. BJOG 2002;109:1235–43.

[10] Zhao H, Strasburger JF, Cuneo BF, et al. Fetal cardiac repolarization abnormalities. Lancet, in review.

[11] Rein AJ, O'Donnell C, Geva T, et al. Use of tissue velocity imaging in the diagnosis of fetal cardiac arrhythmias. Circulation 2002;106:1827–33.

[12] Frommelt PC, Pelech AN, Frommelt MA. Diastolic dysfunction in an unusual case of cardiomyopathy in a child: insights from Doppler and Doppler tissue imaging analysis. J Am Soc Echocardiogr 2003;16:176–81.

[13] Wakai R, Wang M, Martin C. Spaciotemporal properties of the fetal magnetocardiogram. Am J Obstet Gynecol 1994;170:770–6.

[14] Wakai RT, Lengle JM, Leuthold AC. Transmission of electric and magnetic fetal cardiac signals in a case of ectopia cordis: the dominant role of the vermex caseosa. Phys Med Biol, in press.

[15] Leuthold A, Wakai RT, Martin CB. Noninvasive in utero assessment of PR and QRS intervals from the fetal magnetocardiogram. Early Hum Dev 1999;54:235–43.

[16] Frohn-Mulder IM, Stewart PA, Witsenburg M, et al. The efficacy of flecainide versus digoxin in the management of fetal supraventricular tachycardia. Prenat Diagn 1995;15:1297–302.

[17] Simpson J. Fetal tachycardias: management and outcome of 127 consecutive cases. Heart 1998; 79:576–81.

[18] Oudijk MA, Michon MM, Kleinman CS, et al. Sotalol in the treatment of fetal dysrhythmias. Circulation 2000;101:2721–6.

[19] Hansmann M, Grunbruch U, Bald R, et al. Fetal tachyarrhythmias: transplacental and direct treatment of the fetus–a report of 60 cases. Ultrasound Obstet Gynecol 1991;1:162–70.

[20] Van Engelen A, Weijtens O, Brenner J, et al. Management outcome and follow-up of fetal tachycardia. J Am Coll Cardiol 1994;24:1371–5.

[21] Allan L, Chita S, Sharland G, et al. Flecainide in the treatment of fetal tachycardias. Br Heart J 1991;65:46–8.

[22] Sonesson SE, Fouron JC, Wesslen-Eriksson E, et al. Foetal supraventricular tachycardia treated with sotalol. Acta Paediatr 1998;87:584–7.

[23] Jouannic JM, Delahaye S, Fermont L, et al. Fetal supraventricular tachycardia: a role for amiodarone as second-line therapy? Prenat Diagn 2003;23:152–6.

[24] Strasburger JF, Cuneo BF, Michon MM, et al. Amiodarone therapy for drug-refractory fetal tachycardia. Circulation 2004;109:375–9.

[25] Cuneo B, Strasburger JF. Management strategies for fetal tachycardia. Obstet Gynecol 2000; 96:575–81.

[26] Strasburger JF. Fetal arrhythmias. Prog Pediatr Cardiol 2000;11:1–17.

[27] Naheed Z, Strasburger J, Deal B, et al. Fetal tachycardia: mechanisms and predictors of hydrops fetalis. J Am Coll Cardiol 1996;27:1736–40.

[28] Allan L. The normal fetal heart. In: Allan L, Hornberger L, Sharland G, editors. Textbook of fetal cardiology. London: Greenwich Medical Media Limited; 2000. p. 55–102.

[29] Oudijk MA, Ambachtsheer EB, Stoutenbeek P, et al. [Protocols for the treatment of supraventricular tachycardias in the fetus]. Ned Tijdschr Geneeskd 2001;145:1218–9.

[30] Kannenkeril P, Deal B, Johnsrude C, et al. Location of accessory AV connection in fetal tachycardia. Pediatr Cardiol, in review.

[31] Kannankeril PJ, Gotteiner NL, Deal BJ, et al. Location of accessory connection in infants presenting with supraventricular tachycardia in utero: clinical correlations. Am J Perinatol 2003; 20:115–9.

[32] Shiraishi H, Kikuchi Y, Hoshina M, et al. Left atrial tachyarrhythmia in fetal lambs. Pacing Clin Electrophysiol 2002;25:785–90.

[33] Oudijk MA. Fetal tachycardia diagnosis and treatment and the fetal QT interval in hypoxia. Utrecht (NL): Dong UMC, Neoventa Medical AB, Stiefel; 2003.

[34] Simpson J. Fetal arrhythmias. In: Allen L, Hornberger LK, Sharland G, editors. Textbook of fetal cardiology. London: Greenwich Medical Media, Limited; 2000. p. 421–52.

[35] Menendez T, Achenbach S, Beinder E, et al. Magnetocardiography for the investigation of fetal arrhythmias. Am J Cardiol 2001;88:334–6.

[36] Strasburger JF, Wakai RT, Zhimin L, et al. Prenatal preexcitation: magnetocardiographic assessment of Wolff-Parkinson-White Syndrome in the fetus. Pacing Clin Electrophysiol 2002; 24:602.

[37] Li Z, Strasburger JF, Cuneo BF, et al. Giant fetal magnetocardiogram P-waves in congenital atrioventricular block: a marker of cardiac compensation. Circulation 2004;110:2097–101.

[38] Horigome H, Shiono J, Shigemitsu S, et al. Detection of cardiac hypertrophy in the fetus by approximation of the current dipole using magnetocardiography. Pediatr Res 2001;50:242–5.

[39] Till J, Wren C. Atrial flutter in the fetus and young infant: an association with accessory conduction. Br Heart J 1995;67:80–3.

[40] Stevens DC, Schreiner RL, Hurwitz RA, et al. Fetal and neonatal ventricular arrhythmia. Pediatrics 1979;63:771–7.

[41] Casey F, McCrindle B, Hamilton RM, et al. Neonatal atrial flutter: significant early morbidity and excellent long-term prognosis. Am Heart J 1997;133:302–6.

[42] Ferrer PL. Fetal arrhythmias. In: Deal B, Wolff GS, Gelband H, editors. Current concepts in diagnosis and treatment of arrhythmias in infants and children. Armonk (NY): Futura Publishing Company, Inc; 1998. p. 17–63.

[43] Dubin AM, Cuneo BF, Strasburger JF, et al. Congenital junctional ectopic tachycardia and congenital complete atrioventricular block: a shared etiology? Heart Rhythm Journal 2005;2:313–5.

[44] Villain E, Vetter V, Garcia J, et al. Evolving concepts in the management of congenital junctional ectopic tachycardia. A multicenter study. Circulation 1990;81:1544–9.

[45] Johnson W, Dunnigan A, Fehr P, et al. Association of atrial flutter with orthodromic reciprocating fetal tachycardia. Am J Cardiol 1987;59:374–5.

[46] Krapp M, Kohl T, Simpson JM, et al. Review of diagnosis, treatment, and outcome of fetal atrial flutter compared with supraventricular tachycardia. Heart 2003;89:913–7.

[47] Lisowski LA, Verheijen PM, Benatar AA, et al. Atrial flutter in the perinatal age group: diagnosis, management and outcome. J Am Coll Cardiol 2000;35:771–7.

[48] Flack NJ, Zosmer N, Bennett PR, et al. Amiodarone given by three routes to terminate fetal atrial flutter associated with severe hydrops. Obstet Gynecol 1993;82:714–6.

[49] Celiker A, Ceviz N, Ozme S. Effectiveness and safety of intravenous amiodarone in drug-resistant tachyarrhythmias of children. Acta Paediatr Jpn 1998;40:567–72.

[50] Strasburger JF, Wakai RT, Li Z, et al. Clinical and electrophysiologic characteristics of fetal ventricular tachycardia. Pacing Clin Electrophysiol 2003;26:1063.

[51] Teuscher A, Bossi E, Imhof P, et al. Effect of propranolol on fetal tachycardia in diabetic pregnancy. Am J Cardiol 1978;42:304.

[52] Parilla B, Strasburger J, Socol M. Fetal supraventricular tachycardia complicated by hydrops fetalis: a role for direct fetal intramuscular therapy. Am J Perinatol 1996;13:483–6.

[53] Hallak M, Neehof M, Perry R. Fetal supraventricular tachycardia and hydrops fetalis: combined intensive, direct, and transplacental therapy. Obstet Gynecol 1991;78:523–5.

[54] Weiner C, Thompson M. Direct treatment of fetal supraventricular tachycardia after failed transplacental therapy. Am J Obstet Gynecol 1988;158:570–3.

[55] Trotter A, Kaestner M, Pohlandt F, et al. Unusual electrocardiogram findings in a preterm infant after fetal tachycardia with hydrops fetalis treated with flecanide. Pediatr Cardiol 2000;21: 259–62.

[56] Rasheed A, Simpson J, Rosenthal E. Neonatal ECG changes caused by supratherapeutic flecainide following treatment for fetal supraventricular tachycardia. Heart 2003;89:470.

[57] Hall CM, Ward Platt MP. Neonatal flecainide toxicity following supraventricular tachycardia treatment. Ann Pharmacother 2003;37:1343–4.

[58] Raboisson MJ, Fouron JC, Sonesson SE, et al. Fetal Doppler echocardiographic diagnosis and successful steroid therapy of Luciani-Wenckebach phenomenon and endocardial fibroelastosis related to maternal anti-Ro and anti-La antibodies. J Am Soc Echocardiogr 2005;18:375–80.

[59] Villain E, Marijon E, Georgin S. Is isolated congenital heart block with maternal antibiodies a distinct and more severe form of the disease in childhood? Heart Rhythm Journal 2005;2:S45.

[60] Clancy RM, Buyon JP. More to death than dying: apoptosis in the pathogenesis of SSA/Ro-SSB/La-associated congenital heart block. Rheum Dis Clin N Am 2004;30:589–602 [x.].

[61] Jaeggi ET, Fouron JC, Silverman ED, et al. Transplacental fetal treatment improves the outcome of prenatally diagnosed complete atrioventricular block without structural heart disease. Circulation 2004;110:1542–8.

[62] Strasburger JF, Wakai RT, Zhao H, et al. Assessment of fetal heart rhythm and rate in congenital complete heart block by fetal magnetocardiography. Pacing Clin Electrophysiol 2003;26:1126.

[63] Davignon A, Rautaharju P, Boissille E, et al. Normal ECG Standards for infants and children. Pediatr Cardiol 1979–80;1:123–31.

[64] Shinohara K, Miyagawa S, Fujita T, et al. Neonatal lupus erythematosus: results of maternal corticosteroid therapy. Obstet Gynecol 1999;93:952–7.

[65] Breur JM, Visser GH, Kruize AA, et al. Treatment of fetal heart block with maternal steroid therapy: case report and review of the literature. Ultrasound Obstet Gynecol 2004;24:467–72.

[66] Cuneo BF, Strasburger JF, Zhao H, et al. Electrophysiologic patterns of fetal heart rate augmentation with terbutaline in complete AV block. Heart Rhythm Journal 2005;2:S45.

[67] Eronen M, Siren MK, Ekblad H, et al. Short- and long-term outcome of children with congenital complete heart block diagnosed in utero or as a newborn. Pediatrics 2000;106:86–91.

[68] Gregoratos G, Abrams J, Epstein AE, et al. ACC/AHA/NASPE 2002 Guideline update for implantation of cardiac pacemakers and antiarrhythmia devices—summary article: a report of the American College of Cardiology/American Heart Association Task Force on practice guidelines (ACC/AHA/NASPE committee to update the 1998 pacemaker guidelines). J Am Coll Cardiol 2002;40:1703–19.

[69] Fretts RC, Boyd ME, Usher RH, et al. The changing pattern of fetal death, 1961–1988. Obstet Gynecol 1992;79:35–9.

[70] Gardosi J, Badger S, Tonks A, et al. "Unexplained" stillbirths: an investigation of the clinically relevant conditions at the time of fetal death. Am J Obstet Gynecol 2003;189:S158.

[71] Incerpi MH, Miller DA, Samadi R, et al. Stillbirth evaluation: what tests are needed? Am J Obstet Gynecol 1998;178:1121–5.

[72] Schwartz PJ. Stillbirths, sudden infant deaths, and long-QT syndrome: puzzle or mosaic, the pieces of the jigsaw are being fitted together. Circulation 2004;109:2930–2.

[73] Schwartz PJ, Stramba-Badiale M, Segantini A, et al. Prolongation of the QT interval and the sudden infant death syndrome. N Engl J Med 1998;338:1709–14.

[74] Miller TE, Estrella E, Myerburg RJ, et al. Recurrent third-trimester fetal loss and maternal mosaicism for long-QT syndrome. Circulation 2004;109:3029–34.

[75] Rashba EJ, Zareba W, Moss AJ, et al. Influence of pregnancy on the risk for cardiac events in patients with hereditary long QT syndrome. LQTS Investigators. Circulation 1998;97:451–6.

ELSEVIER
SAUNDERS

Clin Perinatol 32 (2005) 913–919

CLINICS IN
PERINATOLOGY

Congenital Heart Disease and Pregnancy: Maternal and Fetal Risks

Michael G. Earing, MD[a],*, Gary D. Webb, MD[b]

[a]*Adult Congenital Heart Disease Program, Herma Heart Center, Medical College of Wisconsin,
9000 West Wisconsin Avenue, Milwaukee, WI 53226, USA*
[b]*Philadelphia Adult Congenital Heart Center, The Children's Hospital of Philadelphia and
University of Pennsylvania Health System, Philadelphia, PA, USA*

The incidence of congenital heart disease (CHD) in the United States is estimated to be 0.5% to 0.8%, or 32,000 new cases per year [1]. This does not include bicuspid aortic valves, occurring in up to 2% to 3% of live births in the United States. As result of medical and surgical advances, approximately 85% of children born with CHD are now surviving into adulthood [2]. This has resulted in a steady increase in the number of girls with CHD reaching childbearing age. In fact, CHD is now the predominant form of heart disease encountered during pregnancy in developed countries [3].

Hemodynamic changes during pregnancy

CHD does not preclude a successful pregnancy; however, the hemodynamic changes that occur during normal pregnancy can have adverse consequences for the at-risk pregnant woman and her fetus. These complications may include heart failure, arrhythmias, stroke, and even death of the mother or fetus [4]. During a normal pregnancy, there is a 20% to 30% increase in red blood cell mass and a 30% to 50% increase in plasma volume, resulting in an increase in total blood volume. In addition, the heart rate increases by 10 beats per minute, and there is a reduction in systemic and pulmonary vascular resistance. As result of these changes, the cardiac output steadily increases until the week 32, when it plateaus at 30% to 50% above the prepregnancy level. During labor and delivery, there are

---

* Corresponding author.
E-mail address: mearing@mcw.edu (M.G. Earing).

0095-5108/05/$ – see front matter © 2005 Elsevier Inc. All rights reserved.
doi:10.1016/j.clp.2005.09.004

further hemodynamic changes. With uterine contractions, an additional 300 to 500 mL of blood can enter the circulation. In addition, the heart rate and blood pressure are increased at the time of labor and delivery. These changes result in the cardiac output at the time of delivery being nearly 80% higher than the prepregnancy level. Immediately after delivery, relief of caval compression results in improved venous return and there is spontaneous diuresis. Most of these physiologic changes resolve by the second postpartum week, but a complete return to baseline may not occur for 6 months [5].

Cardiac contraindications to pregnancy

The task of advising women with CHD with regard to the safety of pregnancy needs to be an integral part of all adult CHD and pediatric cardiology programs. Studies of pregnancy outcomes in women with heart disease have shown that there is an increased risk for maternal cardiovascular and neonatal complications [6]. In general, however, cardiac mortality remains low, and in most cases, one can expect a favorable maternal and fetal outcome [7]. Because of the hemodynamic changes of pregnancy, however, there are certain cardiac conditions that remain a contraindication to pregnancy (Box 1). In general, severe obstructive lesions (eg, mitral and aortic valve stenosis, coarctation of aorta, hypertrophic obstructive cardiomyopathy) and those with advanced pulmonary hypertension (defined as pulmonary artery pressure ≥75% systemic) are poorly tolerated and are considered contraindications to pregnancy [4,8–10]. In contrast, regurgitant lesions and lesions with resting left-to-right shunts in the setting of normal pulmonary artery pressure are typically well tolerated [11]. Other cardiac conditions in which pregnancy should be avoided include class III through IV congestive heart failure attributable to systemic ventricular dysfunction (defined as left ventricular [LV] ejection fraction <40%) and Marfan syndrome with a dilated aortic root of 40 mm or greater [7,11–14].

Box 1. Contraindications to pregnancy

Severe pulmonary hypertension (defined as pulmonary artery pressure ≥75% systemic pressure)
Severe obstructive lesions
    Aortic valve stenosis
    Mitral valve stenosis
    Coarctation of the aorta
    Hypertrophic obstructive cardiomyopathy
Systemic ventricular systolic dysfunction
Class III or IV congestive heart failure
Marfan aortopathy (defined as aortic root diameter ≥40 mm)

Risk stratification and counseling

Risk stratification and counseling of women with CHD is best accomplished before conception and can be obtained by performing a detailed cardiovascular history and physical examination, 12-lead electrocardiogram (ECG), and a transthoracic echocardiogram [4]. In counseling, the underlying cardiac lesion(s) and maternal functional class need to be considered. Classically, patients have been stratified into low-, intermediate-, and high-risk groups based on the nature of their lesion. During the last 10 years, however, it has become increasingly evident that maternal status as defined by New York Heart Association (NYHA) functional class is highly predictive of maternal and fetal prognosis. In an early study of 482 pregnancies in women with CHD, the maternal morbidity rate was significantly less in mothers with NYHA functional class I compared with the others (8% versus 30%) [15]. In this same study, mothers with NYHA functional class I also had a higher fetal survival rate compared with the others (80% versus 68%) [15]. Two subsequent studies involving more than 800 women with heart disease have confirmed maternal status as defined by NYHA functional class as a predictor of outcome for maternal morbidity and mortality and fetal morbidity and mortality [7,11].

In these same two studies, other risk factors for maternal morbidity (defined as maternal heart failure, arrhythmia, stroke, or maternal death) included maternal cyanosis, LV systolic dysfunction (defined as LV ejection fraction ≤40%), left heart obstruction (peak gradient ≥40 mm Hg), and history of prior arrhythmias or cardiac events (eg, arrhythmia, stroke, pulmonary edema) [7,11]. In addition, maternal cyanosis was predictive of neonatal events [7,11]. From these studies, a risk index has been proposed that incorporates these known risk factors along with the patient's specific lesion to predict the maternal risk for experiencing a cardiac event (cardiac death, stroke, pulmonary edema, or arrhythmia) and the risk for a neonatal adverse event (premature death, small for gestational age birth weight, respiratory distress syndrome, intraventricular hemorrhage, or fetal or neonatal death) [7,11]. This system assigns a point score based on the number of risk factors present, with a higher score indicating an increased risk for a cardiac event (Box 2). The estimated risk of a cardiac event in a pregnant woman with heart disease and a score of 0 is estimated to be 5%, whereas the risk rises to 27% with a score of 1 and to 75% with a score of 2 or higher [7,11].

In addition to the underlying cardiac lesion and maternal functional class, it is important during prepregnancy counseling to identify and discuss other associated risk factors that may complicate the pregnancy, such as preexisting arrhythmias, prosthetic valves, chronic anticoagulation, or use of other potentially teratogenic drugs (eg, angiotensin-converting enzyme [ACE] inhibitors). Likewise, the potential for further palliative or corrective surgery before conception, which may improve hemodynamics and reduce maternal and fetal risk as a result, such as in the setting of aortic valve stenosis or cyanosis, should be discussed. Several studies clearly indicate that cardiovascular surgery during pregnancy is less favorable, with a maternal and fetal mortality rate of 6% and 30%, re-

---

Box 2. Risk index for development of cardiac and neonatal event in pregnant women with heart disease

Risk factors for maternal cardiac event
  ≥NYHA functional class II or cyanosis
  Systemic ventricular systolic dysfunction (LV ejection fraction ≤40%)
  Left heart obstruction (aortic or mitral valve stenosis)
  Cardiac event before pregnancy (eg, arrhythmia, stroke, pulmonary edema)
  Other high-risk lesions (eg, pulmonary hypertension, Marfan syndrome with aorta diameter ≥40 mm)
Risk factors for neonatal adverse event
  Presence of maternal heart disease
  Poor maternal functional class (NYHA class II or higher)
  Maternal left heart obstruction
  Maternal age <20 years or >35 years
  Obstetrics risk factors for adverse neonatal events
    Multiple gestations
    Smoking during pregnancy
    Need for anticoagulant therapy during pregnancy

---

spectively [16]. Therefore, cardiac surgery during pregnancy should be reserved for patients refractory to medical therapy in whom further delay would be detrimental to maternal health.

Finally, during counseling, the risk of CHD in the offspring of a woman with heart disease needs to be discussed. In general, the risk of CHD is considered to be 0.5% to 0.8% in the general population [1]. In the setting of a first-degree relative with CHD, however, the risk increases 10-fold, with an estimated incidence of 5% to 7% [17]. Left heart obstructive lesions may have a slightly higher recurrence rate [3]. Often, the cardiac lesion in the offspring is not the same as that in the mother. The exception to this is in the setting of a lesion inherited in an autosomal dominant fashion (conferring a 50% risk of recurrence in the offspring), such as Marfan syndrome and 22q11.2 microdeletion syndrome [3].

Management

Management of pregnant women with CHD depends on the underlying cardiac condition and their maternal functional class. In general, women considered to have a low-risk lesion and who are in NYHA class I before pregnancy are followed with fetal ultrasound and fetal cardiac ultrasound and can be safely delivered in a community hospital. These patients should limit their strenuous exercise and obtain adequate rest. Maintaining an adequate hemoglobin concentration (hemoglobin concentration ≥ 11 g/dL) is also important [18]. Finally, although pregnancy is typically well tolerated in this patient group, the hemodynamic consequences of pregnancy can exacerbate or promote the development of arrhythmias [7,11]. As result, monitoring for arrhythmias should be an integral part of regular cardiovascular and obstetric prenatal visits.

When an arrhythmia occurs in the setting of pregnancy and heart disease, it is preferable to avoid pharmacologic treatment. In situations in which the arrhythmias become symptomatic or recurrence carries significant risk to the mother or fetus, however, medical therapy may be needed. In the setting of atrial fibrillation or flutter, digoxin and beta-blockers are preferred, given their safety profile [19]. Elective and emergent cardioversion has been performed safely during pregnancy [18,19]. In settings in which oral antiarrhythmic agents are necessary, quinidine has been used most frequently, without clear adverse fetal effects [18]. The use of other antiarrhythmics, such as adenosine, sotalol, and lidocaine, has been reported in the literature and generally seems to be well tolerated; however, data with regard to their safety profile remain limited [4,18]. The use of amiodarone during pregnancy has also been reported [20,21]. These recent studies indicate that the risk for teratogenicity may be lower than previously reported but that there continues to be a significant risk for impaired neonatal thyroid function [20].

With few exceptions, vaginal delivery with a facilitated second stage of labor (forceps delivery or vacuum extraction) is the preferred route of delivery in patients with CHD. Cesarean delivery is indicated when obstetric reasons are present, in those patients on coumadin, and in those patients with acute aortic dissection, Marfan syndrome with a dilated aortic root, or severe pulmonary hypertension and severe cardiac obstructive lesions. Labor should be conducted in the left lateral decubitus position to attenuate hemodynamic fluctuations associated with contractions. Epidural anesthesia with adequate volume preload is the preferred method of pain control in women with CHD, particularly in patients with single-ventricle physiology [4,18,22,23].

The American Heart Association currently does not recommend endocarditis prophylaxis for women with CHD expected to have an uncomplicated delivery. Nevertheless, many centers with significant experience with CHD and pregnancy continue to recommend endocarditis prophylaxis, given that it can often be difficult to predict which delivery may become complicated. Typically, antibiotic therapy using the gastrointestinal and genitourinary regimen is given 30 to 60 minutes before delivery is expected and is repeated 8 hours later [18].

Pregnant women with high-risk lesions who are in NYHA class III through IV should be managed in a high-risk pregnancy center experienced with CHD by a multidisciplinary team, including personnel from obstetrics, cardiovascular anesthesia, cardiology, and pediatrics. Once fetal maturity is confirmed, elective induction of labor is often preferred. Invasive hemodynamic monitoring in these difficult patients with intra-arterial monitoring with or without a central venous catheter is often helpful and allows for rapid intervention if complications arise.

In the immediate postpartum period, large fluctuations in hemodynamics continue. As a result, during the postpartum period, these patients should be monitored for a minimum of 72 hours in the hospital [4,18,22].

Summary

Women with CHD now comprise most patients with heart disease seen during pregnancy, accounting for 80% of all patients. In general, pregnancy is well tolerated in patients with CHD. For some women with particularly high-risk lesions and poor functional class, however, pregnancy poses significant risk for cardiovascular complications, including premature death. As result, preconception counseling and risk stratification are mandatory and should be done in all women of childbearing age with CHD.

References

[1] Perloff JK, Warnes CA. Congenital heart disease in adults: a new cardiovascular specialty. Circulation 2001;84:1881–90.

[2] Warnes CA. The adult with congenital heart disease: born to be bad? J Am Coll Cardiol 2005; 46:1–8.

[3] Siu SC, Colman JM. Congenital heart disease: heart disease and pregnancy. Heart 2001;85: 710–5.

[4] Colman JM, Siu SC. Pregnancy in adult patients with congenital heart disease. Prog Pediatr Cardiol 2003;17:53–60.

[5] Hunter S, Robson SC. Adaptation of the maternal heart in pregnancy. Br Heart J 1992;68:540–3.

[6] Siu SC, Colman JM, Sorensen S, et al. Adverse neonatal and cardiac outcomes are more common in pregnant women with cardiac disease. Circulation 2002;105:2179–84.

[7] Siu SC, Sermer M, Colman JM, et al. Prospective Multicenter Study of Pregnancy Outcomes in Women with Heart Disease. Circulation 2001;104:515–21.

[8] Elkayam U, Bitar F. Valvular heart disease and pregnancy part I: native valves. J Am Coll Cardiol 2005;46:223–30.

[9] Weiss B, Zemp L, Seifert B, et al. Outcome of pulmonary vascular disease in pregnancy: a systemic overview from 1978–1996. J Am Coll Cardiol 1998;31:1650–7.

[10] Avila W, Grinberg M, Snitcowsky R, et al. Maternal and fetal outcome in pregnant women with Eisenmenger's syndrome. Eur Heart J 1995;16:460–4.

[11] Siu SC, Sermer M, Harrison DA, et al. Risks and predictors for pregnancy-related complications in women with heart disease. Circulation 1997;96:2789–94.

[12] Ceci O, Berardesca C, Caradonna F, et al. Recurrent peripartum cardiomyopathy. Eur Heart J 1998;76:29–30.

[13] Sutton MS, Cole P, Plappert M, et al. Effects of subsequent pregnancy on left ventricular function in peripartum cardiomyopathy. Am Heart J 1991;121:1776–8.

[14] Rossiter J, Repke J, Morales A, et al. A prospective longitudinal evaluation of pregnancy in the Marfan syndrome. Am J Obstet Gynecol 1995;173:1599–606.

[15] Whittemore R, Hobbins J, Engle M. Pregnancy and its outcome in women with and without surgical treatment of congenital heart disease. Am J Cardiol 1982;50:641–51.

[16] Weiss BM, von Segesser LK, Alon E, et al. Outcome of cardiovascular surgery and pregnancy: a systemic review of the period of 1984–1996. Am J Obstet Gynecol 1998;179:1643–53.

[17] Romano-Zelekha O, Hirsch R, Blieden L, et al. The risk for congenital heart defects in off-spring of individuals with congenital heart defects. Clin Genet 2001;59:325–9.

[18] Connolly HM, Warnes CA. Pregnancy and conception. In: Gatzoulis MA, Webb GO, Daubeney PEF, editors. Diagnosis and management of adult congenital heart disease. Edinburgh, Scotland: Churchill Livingstone; 2003. p. 135–44.

[19] Lee JC, Wetzel G, Shannon K. Maternal arrhythmia management during pregnancy in patients with structural heart disease. Prog Pediatr Cardiol 2004;19:71–82.

[20] Bartalena L, Bogazzi F, Braverman LE, et al. Effects of amiodarone administration during pregnancy on neonatal thyroid function and subsequent neurodevelopment. J Endocrinol Invest 2001;24(2):116–30.

[21] Widerhorn J, Bhandari AK, Bughi S, et al. Fetal and neonatal adverse effects profile of amio-darone treatment during pregnancy. Am Heart J 1991;122:1162–6.

[22] Koos BJ. Management of uncorrected, palliated, and repaired cyanotic congenital heart disease in pregnancy. Prog Pediatr Cardiol 2004;19:25–45.

[23] Elkayam U, Bitar F. Valvular heart disease and pregnancy: part II: prosthetic valves. J Am Coll Cardiol 2005;46:403–10.

CLINICS IN
PERINATOLOGY

Clin Perinatol 32 (2005) 921–946

Delivery Room and Early Postnatal Management of Neonates Who Have Prenatally Diagnosed Congenital Heart Disease

Beth Ann Johnson, MD, MA[a],*, Anne Ades, MD[b]

[a]Herma Heart Center, Children's Hospital of Wisconsin, 9000 West Wisconsin Avenue,
Milwaukee, WI 53226, USA
[b]Division of Neonatology, The Children's Hospital of Philadelphia, 34th and Civic Center Boulevard,
Philadelphia, PA 19104, USA

Advances in fetal echocardiography have led to increasing numbers of infants being diagnosed prenatally as having congenital heart disease (CHD). Consequently, neonatologists are more commonly asked to attend the deliveries of infants who have prenatally diagnosed CHD. Optimal care of infants who have significant CHD begins before delivery with in utero management by perinatologists and continues with skilled resuscitation in the delivery room and subsequent timely admission to an intensive care unit. Prenatal diagnosis allows for coordination of care surrounding delivery and during the early postnatal hours. Knowledge of the expected transitional circulation occurring with birth and the pathophysiologic implications of CHD increases the likelihood of providing efficient and effective therapies anticipating improved neonatal care and outcomes.

Fetal echocardiography

Because the prenatal diagnosis can have a profound impact on decisions surrounding pregnancy, delivery, and postnatal management, accuracy in diagnosis is important. Several studies have evaluated the accuracy of prenatal echocardiographic diagnoses. In a study by Forbus and colleagues [1] published

---

* Corresponding author.
E-mail address: bajohnson@chw.org (B.A. Johnson).

0095-5108/05/$ – see front matter © 2005 Elsevier Inc. All rights reserved.
doi:10.1016/j.clp.2005.09.014   *perinatology.theclinics.com*

in 2004, the prenatal diagnosis of 133 infants was accurate in 119 (89.5%). In only 5 of the 14 patients who had postnatal discrepancies would the initial neonatal management have been different had the prenatal diagnosis been more accurate. Continuing to support the high accuracy of prenatal diagnosis, a 2001 series by Perolo and colleagues [2] calculated prenatal diagnostic accuracy to be 91% (236 of 260 cases). Of the fifteen discrepancies reported in this series, in 6 cases the lesion was different than the prenatal diagnosis and in 9 cases the infant had normal intracardiac anatomy. Rychik and colleagues [3] investigated the accuracy of fetal echocardiography specifically in regards to the fetus diagnosed as having single-ventricle anatomy. They reviewed 57 fetuses that had been identified on multiple prenatal scans to have single-ventricle anatomy between 1990 and 1995. Of the 43 fetuses carried to term, the prenatal diagnosis of single-ventricle heart was accurate in 93% (40 of 43); and in 70% of the neonates (30 of 43), the postnatal diagnosis was identical to the prenatal prediction. The initial management or surgical strategy did not change in 9 of the 13 newborns in this series in whom the postnatal diagnosis differed from prenatal diagnosis. Based on the literature discussed above, a prenatal diagnosis of CHD is accurate approximately 90% of the time; and the discrepancies that do occur rarely have a significant impact on the initial neonatal management. Despite some forms of CHD being difficult to visualize in utero, such as coarctation of the aorta [4–6], and despite other factors that complicate fetal echocardiography, such as maternal obesity, multiple gestations, and fetal lie or movements [6–9], prenatal diagnoses of CHD are highly accurate.

Prenatal diagnosis: impact on preoperative condition

Ideally, a prenatal diagnosis of complex CHD improves the preoperative condition and the clinical and neurodevelopmental outcomes of infants requiring neonatal cardiac surgery by preventing postnatal hemodynamic instability and hypoxemia. In theory, the hypoxemia, hypoperfusion, and acidosis associated with the cardiogenic shock that may accompany postnatally diagnosed CHD could be avoided and outcomes accordingly improved. Many investigators have studied the impact of a prenatal diagnosis on outcome variables. Despite similar surgical mortality, overall hospital mortality, duration of mechanical support, or length of hospital stay between infants diagnosed prenatally and infants diagnosed postnatally, decreased preoperative morbidity has been reported in infants diagnosed prenatally [10–13]. Between 1991 and 2000, Verheijen and colleagues [13] compared preoperative variables of 21 infants who had prenatally diagnosed CHD to those of 188 patients diagnosed postnatally. Those diagnosed prenatally had significantly lower lactate levels compared with infants diagnosed postnatally. The investigators suggested that the elevated lactate levels in the postnatally diagnosed group may contribute to an increased incidence of neurodevelopmental impairment and neuronal damage. They concluded that prenatal diagnosis may have an important role in the prevention of neurologic sequelae

[13]. Eapen and colleagues [10] also noted improved preoperative condition in infants diagnosed prenatally. In this series, only 7% of prenatally diagnosed infants had a base deficit less than -8 mEq/L as compared with 44% of the infants diagnosed postnatally [10]. Similarly, Kumar and colleagues [12] found that infants who had prenatally diagnosed CHD had a higher pH, and a lower maximum blood urea nitrogen and creatinine before surgery compared with infants diagnosed postnatally.

Fetal circulation

To appropriately care for infants who have prenatally diagnosed CHD appropriately in the delivery room and during the first days of life, it is important to understand the cardiovascular physiology of transitioning to extrauterine life and how this process is altered in the fetus and newborn who have CHD. Circulatory patterns in the fetus differ greatly from those of the newborn who has successfully transitioned to extrauterine life (Fig. 1). Both intrauterine and postnatal cardiovascular systems seek to deliver oxygen and remove wastes [14]. The source of oxygenated blood for the fetus is the placenta, rather than the lungs. Blood high in oxygen returns to the fetus from the placenta by way of the umbilical vein. A portion of the umbilical venous blood joins the inferior vena cava via the ductus venosus. This highly oxygenated blood from the placenta is returned to the right atrium, where the eustachian valve creates preferential

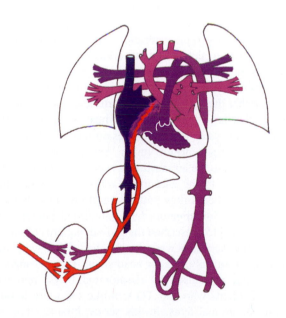

Fig. 1. Normal fetal circulation.

streaming, directing the oxygenated blood across the foramen ovale into the left atrium. This blood crosses the mitral valve and is ejected from the left ventricle to the ascending aorta, thus supplying the head and upper torso with the body's most highly oxygenated blood. During diastole, the left ventricle also serves the myocardium, delivering similarly highly oxygenated blood through the coronary arteries [14]. The effective summation of the fetal flow patterns achieves high levels of oxygen saturation in the developing brain and contracting myocardium.

The deoxygenated blood returning from the lower extremities by way of the inferior vena cava is joined in the right atrium by venous return from the superior vena cava and from the myocardium by way of the coronary sinus. This right atrial deoxygenated blood crosses the tricuspid valve and is ejected by the right ventricle. Because of the high pulmonary vascular resistance in utero, only a small portion of the right ventricular output (approximately 12%) enters the pulmonary circulation [14]. The remainder of the right ventricular outflow crosses the ductus arteriosus to provide blood flow to the lower portion of the body. Of the descending aortic blood flow, two-thirds returns to the placenta for oxygenation while the remaining one-third serves the lower body [14].

Changes in fetal circulation associated with congenital heart disease

Normal anatomic pathways of fetal cardiac shunting permit redistribution of blood flow in structural heart disease, so much so that most forms of CHD are well-tolerated in utero [14]. The exceptions are CHD associated with myocardial dysfunction or severe atrioventricular (AV) valve regurgitation. In fetuses that have transposition of the great arteries (TGA), the ascending aorta is aligned with and receives blood from the right ventricle. The usual fetal intracardiac shunts (ductus venosus, foramen ovale, and ductus arteriosus) are still present, therefore the fetal blood with the lowest oxygen saturation is directed—as in the normal fetus—to the right ventricle, but then is ejected into the ascending aorta, coronary arteries, and brain, rather than into the ductus arteriosus, lower body, and placenta (Fig. 2). In fetuses that have hypoplastic left heart syndrome (HLHS), there is complete mixing of fetal systemic venous (desaturated) and umbilical vein (more highly saturated) in the right atrium, rather than the preferential streaming of more oxygenated blood into the left atrium as seen in the normal fetus. The result is lower oxygen delivery to the ascending aorta, brain, and coronary arteries (Fig. 3). Although these altered flow patterns rarely result in hemodynamic concerns for the fetus, some investigators have suggested potential consequences. Rosenthal and colleagues [15] described the growth patterns observed in neonates who had CHD. In this series, newborns who had TGA were mildly growth-retarded with disproportionately smaller head sizes. The investigators speculated that this finding could be caused by desaturated blood perfusing the heads and upper torsos of infants who had TGA unlike the more highly oxygenated placental blood in the normal fetus. In this series, infants who had HLHS also had smaller head sizes, again postulated to be caused by altered flow patterns.

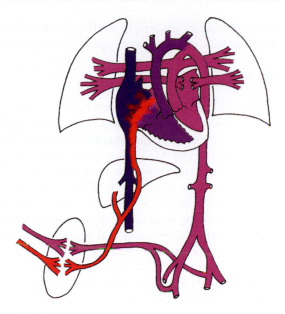

Fig. 2. Fetal circulation in transposition of the great arteries.

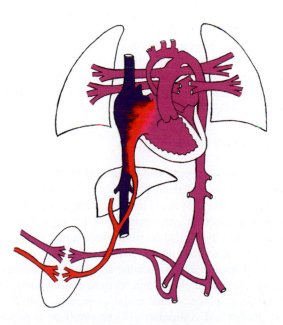

Fig. 3. Fetal circulation in hypoplastic left heart syndrome.

Variations of in utero circulatory patterns in CHD may alter the normal growth and development of the fetus and may have significant long-term effects.

Changes occurring with delivery

At delivery, the fetal circulation must undergo significant changes. Transition from intrauterine circulatory patterns to postnatal circulatory patterns involves elimination of the low-resistance placenta from the circulation, expansion of the lungs, increased pulmonary artery blood flow and closure of the intrauterine shunts. Closure of the ductus venosus and the foramen ovale rely heavily on the hemodynamic changes that occur after birth. With delivery and initiation of respiration, pulmonary resistance decreases, blood flow across the pulmonary circuit multiplies, and blood volume returning to the left atrium increases. All these factors serve to increase left atrial pressures and lead to closure of the foramen ovale as the flap valve is pushed against the atrial septum. After placental separation and loss of umbilical venous flow, the ductus venosus passively closes, with complete closure common by the end of the first week of life [14]. Closure of the ductus arteriosus usually occurs over hours to days and depends on the interplay among vascular mediators, such as oxygen, prostaglandins, and possibly hormones [14].

Ductus arteriosus

Infants who have CHD may have lesions that restrict either blood flow to the lungs or blood flow to the body. Maintaining ductal patency is vital for infants who have obstructive CHD because it provides an alternate source of blood flow distal to the obstruction. Postnatal closure of the ductus arteriosus may lead to acute decompensation in the newborn period with either profound cyanosis in right-sided obstructive lesions or low cardiac output and cardiogenic shock in left-sided obstructive lesions.

Postnatal timing of ductal closure

Several researchers have investigated the timing of physiologic ductal closure; and in all published reports, ductal closure has been found rarely to be immediate, but nearly universal by 4 days of age. Lim and colleagues [16] studied 51 healthy term infants who had birth weights appropriate for gestational age. Infants in whom functional ductal closure had occurred were noted as follows: on day one (age 5–23 hours) 20% of infants; on day two (age 24–47 hours) 82% infants; on day three (age 51–71 hours) 96% of infants; and by day four (age 72–91 hours) 100% of infants demonstrated physiologic closure of the ductus. This study also documented intermittent patency after initial closure in 6 of 20 infants studied for 7 days [16]. Reller and colleagues [17] reported on a series of 63 infants born at 30 weeks gestation or later. In his study, on day one, 8% of infants had

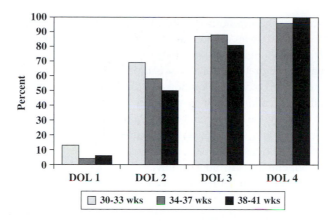

Fig. 4. Rate of ductal closure by gestational age and day-of-life. DOL, day-of-life; wks, weeks. (*Data from* Reller M, Rice M, McDonald R. Review of studies evaluating ductal patency in the premature infant. J Pediatr 1993;122:S59–62.)

spontaneous closure; on day two, 60% of infants; on day three, 86% of infants; and on day four all but 1 infant had acquired spontaneous ductal closure (Fig. 4) [17]. Lastly, Gentile and colleagues [18] reported similar findings. In this study, all infants evaluated during the first 8 hours of life had a patent ductus arteriosus. Spontaneous closure had occurred in 42% at 24 hours of age, in 90% at 48 hours of age, and in all infants at 96 hours [18].

Delivery room resuscitation

Five to 10% of infants who do not have CHD require more than routine care at birth and 1% to 10% require assisted ventilation [19–22]. Among infants who have CHD, a similar proportion does well at delivery, requiring no more than routine assistance, such as drying, warming, and stimulating. Mirlesse and colleagues [23] reported on 110 infants who had prenatally diagnosed CHD. Neonatologists were present for every delivery, but additional resuscitation was necessary in only 11 cases.

General principles of delivery room resuscitation

Readiness of equipment and trained providers is essential for effective neonatal resuscitation whether CHD is present or not. Equipment should be readily available, easy to find, and routinely inspected and tested before each delivery. Planning for the delivery of an infant who has prenatally diagnosed CHD may also include preparation for prostaglandin infusion, isoproterenol administration, or external pacing. Although intervention beyond routine care is only occasionally required for infants who have prenatally diagnosed CHD, supplies and trained personnel should be ready.

Resuscitation of the newborn who has CHD includes the same algorithm as resuscitation of infants who do not have CHD [19,24]. Additionally, the team in the delivery room should have knowledge of the underlying cardiac anatomy, expected changes with transitional circulation, the need for postnatal ductal patency, and expected oxygen saturations (Table 1). In general, newborns should receive initial interventions, such as warming, drying, positioning to create airway patency, clearing the airway, and stimulating. These initial actions should be completed quickly; and subsequent resuscitative steps rely on rapid, accurate assessment of respirations, heart rate, and color [20]. With the notable exception of complete congenital heart block, a newborn's heart rate should generally be greater than 100 beats/min. In the absence of coexisting conduction-system disease, the presence of structural heart disease should not preclude the heart rate being in the normal range. If the infant is breathing comfortably, has a heart rate greater than 100 beats/min, and has adequate color centrally, no further intervention is required. If the heart rate is less than 100 beats/min, respiratory effort should be evaluated and effective positive pressure ventilation (PPV) initiated if respiratory effort is ineffective. Neonatal bradycardia, even in the presence of structural heart disease, is most likely secondary to inadequate respiratory patterns and therefore should improve with effective PPV. Most commonly, PPV leads to improved heart rate and perfusion, followed by improvement in tone and respirations. If significant bradycardia (<60 beats/min) is not conduction-

Table 1
Lesion-specific considerations

Cardiac lesion	Special considerations
Left-to-right shunt lesions (ventricular septal defect, atrioventricular canal, truncus arteriosus)	None
Tetralogy of Fallot	None, may require PGE_1 if severe right ventricular outflow tract obstruction is present.
Transposition of the great arteries	Lower than normal saturations expected. Deliver in a center that can do balloon atrial septostomy (BAS) if atrial septal restriction suspected. PGE_1 in most cases.
Total anomalous pulmonary venous return	Lower than normal saturations expected. Deliver in a center that can perform urgent cardiac surgery if obstruction expected.
Single ventricle with ductal-dependent pulmonary blood flow	Lower than normal saturations expected. PGE_1 to be started.
Single ventricle with ductal-dependent systemic blood flow	Lower than normal saturations expected. PGE_1 to be started. Deliver in a center that can perform urgent cardiac surgery or BAS if atrial septum restrictive.
Ebstein's anomaly of the tricuspid valve	Variable course depending on severity of tricuspid regurgitation, and degree of right ventricular outflow tract obstruction.

Abbreviations: BAS, balloon atrial septostomy; PGE_1, prostaglandin E_1.

system-related and does not respond to PPV, chest compressions should be initiated concurrent with preparation of resuscitation medications. Endotracheal intubation should occur if the resuscitation becomes prolonged or if PPV is ineffective. Complete directions for administering chest compression and performing endotracheal intubation are beyond the scope of this review but are taught in the Neonatal Resuscitation Program (NRP) [24]. The unique complexities of meconium aspiration or prematurity should be given priority in the delivery room, and management of these problems should follow established guidelines regarding intubation, temperature regulation, and surfactant administration. The use of 100% oxygen (as currently recommended by NRP), volume, and certain medications deserve further consideration, because their appropriateness may be altered in the presence of CHD.

Oxygen and congenital heart disease

Oxygen must be used with caution in infants who have HLHS and other forms of single-ventricle physiology in whom a rapid decrease in pulmonary vascular resistance may compromise systemic blood flow. Rarely, infants who have HLHS do have lung disease in concert with structural heart disease; and these particular infants may benefit from supplemental oxygen. Providers must be aware, however, of the unique cardiac anatomy and physiology of infants who have HLHS and the possible deleterious effects of the use of supplemental oxygen in these patients. In single-ventricle physiology, the ratio of pulmonary to systemic resistances in the vascular beds determines the relative proportion of blood flow to each circuit. Supplemental oxygen acts as a potent vasodilator in the pulmonary bed. When pulmonary vascular resistance decreases in an infant who has HLHS, blood ejected from the single right ventricle preferentially enters the pulmonary circuit rather than the systemic circuit by way of the patent ductus arteriosis (PDA) to the descending aorta, thus impairing systemic cardiac output [25]. In this manner, supplemental oxygen can worsen systemic output, as indicated in the newborn by poor urine output, metabolic acidosis, and poor perfusion. This low-cardiac-output state can increase the risk for end-organ damage, such as renal injury, brain injury, and necrotizing enterocolitis. An arterial saturation (SaO_2) of 80% to 85% usually corresponds to adequate pulmonary and systemic blood flow and thus optimizes oxygen delivery. Because the goal of managing patients who have single-ventricle physiology preoperatively is to maximize oxygen delivery and not arterial saturation, supplemental oxygen, if indicated, may be titrated, typically to achieve an arterial saturation of 80% to 85%.

Pulse oximetry

Although pulse oximetry is not routinely used in the delivery room for normal healthy infants, it may be more commonly used in the delivery-room resuscitation of newborns who have CHD. Normal pulse oximetry values in the first minutes of life for infants who do not have structural heart disease may not be well-known; and as a result, providers may become overly concerned with desaturation in the first minutes of life. To evaluate arterial saturations immediately following delivery, SaO_2 was measured in 50 healthy neonates of 35 weeks gestation or greater. The pre- and postductal SaO_2 values ranged from 67% to 73% after 2 minutes of life, with increases to normal levels by 15 minutes of age [26]. The threshold of 95% saturation was not routinely achieved until 12 minutes preductally and 14 minutes postductally. Additionally, at 2 minutes of age, the preductal saturations were significantly higher than the postductal saturations in these healthy newborns; and the difference remained statistically significant until 10 minutes of age [26]. These findings were confirmed by other investigators, Harris and colleagues [27], who studied 32 infants delivered vaginally. The mean arterial saturation at 1 minute of life was found to be 61% and at 7 minutes, the mean value was 82%. In this same series, 44 infants delivered by cesarean section had a mean arterial saturation at 1 minute of age of 46% and at 7 minutes of life, 82% [27]. This cumulative data suggests that even healthy newborn infants remain relatively desaturated in the immediate postpartum period and that saturations as low as 50% can be normal in the first minute of life [28]. This knowledge should permit more accurate interpretation of oxygen saturations in newborns who have and who do not have CHD, leading to more judicious use of supplemental oxygen.

Volume

Without easily identified sources of fluid loss, hypovolemia is rarely the cause of hypotension in the newborn who does not have CHD. Therefore, careful use of fluid resuscitation is generally warranted. Prostaglandin therapy, however, commonly causes vasodilatation and relative hypovolemia in neonates who have CHD. Additionally, in parallel circulation, the capacitance of the pulmonary circulation "steals" blood from the systemic circulation, also leading to relative hypovolemia. Thus, newborns who have CHD, particularly ones receiving a prostaglandin infusion, may benefit from volume resuscitation. Nonspecific signs of hypovolemia include pale, mottled skin; cool extremities; hypotension; tachycardia; and prolonged capillary refill [29]. If concern exists regarding the infant's hemodynamic status, 10 mL/kg of isotonic volume should be given and response monitored. If, however, hemodynamic compromise is caused by myocardial depression from hypoxemia or acidosis, volume loading the ventricle may actually be detrimental. If the infant's response to volume is paradoxic or little improvement is seen, echocardiography should be considered to assess myocardial function, to rule out pericardial effusion, and to assess ductal patency.

Medications

In the newborn who does not have CHD, epinephrine and bicarbonate are currently the only recommended medication in the delivery room in the event of cardiopulmonary resuscitation. Resuscitation of the neonate who has complex CHD has not been studied in detail. In an animal model of single-ventricle physiology, however, the effect of epinephrine on the ratio of pulmonary blood flow to systemic blood flow (Q_p/Q_s) and on oxygen delivery was tested [30]. The effect of epinephrine was tested while providing 50% and 100% oxygen. Epinephrine increased cardiac output at 50% and 100% oxygen. Epinephrine decreased Q_p/Q_s at high and low FiO_2. In newborns who have ductal-dependent CHD and who are frequently prone to excessive pulmonary blood flow and inadequate systemic perfusion, a decrease in the Q_p/Q_s ratio represents improved systemic blood flow. In addition, epinephrine increased oxygen delivery as measured by a significant increase in systemic venous saturation (SVO_2). With 100% oxygen, epinephrine significantly lowered the arteriovenous difference (AVO_2), another measure of cardiac output and oxygen delivery. Epinephrine improved oxygen delivery by increasing cardiac output and by moving the Q_p/Q_s ratio closer to one [30]. These data support the use of epinephrine if needed in patients who have CHD.

Another medication occasionally used in the perinatal period is sodium bicarbonate, though its use and benefits are controversial. Some providers use it to improve the lactic acidosis that may accompany poor cardiac output and poor peripheral perfusion. The acidemia present perinatally in infants who do not have CHD is often respiratory in nature and corrects rapidly with ventilation, which may also be the case in infants who have CHD who suffer a period of asphyxia at delivery. Persistent metabolic acidosis, after respiratory clearance, suggests poor oxygen delivery or inadequate perfusion to tissues because of poor cardiac output; and therapies should be aimed at improving systemic blood flow. Effective resuscitation, by improving cardiac output, allows for the hepatic conversion of lactate to bicarbonate, restoring serum-buffering abilities and improving acidemia. Administration of bicarbonate is a temporizing measure that may permit physiologic survival until specific therapy is provided, but it does not correct the underlying disturbance.

Prostaglandin E_1

Though not a recommended medication in NRP, for many prenatally diagnosed neonates who have CHD, prostaglandin E_1 (PGE_1) is useful to start in the immediate postnatal period. Aprostadil (Prostin VR Pediatric Sterile Solution, Upjohn) was approved by the Food and Drug Administration (FDA) in 1981 for use in infants who had CHD and required ductal patency until palliative surgery [31]. PGE_1 is biosynthesized and is quickly metabolized. Sixty to 80% of PGE_1 is metabolized on first pass through the lungs. Thus, it must be administered by way of continuous infusion [31,32]. PGE_1 metabolites, produced by oxidative processes, have less bioactivity and are excreted primarily by the kidney [31]. Elimination from the body is complete within 24 hours after administration [32].

Common side effects

Common side effects of prostaglandin therapy include: vasodilatation with resultant hypotension, apnea, rash, and fever (Box 1) [31]. In 1981, Lewis and colleagues [33] reported on the PGE_1 side-effect profile as collected from all 56 investigators in the United States who administered the drug under the investigational new drug protocol of Upjohn Company between 1976 and 1979. This study included data from 492 infants treated with PGE_1. The most common side effect was respiratory depression in 12% of the infants. PGE_1 was stopped in 22 of 58 infants who experienced respiratory depression but was restarted in seven instances without any recurrences reported. The investigators reported respiratory depression more commonly in infants weighing less than 2 kg. At that time the dosage commonly used was 0.1 mcg/kg/min [33].

Kramer and colleagues [34] treated 91 newborns with PGE_1 for a total treatment time of 394 hours. Even though the original data suggested dosing at 0.1 mcg/kg/min, of the total treatment time during Kramer's study, doses less than 0.01 mcg/kg/min were used 43% of the time and doses greater than 0.02 mcg/kg/min were used only 5% of the time [34]. All infants who had ductal-dependent systemic blood flow showed improvement in lower body perfusion, even at these much lower doses. Regarding side effects, 38% of infants who had TGA and 35% of infants who had obstructed pulmonary blood flow showed periods of hypotension (systolic pressures more than 2 SD below normal values for more than 30 minutes) that were easily treated with volume. In this study 38% of spontaneously breathing patients developed apneas. When comparing the spontaneously breathing infants receiving high-dose PGE_1

Box 1. Side effects of prostaglandin E_1

Common side effects:

Apnea
Hypotension/capillary leak
Fever
Rash

Less common side effects:

Gastric outlet obstruction
Cortical hyperostosis
Leukocytosis
Seizures

(>0.01 mcg/kg/min) and those receiving low dose PGE_1 (<0.01 mcg/kg/min), twice as many infants developed apnea on high dose as compared with low dose, suggesting that although clinical response is not dose-dependent, the presence of side effects may be. Importantly, prostaglandin therapy alone does not mandate mechanical ventilation, as during 86% of the treatment time in Kramer's study, infants were spontaneously ventilating [34]. Saxena and colleagues [35] reported apnea requiring mechanical ventilation in only 5 of 56 spontaneously breathing neonates treated with PGE_1. The apneic events reported by Saxena occurred in the first hour of treatment in all cases.

Less common side effects

Less common side effects attributed to PGE_1, especially after chronic therapy, include cortical hyperostosis, leukocytosis, and gastric outlet obstruction. Teixeira and colleagues [36] reported on cortical hyperostosis occurring in 5 infants receiving PGE_1 for more than 21 days. The patients were irritable and had swelling of the limbs. The periosteal lesions regressed over months after discontinuing PGE_1 [36]. Leukocytosis has also been reported with prostaglandin infusion. Arav-Boger and colleagues [37] described a newborn who had temporally related leukocytosis with PGE_1 infusion. When 16 infants were retrospectively evaluated, they found that white blood cell counts increased 39% on average with PGE_1 infusion [37]. Administration of PGE_1 has also been associated with gastric outlet obstruction secondary to antral mucosal thickening. Symptoms include poor feeding, vomiting, diarrhea, and abdominal distention [38] and may mimic those of pyloric stenosis with projectile vomiting and weight loss [39]. In all reports the antral thickening was noted to resolve over a period of weeks after discontinuation of therapy [39,40].

Dose

As mentioned above, the initial studies recommended a PGE_1 starting dose of 0.1 mcg/kg/min [70]. More recent studies, however, have reported clinical success with lower doses and fewer associated side effects. Hallidie-Smith [41] studied infants at various PGE_1 doses between 0.1 and 0.005 mcg/kg/min. She reported no failures of response to prostaglandin infusion in CHD, even at the very low doses. More important, no side effects were recorded in infants given doses between 0.01 and 0.005 mcg/kg/min [41]. The authors strongly support the view that apneic events and other major side effects are dose related. Reddy recommends any initial dosage employed be decreased to 0.01 mcg/kg/min as soon as the desired effect is achieved, again reporting that side effects are more common at higher doses [42]. In some cases, clinicians may wish to assess ductal patency by echocardiography before using lower doses. Kramer and colleagues [34] recommend a starting dose of 0.015 mcg/kg/min and increasing the dose if the clinical improvement is inadequate. Box 2 contains information on one accepted mixing strategy for the preparation of PGE_1 infusion.

Box 2. Preparing PGE$_1$ solution

1. 6 × birth weight = "X"
2. Divide 500 (mcg/cc; concentration of commercially prepared vial) by "X" = "Y"
3. To commercially prepared vial (1cc of 500 mcg/cc) add "Y" cc of normal saline.
4. The dose of 0.01 mcg/kg/min = 0.1 cc/hr intravenous drip rate
5. Solution has shelf life of 72 hours when prepared in normal saline

Drip Chart

Dose		IV Drip rate of prepared solution
0.01 mcg/kg/min	=	0.1 cc/hr
0.02 mcg/kg/min	=	0.2 cc/hr
0.03 mcg/kg/min	=	0.3 cc/hr
0.04 mcg/kg/min	=	0.4 cc/hr
0.05 mcg/kg/min	=	0.5 cc/hr

Prevention of associated apnea

In 2003, Lim and colleagues [43] reported on the efficacy of aminophylline in preventing the apnea associated with PGE$_1$ administration. They evaluated 42 infants receiving PGE$_1$ at a starting dose of 0.01 mcg/kg/min. The infants received either aminophylline or placebo. Serum levels of aminophylline were obtained and no deleterious side effects were attributed to aminophylline. The investigators found that aminophylline reduced the incidence of apnea and the need for intubation associated with PGE$_1$ therapy [43]. In the group of 21 infants receiving aminophylline, no infant required intubation for apnea and only 2 infants had apneic events. Of the 21 infants receiving placebo, 11 had apneic events and 6 required intubation for apnea. Furthermore, infants receiving aminophylline did not become apneic with sedation, whereas 4 of 6 infants receiving sedation while on placebo became apneic [43]. The administration of aminophylline with PGE$_1$ decreases the incidence of intubation while receiving prostaglandin therapy and the potential complications of mechanical ventilation.

Lesions that may result in physiologic compromise soon after birth

Three lesions are well known to cause significant hemodynamic compromise after separation from the placenta: TGA with intact ventricular septum and a restrictive atrial septum, HLHS with an intact atrial septum, and obstructed total anomalous pulmonary venous return (TAPVR) (Table 2). These three lesions are different anatomically, but share the common feature of the inability to provide pulmonary venous blood to the systemic circulation, resulting in severe hypoxemia. In TGA with intact ventricular septum and intact or restrictive atrial septum, the only means of mixing pulmonary and systemic blood flow is by way of the PDA. The PDA, although beneficial, often does not provide adequate intercirculatory mixing; and the saturations can be extremely low, especially in the ascending aorta. Such infants benefit from a balloon atrial septostomy, a catheter procedure that creates a communication between the atria and can lead to an immediate and significant increase in atrial level mixing, with a subsequent increase in systemic oxygen saturation.

Similarly, in HLHS with intact atrial septum, the pulmonary venous blood cannot cross to the systemic circulation, as there is no egress from the left atrium. Infants who have HLHS are dependent on a patent atrial communication to allow pulmonary venous return to cross from the left atrium to the right atrium, entering both the pulmonary circuit and the systemic circuit by way of the PDA. Infants who have HLHS and intact atrial septum present with severe cyanosis as pulmonary venous flow cannot reach the systemic circulation.

In obstructed TAPVR, the pulmonary veins, instead of returning to the left atrium, connect with venous structures either above the heart (supracardiac) or below the diaphragm (infradiaphragmatic). Because of venous obstruction, the pulmonary vasculature quickly becomes congested; and as blood does not return to the heart, left-sided filling is quickly compromised, as is cardiac output. The

Table 2
Cardiac lesions likely to require urgent intervention

Cardiac lesion	Anatomy/Physiology	Intervention
Hypoplastic left heart syndrome with intact atrial septum	Inability to provide pulmonary venous return (oxygenated blood) to systemic circulation	Surgical atrial septectomy or balloon atrial septostomy
Transposition of the great arteries with restrictive atrial septal defect	Inability to provide pulmonary venous return (oxygenated blood) to systemic circulation	Balloon atrial septostomy
Total anomalous pulmonary venous return with obstruction	Inability to provide pulmonary venous return (oxygenated blood) to systemic circulation	Surgical repair
Tetralogy of Fallot with absent pulmonary valve	Severely dilated main and branch pulmonary arteries causing external bronchial compression	Prone positioning, continuous positive airway pressure, or intubation
Complete congenital heart block	Poor cardiac output due to lack of atrioventricular synchrony or low ventricular rate	Increase ventricular rate with isoproterenol or pacing

infants present with limited cardiac output and extreme hypoxemia. Urgent surgical intervention is required to relieve the obstruction and correct the lesion.

An additional lesion that can present with early decompensation in the delivery room is tetralogy of Fallot with absent pulmonary valve. In this congenital lesion, there is a rudimentary pulmonary valve with severe regurgitation from the branch pulmonary arteries back into the main pulmonary artery and right ventricle. This regurgitation results in severely dilated proximal branch pulmonary arteries and proximal and distal compression of the airway. Infants who have tetralogy of Fallot with absent pulmonary valve can present with significant respiratory distress after delivery. Patency of the infant's airway is sometimes maintained with prone positioning; other times continuous positive airway pressure or intubation is required. Once the airway has been secured, the infant is usually stable hemodynamically.

Ex utero intrapartum treatment procedure

In severe cases of CHD or lung or airway disease expected to cause immediate deterioration after separation from the placenta, rapid invasive intervention may be necessary. The ex utero intrapartum treatment (EXIT) procedure is a surgical procedure designed with the goal of creating hemodynamic stability at delivery for infants who are predicted to have cardiopulmonary failure on separation from the placenta. The EXIT procedure seeks to create a controlled situation out of a potentially catastrophic emergency. In the EXIT procedure, the mother is provided deep inhalation anesthesia to decrease uterine tone and to prevent placental separation. The uterus is exposed, a stapled hysterotomy is performed and the head, neck, and shoulders of the infant are delivered. After partial delivery, the neonate is closely monitored with pulse oximetry and echocardiography throughout the subsequent surgical procedure or airway stabilization. The EXIT procedure has been successfully applied to fetuses that have several abnormalities with which cardiopulmonary compromise is expected immediately following delivery, such as large cystic adenomatoid malformations, large neck masses with suspected airway compromise, or congenital high airway obstructive syndrome (CHAOS). The Children's Hospital of Philadelphia has reported a series of 31 neonates treated with the EXIT procedure between 1996 and 2001 [44,45]. The series included an infant who had congenital diaphragmatic hernia and tetralogy of Fallot who underwent an EXIT-to-Extracorporeal Membrane Oxygenation (ECMO) procedure at 36 weeks gestation. The neonate remained hemodynamically stable on placental bypass for 90 minutes without acidosis or hypoxemia while transitioned to ECMO. In the case of EXIT-to-ECMO, after delivering the fetal head, neck, and shoulders, the neck dissection was performed and arterial and venous ECMO cannulas were placed. This radical surgical procedure is currently only performed in select fetal centers and has been attempted to be used with lesions such as HLHS with intact atrial septum to avoid the potential immediate cardiopulmonary failure that may occur and is commonly fatal.

Location of delivery

Decisions regarding location of delivery will depend on the expected immediate postnatal course. There is a report by Kelsall and colleagues [46] that suggests infants can be safely delivered outside regional cardiac centers and uneventfully transported while receiving PGE_1 therapy. Other investigators suggest that delivery in tertiary centers may be especially beneficial for certain structural cardiac lesions [23,47,48]. In a series of 110 prenatally diagnosed infants by Mirlesse and colleagues in 2001 [23], researchers found that infants who had TGA frequently required invasive resuscitation not readily available except at tertiary centers. These investigators recommended that infants prenatally diagnosed with TGA be delivered where providers are available to perform an urgent balloon atrial septostomy, if indicated.

Intact atrial septum is rare in HLHS and is associated with hydrops fetalis and pulmonary lymphangectasia. In a series from The Children's Hospital of Philadelphia between 1990 and 1997, 316 infants who had HLHS were referred for care [49]. Eighteen, or 5.7%, of these neonates had an intact atrial septum diagnosed by echocardiography. Of the 18 infants who had HLHS and intact atrial septum, 17 received stage one palliation; and of this group of 17, there were eleven in-hospital deaths. All neonates presented and received intervention within 36 hours of age. One prenatally diagnosed infant was delivered by induced vaginal delivery and received a surgical atrial septectomy by 1 hour of age. A second prenatally diagnosed infant was delivered by way of cesarean section and placed on bypass by 30 minutes of age, followed by stage one palliation. This particularly lethal cardiac lesion causes severe and immediate hemodynamic compromise that requires rapid intervention if the infant is to survive. Fetal interventional procedures to open the atrial septum may show promise for this lesion.

Infants who have obstructed TAPVR can present with immediate physiologic compromise after delivery. These infants do not improve with PGE_1 and may actually deteriorate if the pulmonary bed vasodilates or receives more flow from a patent ductus arteriosus becoming further congested [35,41]. Obstructed TAPVR is a lesion requiring urgent surgical intervention to decompress the pulmonary veins. For these three lesions in particular—TGA with restrictive or intact atrial septum, HLHS with intact atrial septum, and obsructed TAPVR—consideration should be made for delivery to occur in facilities that can rapidly provide the necessary interventions.

Complete congenital heart block

The bulk of this review has focused on structural heart disease. Fetal rhythm abnormalities, however, may also be diagnosed prenatally and may require more invasive resuscitation in the delivery room. The most common fetal arrhythmia requiring intervention in the delivery room is complete congenital heart block

(CCHB). This dysrhythmia can necessitate premature delivery because of developing hydrops fetalis and can cause significant symptomatology immediately following delivery. The resulting bradycardia of CCHB can lead to poor cardiac output, heart failure, pericardial effusion, and, in the most extreme condition, hydrops fetalis. The incidence of CCHB is 1/20,000 live births [50–53], and it is diagnosed in the presence of persistent bradycardia by auscultation or sonography [52]. Asyncrony between atrial and ventricular contractions can be seen by fetal echocardiography [53]. CCHB has often been associated with maternal auto-immune disease. The cause of CCHB is usually transplacental transfer of anti-bodies (anti-Ro and anti-La) in mothers who have connective tissue disorders. The anti-Ro and anti-La antibodies have an unexplained predilection for the AV node, which leads to fibrous replacement of the AV nodal conducting system [51,54,55]. In a reported series of 91 fetuses who had CCHB, the median age at diagnosis was 29 weeks gestation [51].

One-quarter to one-third of patients who have CCHB have associated structural heart disease [56]. Infants who have CCHB and structural heart disease are especially at risk for cardiac decompensation because their ability to maintain adequate cardiac output is limited by structural abnormalities and low heart rate [56]. The diagnosis of complete congenital heart block in the fetus should prompt a complete cardiac evaluation to rule out the presence of structural heart disease [53]. The prognosis of infants who have CCHB is worsened by poor fetal growth, associated structural anomalies, or a ventricular rate of less than 55 beats/min (which is associated with the development of hydrops) [52,54,57–59]. The development of hydrops is ominous and often approached by early delivery of the neonate followed by therapies to increase heart rate [8]. In the series reported by Eronen and colleagues [51], the fetal heart rate was significantly lower in fetuses that had hydrops than in fetuses that did not have hydrops (50 beats/min versus 61 beats/min); and hydrops was present in 27% of infants who had complete heart block. Complications such as premature delivery secondary to hydrops and the associated problems of prematurity add even more complexity to the neonate's condition at delivery [60].

The symptoms of CCHB at delivery vary in relationship to the underlying ventricular rate and to the myocardial adaptations made to meet the infant's metabolic requirements. The neonatal heart is somewhat able to compensate for the decreased rate of CCHB by increasing the stroke volume by way of increasing ventricular size and fractional shortening [54,57]. The infant, however, has less ability to increase stroke volume as compared with the adult. Newborns may be asymptomatic or may present in varying degrees of low cardiac output or even congestive heart failure [50]. Hydrops fetalis and intrauterine demise are not uncommon in fetuses that have CCHB. Infants surviving to delivery who have hydrops require the presence in the delivery room of personnel who can emergently drain fluid collections, if present and compromising physiologic stability, as well as someone who can provide appropriate cardiac interventions [56].

Infants who have CCHB tend to tolerate vaginal delivery fairly well unless they are in distress or in heart failure [50]. Arrangements for treatment of CCHB, neonatal bradycardia, and congestive heart failure with inotropic and chronotropic agents and temporary or permanent pacing soon after birth should be made prior to delivery [50,56,61]. As with structural heart disease, a team of providers skilled in resuscitation and capable of rapid assessment and intervention should be present in the delivery room. Severe symptoms or hydrops fetalis suggest an urgent need for pacing. If the patient is suffering from poor cardiac output, chronotropic agents such as isoproterenol or atropine may be given while arrangements are made for pacing [50,56,60]. Data support starting isoproterenol at 0.2 mcg/kg/min and gradually increasing the dose to 0.6 mcg/kg/min as required for effect. In a report by Quek and colleagues [60], isoproterenol was effective in bringing the baseline ventricular rate up to a maximum of 65 beats/min. Transcutaneous pacing may also be considered in the infant who presents in extremis [50,56]. Mirlesse and colleagues [23] reported 17 cases of intrauterine arrhythmias. In this series, five of the infants who had complete heart block required placement of a pacing electrode within hours of birth. Infants who are asymptomatic and have a heart rate greater than 50 to 55 beats/min, the level considered to place one at risk for sudden death in the absence of structural heart disease, do not require immediate intervention but should be transferred and closely monitored in an intensive care unit setting. According to several published studies, more than 50% of neonates who have CCHB require permanent pacemakers in the newborn period [51,60].

Supraventricular tachycardia

A common arrhythmia of infancy is supraventricular tachycardia (SVT), with an estimated incidence of 1/25,000 infants [62]. SVT can be caused by several different mechanisms: accessory pathway mediated, AV nodal reentry, atrial flutter, and atrial ectopic tachycardia, to name a few. Accessory-pathway–mediated SVT is the most common form of SVT in infants. Accessory pathways are bands of specialized muscle tissue that form an electrical connection, in addition to the AV node, between the atrium and the ventricle [62]. Wolff-Parkinson-White syndrome (WPW) is a form of accessory- pathway–mediated SVT in which preexcitation is visible on electrocardiogram in the form of a delta wave or slurring of the upstroke of the QRS complex.

SVT in neonates is a narrow-complex tachycardia with heart rates typically greater than 200 beats/min. SVT can be well-tolerated in infancy, and the urgency of intervention depends on the infant's hemodynamic condition. Most neonates can tolerate SVT for several hours before becoming symptomatic. In such instances, the newborn may develop irritability, lethargy, and poor feeding after hours of SVT. Conversely, some SVT may cause immediate hemodynamic compromise with low blood pressure and poor perfusion. Vagal maneuvers may be attempted if the patient is clinically stable or while preparing for direct current (DC) cardioversion or transesophageal pacing. A slurry of ice and water in a plastic bag might successfully break the SVT. The ice slurry must be applied vigorously and cover the mouth and nose. Adenosine is successful in converting most infants from SVT to normal sinus rhythm. To increase the likelihood of success, the medication should be given as centrally as possible and given quickly, followed immediately by a saline flush. The initial dose of adenosine is 100 mcg/kg. This dose can be increased to 200 mcg/kg if the lower dose is unsuccessful. If the patient does not respond to adenosine, but is stable hemodynamically, consultation with a pediatric electrophysiologist may be helpful in guiding the next steps in medical management. Most typically, the patient may be started on propranolol, 2 to 3 mg/kg, divided three times a day, and adenosine conversion can be reattempted after the initial dose of propranolol. If the patient is clinically compromised by the tachycardia, synchronized DC cardioversion is indicated starting at 1 to 2 j/kg or transesophageal pacing. If the patient does not respond to any of these therapies, the diagnosis of reentrant SVT should be reevaluated. Sinus tachycardia can present with similar heart rates in neonates and is most often caused by hypovolemia, fever, anemia, or pain [62]. Additionally, ventricular tachycardia may occasionally appear as a narrow-complex tachycardia in infancy [62].

Maternal–infant bonding

Given that many infants who have prenatally diagnosed CHD are rapidly transferred from the delivery room to the intensive care unit, the usual mother–infant bonding process may not be initiated. The issue of maternal–infant bonding has received much attention recently; and many newborn nurseries are moving away from centralized nurseries, having healthy infants room-in with the mother at all times. Researchers have studied the importance of the maternal–infant bonding process even as it has to do with time spent together in the first hours of the newborn's life. Several studies of healthy term newborns have shown benefits of early contact for the mother and the infant, with mothers appearing more attached and affectionate at 36 hours, and infants appearing happier at 3 months and more advanced neurodevelopmentally at 1 year as measured by the Gesell Developmental Test [63–66]. A recent study confirmed the importance of early maternal–infant interaction, reporting that the development of feelings of maternal attachment to the newborn was significantly related to the time of first holding the infant. The sooner the mother held the infant, the sooner she began to experience feelings of maternal attachment [67]. Although neonates who have prenatally diagnosed CHD have not been specifically studied to assess similar beneficial effects, this data supports the view that for infants who have CHD who do well at delivery, it is appropriate and arguably important to allow a period of time of interaction between the mother and infant before invasive therapies and before taking the newborn to the intensive care unit. Data on the natural history of patent ductus arteriosus (see the discussion above) and predicted hemodynamic stability in the presence of a PDA, suggest that a brief period of mother–infant interaction should also be safe.

The literature does demonstrate that infants who have CHD are especially at risk for poor mother–infant interactions, suggesting this early period of interaction immediately following delivery may be even more important for infants who have CHD. Gardner and colleagues [68] filmed 20 mother–infant dyads for 30 minutes 2 days before surgery and 6 months after surgery. These dyads were compared with noncardiac mother–infant pairs [68]. Mothers and their infants who had CHD showed less positive affect and engagement than the comparison group at both sessions. Mothers of babies who had CHD were psychologically distressed at both sessions, reporting high levels of frustration in feeling unable to care for and calm their infants. Goldberg also showed poor attachment between cardiac infants and their mothers in follow-up at 12 and 18 months after birth. Infants who had CHD were less likely to have secure attachment behaviors than the comparison group free of major health problems [69]. Additionally, Goldberg found that the small number of cardiac infants who were in the securely attached group showed more subsequent improvement in health than insecurely attached cardiac peers. This study suggests that improving infant–mother relationships also may benefit the infant's physical health also.

Practical experience and current recommendations

Most infants who have CHD do well at delivery, rarely requiring any resuscitative effort other than that which is common for healthy newborns. A select group, perhaps 20% to 30% of all infants who have CHD, require patency of the ductus arteriosus for postnatal survival, and therefore are in need of intravenous access and prostaglandin therapy shortly after birth. A very small subgroup requires urgent catheter or surgical intervention. Communication and coordination among the obstetric, neonatal, and cardiovascular teams are essential to plan the location of delivery, immediate postnatal physiologic expectations, and medical management.

At Children's Hospital of Wisconsin, families of infants prenatally diagnosed as having CHD meet with providers of the Fetal Concerns Program shortly after diagnosis. The mother and father (or other support systems) meet with a perinatologist, a cardiologist, a neonatologist, and a representative from the cardiovascular surgical team. Parents are provided education and opportunities to tour the hospital facilities. Delivery is encouraged at the adjoining adult hospital, not only to benefit the newborn but also to allow the mother to be close to the neonate after admission to the neonatal intensive care unit (NICU). For each delivery of a neonate who has prenatally diagnosed CHD, a neonatal resuscitation team is in attendance. The usual practice is that immediately following delivery, the infant is brought to the warmer where he or she is resuscitated and evaluated by the neonatal team. This resuscitation usually requires little more than drying the infant and clearing the airway. As the ductus arteriosus is patent at the time of delivery, these infants are nearly always hemodynamically stable; and only rarely is additional assistance required by the newborn in the delivery room.

After confirming cardiopulmonary stability, the objective is to allow the parents to see and hold the newborn. From the delivery room in the adult hospital, the infant is monitored and transported to the NICU in the adjoining Children's Hospital. On arrival in the NICU, umbilical lines are placed, PGE_1 is started, and a postnatal confirmatory echocardiogram is performed. This process is usually completed during the infant's first two hours of life. After confirming ductal patency, the usual dose of PGE_1 is 0.01 mcg/kg/min. Because of the potential complications of central line placement and prostaglandin infusion, for lesions in which the necessity of neonatal surgical intervention is not certain prenatally (eg, mild forms of coarctation of the aorta, tetralogy of Fallot), the postnatal echocardiogram is performed before line placement to confirm the probable necessity of neonatal surgery. Intravenous caffeine is often useful in preventing prostaglandin-related apnea and subsequent intubation in the preoperative period. The caffeine citrate dose employed is a single loading dose of 20 mg/kg followed by 5 mg/kg daily.

At The Children's Hospital of Philadelphia (CHOP), the approach to medical management in the immediate perinatal period is slightly different. Similar preoperative meetings with the multiple care providers are arranged following the diagnosis. Before planned and expected deliveries, the fetal cardiology team contacts the neonatal team and a plan is made regarding the need for PGE_1, umbilical lines, and planned admitting unit (some infants may stay at the NICU at either the delivery hospital or at CHOP; alternatively they may be transferred to the cardiac intensive care unit at CHOP). In the case of infants whose physiology may be adversely affected by oxygen supplementation, the blenders for oxygen flow are set on room air before delivery. If the infant does not respond to initial room air resuscitation, then the oxygen will be incrementally increased as needed. The deliveries currently occur at the adjoining adult hospital. In general, if the infants are expected to be stable and delivered vaginally, they are delivered in the labor room with initial resuscitation there as needed. Then the parents are given a chance to hold the infant if he or she is stable. In patients in whom it is determined prenatally that neonatal surgical management will be necessary, they are taken to an infant resuscitation room and umbilical lines are placed, as well as a peripheral intravenous line for institution of PGE_1 until confirmation of correct umbilical venous catheter (UVC) placement. In most cases PGE_1 is started at 0.025 mcg/kg/min in the first 15 to 20 minutes of life and titrated down to 0.01 mcg/kg/min once ductal patency has been established by postnatal echocardiography. In addition, a blood gas from one of the umbilical lines is obtained before transfer; and treatment is given as needed. The infant is then transferred directly to the cardiac intensive care unit.

Summary

Increasingly, advances in fetal echocardiography are providing highly accurate diagnoses of CHD before delivery. Planning for the delivery-room management of infants who have prenatally diagnosed CHD should include the availability of trained personnel and readiness of appropriate supplies. Most neonates who have CHD will not require delivery room resuscitation in excess of routine care; however, a small number of prenatally diagnosed cardiac lesions will likely require more invasive medical and surgical intervention immediately following delivery. These lesions should inspire even greater attention to postnatal clinical condition and prompt resuscitation. TGA with intact ventricular septum and restrictive atrial septum, HLHS with intact atrial septum, obstructed TAPVR, and CCHB are lesions that commonly require urgent postnatal intervention; and medical preparation before delivery should be a priority to produce the best possible outcomes. For all neonates who have ductal-dependent blood flow, PGE_1 administration in the early postnatal period permits preoperative stabilization. PGE_1 administration, however, is accompanied by predictable side effects that need to be monitored for and treated, if necessary.

Acknowledgments

With special recognition and deep appreciation to L. Eliot May, PA-C who created the color diagrams in this article.

References

[1] Forbus GA, Atz AM, Shirali GS. Implications and limitations of an abnormal fetal echocardiogram. Am J Cardiol 2004;94:688–9.

[2] Perolo A, Prandstraller D, Ghi T, et al. Diagnosis and management of fetal cardiac anomalies: 10 years of experience at a single institution. Ultrasound Obstet Gynecol 2001;18:615–8.

[3] Rychik J, Tian ZY, Fogel MA, et al. The single ventricle heart in the fetus: accuracy of prenatal diagnosis and outcome. J Perinatol 1997;17:183–8.

[4] Shub A, Ward C, Lee-Tannock A, et al. Fetal echocardiography: are we getting it right? Prenat Diagn 2004;24:972–6.

[5] Bromley B, Estroff JA, Sanders SP, et al. Fetal echocardiography: accuracy and limitations in a population at high and low risk for heart defects. Am J Obstet Gynecol 1992;166: 1473–81.

[6] Chang AC, Huhta JC, Yoon GY, et al. Diagnosis, transport, and outcome in fetuses with left ventricular outflow tract obstruction. J Thorac Cardiovasc Surg 1991;102:841–8.

[7] Strauss A, Toth B, Schwab B, et al. Prenatal diagnosis of congenital heart disease and neonatal outcome—a six years experience. Eur J Med Res 2001;6:66–70.

[8] Rowland D, Wheller J. Congenital heart disease and arrhythmias in the fetus. In: Allen H, Clark E, Gutsell H, Driscoll D, editors. 6th edition. Moss and Adams' heart disease in infants, children and adolescents including the fetus and young adult, Vol 1. Philadelphia: Lippincott, Williams and Wilkins; 2001. p. 570–81.

[9] DeVore GR, Medearis AL, Bear MB, et al. Fetal echocardiography: factors that influence imaging of the fetal heart during the second trimester of pregnancy. J Ultrasound Med 1993; 12:659–63.

[10] Eapen RS, Rowland DG, Franklin WH. Effect of prenatal diagnosis of critical left heart obstruction on perinatal morbidity and mortality. Am J Perinatol 1998;15:237–42.

[11] Mahle WT, Clancy RR, McGaurn SP, et al. Impact of prenatal diagnosis on survival and early neurologic morbidity in neonates with the hypoplastic left heart syndrome. Pediatrics 2001;107: 1277–82.

[12] Kumar RK, Newburger JW, Gauvreau K, et al. Comparison of outcome when hypoplastic left heart syndrome and transposition of the great arteries are diagnosed prenatally versus when diagnosis of these two conditions is made only postnatally. Am J Cardiol 1999;83:1649–53.

[13] Verheijen PM, Lisowski LA, Stoutenbeek P, et al. Lactacidosis in the neonate is minimized by prenatal detection of congenital heart disease. Ultrasound Obstet Gynecol 2002;19:552–5.

[14] Friedman AH, Fahey JT. The transition from fetal to neonatal circulation: normal responses and implications for infants with heart disease. Semin Perinatol 1993;17:106–21.

[15] Rosenthal GL, Vargo TA, Ferencz C. Differences in fetal somatic growth may be due to abnormal intrauterine hemodynamics. Pediatrics 1997;100:435A.

[16] Lim MK, Hanretty K, Houston AB, et al. Intermittent ductal patency in healthy newborn infants: demonstration by colour doppler flow mapping. Arch Dis Child 1992;67:1217–8.

[17] Reller MD, Rice MJ, McDonald RW. Review of studies evaluating ductal patency in the premature infant. J Pediatr 1993;122:S59–62.

[18] Gentile R, Stevenson G, Dooley T, et al. Pulsed doppler echocardiographic determination of time of ductal closure in normal newborn infants. J Pediatr 1981;98:443–8.

[19] Wolkoff LI, Davis JM. Delivery room resuscitation of the newborn. Clin Perinatol 1999;26: 641–58.

[20] Contributors and Reviewers for the Neonatal Resuscitation Guidelines. International guidelines for neonatal resuscitation: an excerpt from the guidelines 2000 for cardiopulmonary resuscitation and emergency cardiovascular care: International Consensus on Science. Pediatrics 2000;106:29–44.

[21] Saugstad OD, Ramji S, Vento M. Resuscitation of depressed newborn infants with ambient air or pure oxygen: a meta-analysis. Biol Neonate 2005;87:27–34.

[22] Vento M, Asensi M, Sastre J, et al. Six years of experience with the use of room air for the resuscitation of asphyxiated newly born term infants. Biol Neonate 2001;79:261–7.

[23] Mirlesse V, Cruz A, Le Bidois J, et al. Perinatal management of fetal cardiac anomalies in a specialized obstetric-pediatrics center. Am J Perinatol 2001;18:363–71.

[24] Textbook of Neonatal Resuscitation. 4th edition. American Academy of Pediatrics; 1994.

[25] Satomi G, Yasukochi S, Shimizu T, et al. Has fetal echocardiography improved the prognosis of congenital heart disease? comparison of patients with hypoplastic left heart syndrome with and without prenatal diagnosis. Pediatr Int 1999;41:728–32.

[26] Toth B, Becker A, Seelbach-Gobel B. Oxygen saturation in healthy newborn infants immediately after birth measured by pulse oximetry. Arch Gynecol Obstet 2002;266:105–7.

[27] Harris AP, Sendak MJ, Donham RT. Changes in arterial oxygen saturation immediately after birth in the human neonate. J Pediatr 1986;109:117–9.

[28] Rao R, Ramji S. Pulse oximetry in asphyxiated newborns in the delivery room. Indian Pediatr 2001;38:762–6.

[29] Evans N. Volume expansion during neonatal intensive care: do we know what we are doing? Semin Neonatol 2003;8:315–23.

[30] Reddy VM, Liddicoat JR, McElhinney DB, et al. Hemodynamic effects of epinephrine, bicarbonate and calcium in the early postnatal period in a lamb model of single-ventricle physiology created in utero. J Am Coll Cardiol 1996;28:1877–83.

[31] Roehl SL, Townsend RJ. Alprostadil (Prostin VR pediatric sterile solution, the Upjohn Company). Drug Intelligence and Clinical Pharmacy 1982;16:823–32.

[32] Rikard DH. Nursing care of the neonate receiving prostaglandin E_1 therapy. Neonatal Netw 1993;12:17–22.

[33] Lewis AB, Freed MD, Heymann MA, et al. Side effects of therapy with prostaglandin E_1 in infants with critical congenital heart disease. Circulation 1981;64:893–8.

[34] Kramer HH, Sommer M, Rammos S, et al. Evaluation of low dose prostaglandin E_1 treatment for ductus dependent congenital heart disease. Eur J Pediatr 1995;154:700–7.

[35] Saxena A, Sharma M, Kothari SS, et al. Prostaglandin E$_1$ in infants with congenital heart disease: Indian experience. Indian Pediatr 1998;35:1063–9.

[36] Teixeira OH, Carpenter B, MacMurray SB, et al. Long-term prostaglandin E$_1$ therapy in congenital heart defects. J Am Coll Cardiol 1984;3:838–43.

[37] Arav-Boger R, Baggett HC, Spevak PJ, et al. Leukocytosis caused by prostaglandin E$_1$ in neonates. J Pediatr 2001;138:263–5.

[38] Peled N, Dagan O, Babyn P, et al. Gastric-outlet obstruction induced by prostaglandin therapy in neonates. N Engl J Med 1992;327:505–10.

[39] Merkus PJ, Cromme-Dijkhuis AH, Robben SG, et al. Prostaglandin E$_1$ and gastric outlet obstruction in infants. Lancet 1993;342:747.

[40] Hammerman C. Patent ductus arteriosus: clinical relevance of prostaglandins and prostaglandin inhibitors in PDA pathophysiology and treatment. Clin Perinatol 1995;22:457–79.

[41] Hallidie-Smith KA. Prostaglandin E$_1$ in suspected ductus dependent cardiac malformation. Arch Dis Child 1984;59:1020–6.

[42] Reddy SC, Saxena A. Prostaglandin E$_1$: First stage palliation in neonates with congenital cardiac defects. Indian J Pediatr 1998;65:211–6.

[43] Lim DS, Kulik TJ, Kim DW, et al. Aminophylline for the prevention of apnea during prostaglandin E$_1$ infusion. Pediatrics 2003;112:e27–9.

[44] MacKenzie TC, Crombleholme TM, Flake AW. The ex-utero intrapartum treatment. Curr Opin Pediatr 2002;14:453–8.

[45] Bouchard S, Johnson MP, Flake AW, et al. The EXIT procedure: experience and outcome in 31 cases. J Pediatr Surg 2002;37:418–26.

[46] Kelsall A, Yates R, Sullivan I. Antenatally diagnosed cardiac disease: where to deliver. Arch Dis Child 2000;82:A1.

[47] Penny DJ, Shekerdemian LS. Management of the neonate with symptomatic congenital heart disease. Arch Dis Child Fetal Neonatal Ed 2001;84:F141–5.

[48] Bonnet D, Coltri A, Butera G, et al. Detection of transposition of the great arteries in fetuses reduces neonatal morbidity and mortality. Circulation 1999;99:916–8.

[49] Rychik J, Rome JJ, Collins MH, et al. The hypoplastic left heart syndrome with intact atrial septum: Atrial morphology, pulmonary vascular histopathology and outcome. J Am Coll Cardiol 1999;34:554–60.

[50] Ross B, Gillette P. Atrioventricular block and bundle branch block. In: Gillette P, Garson A, editors. Clinical pediatric arrhythmias. 2nd edition. Philadelphia: WB Saunders Company; 1999. p. 68–70.

[51] Eronen M, Siren MK, Ekblad H, et al. Short- and long-term outcome of children with congenital complete heart block diagnosed in utero or as a newborn. Pediatrics 2000;106:86–91.

[52] Baschat AA, Gembruch U, Knopfle G, et al. First-trimester fetal heart block: a marker for cardiac anomaly. Ultrasound Obstet Gynecol 1999;14:311–4.

[53] Sherman SJ, Featherstone LS. Congenital complete heart block and successful vaginal delivery. J Perinatol 1997;17:489–91.

[54] Eronen M, Heikkila P, Teramo K. Congenital complete heart block in the fetus: hemodynamic features, antenatal treatment, and outcome in six cases. Pediatr Cardiol 2001;22: 385–92.

[55] Cohen M, Jedeikin R. Arrhythmias in the fetus and newborn. In: Taeusch H, Ballard R, Gleason C, Avery M, editors. Avery's diseases of the newborn. 8th edition. Philadelphia: WB Saunders Company; 2005. p. 873–87.

[56] Ross B, Tripple D. Atrioventricular block. In: Garson A, Bricker J, Neish S, editors. The science and practice of pediatric cardiology. 2nd ed. Baltimore (MD): Williams and Wilkins; 1998. p. 2047–57.

[57] Minassian VA, Jazayeri A. Favorable outcome in a pregnancy with complete fetal heart block and severe bradycardia. Obstet Gynecol 2002;100:1087–9.

[58] Groves AM, Allan LD, Rosenthal E. Outcome of isolated congenital complete heart block diagnosed in utero. Heart 1996;75:190–4.

[59] Schmidt KG, Ulmer HE, Silverman NH, et al. Perinatal outcome of fetal complete atrio-ventricular block: a multicenter experience. J Am Coll Cardiol 1991;17:1360–6.

[60] Quek SC, Low KT, Sim EK, et al. A case report on the perinatal management of a 30-week preterm baby with congenital complete heart block. Ann Acad Med Singapore 2000;29:510–3.

[61] Kovalchin JP, Silverman NH. The impact of fetal echocardiography. Pediatr Cardiol 2004; 25:299–306.

[62] Artman M, Mahony L, Teitel D. Neonatal cardiology. New York: The McGraw-Hill Companies; 2002.

[63] De Chateau P. The interaction between the infant and the environment: the importance of mother-child contact after delivery. Acta Paediatr Scand Suppl 1988;344:21–30.

[64] de Chateau P, Wiberg B. Long-term effect on mother-infant behaviour of extra contact during the first hour post partum. III. follow-up at one year. Scand J Soc Med 1984;12:91–103.

[65] de Chateau P. The first hour after delivery—its impact on synchrony of the parent-infant relationship. Paediatrician 1980;9:151–68.

[66] Anisfeld E, Lipper E. Early contact, social support, and mother–infant bonding. Pediatrics 1983; 72:79–83.

[67] Troy NW. Early contact and maternal attachment among women using public health care facilities. Appl Nurs Res 1993;6:161–6.

[68] Gardner FV, Freeman NH, Black AM, et al. Disturbed mother–infant interaction in association with congenital heart disease. Heart 1996;76:56–9.

[69] Goldberg S, Simmons RJ, Newman J, et al. Congenital heart disease, parental stress, and infant–mother relationships. J Pediatr 1991;119:661–6.

[70] Freed MD, Heyman MA, Lewis AB, et al. Prostaglandin E_1 in infants with ductus arteriosus–dependent congenital heart disease. Circulation 1981;64:899–905.

CLINICS IN
PERINATOLOGY

Clin Perinatol 32 (2005) 947–961

The Neonate with Congenital Heart Disease: What the Cardiac Surgeon Needs to Know from the Neonatologist and the Cardiologist

Robert D.B. Jaquiss, MD[a,b,*], James S. Tweddell, MD[a,b]

[a]Medical College of Wisconsin, 9000 West Wisconsin Avenue, MS 715, Milwaukee, WI 53221, USA
[b]Children's Hospital of Wisconsin, Milwaukee, WI, USA

A cardiac surgeon planning an operation for a neonate with congenital heart disease (CHD) is likely to be most successful if he or she is maximally informed about the patient by his or her colleagues in cardiology and neonatology. Beyond the self-evident need to have the exact anatomic diagnosis clearly outlined, there are a number of other pieces of physiologic, historic, and even social information that can help the surgeon to provide the best outcome. The information required varies with the individual patient but in all cases must include prenatal details, circumstances of birth, postnatal complications, coexistent congenital malformations, the presence of any identifiable syndromes or other genetic abnormalities, and the identification of any consequential electrolyte or hematologic abnormalities. In this article, we discuss each of these areas in more detail and then discuss some specific congenital cardiac malformations to emphasize the unique anatomic and surgical issues that each malformation presents. We also review some of the management and monitoring techniques that we believe are helpful in optimizing the preoperative condition of the neonate with CHD, which, in turn, offers the best chance for a successful postsurgical result.

* Corresponding author. Medical College of Wisconsin, 9000 West Wisconsin Avenue, MS 715, Milwaukee, WI 53221.
    E-mail address: rjaquiss@chw.org (R.D.B. Jaquiss).

0095-5108/05/$ – see front matter © 2005 Elsevier Inc. All rights reserved.
doi:10.1016/j.clp.2005.09.002

Prenatal information

With the widespread application of prenatal ultrasound and fetal echocardiography, it is increasingly the case that the neonate with surgically significant CHD has been diagnosed in utero [1]. This early diagnosis is broadly beneficial to the parents, the heath care team, and, most importantly, the baby [2]. The advantages to the parents include the opportunity for education and preparation by knowledgeable perinatologists and cardiac specialists. In many instances, the parents may be introduced to the surgeon, which allows for a relatively relaxed and thorough discussion of the upcoming surgery. The prospect of the surgery is doubtless still quite daunting for the parents, but the preparation allowed by prenatal diagnosis and discussion may return some sense of control to them.

For the health care team, prenatal diagnosis allows for the preparation of parents as described but also allows for the prevention of complications that may arise from delayed diagnosis of important CHD. This often takes the form of tailoring the circumstances of delivery in terms of timing and location. The timing of delivery is controllable by tocolytic agents to some extent if it is thought that additional pulmonary maturation may be helpful. Alternatively, if additional gestation is thought to be unnecessary or even harmful, elective cesarean section may be performed. In either case, the delivery should be arranged so as to occur in a location with a neonatal intensive care unit and the facility to perform neonatal cardiac surgery. The presence of a neonatologist in the delivery room should also be planned in case immediate intervention is required.

From the perspective of the infant with CHD, prenatal diagnosis allows for a much smoother transition to postnatal life. In particular, the immediate application of respiratory support and prostaglandin infusions, if needed, can prevent or minimize any physiologic derangements that might otherwise occur. At a minimum, if "preemptive" resuscitation is not necessary, appropriate and more intensive monitoring, including umbilical vascular catheter placement, can be established immediately after delivery.

Birth history

Whether the diagnosis of CHD is made in utero or later, the history of the circumstances of birth may be extremely important, particularly if the delivery is difficult or prolonged or involves significant resuscitative efforts. The newborn with a significant cardiac malformation is remarkably tolerant to extreme stress, at least in comparison to older children, but nonetheless requires time to recover from a difficult entry into the world. In the best of circumstances, this may mandate a few hours; however, much more frequently, it means delaying surgery for several days. Although this period of stabilization and recovery postpones an operation that anxious parents may have anticipated for months, it certainly makes for a better surgical candidate. Moreover, as a practical matter, it often means that both parents are able to be with the baby before and immediately after surgery rather than the mother still recovering in her own hospital bed while her newborn is undergoing surgery at a location remote from her own.

Complete postnatal evaluation

Once an infant has been identified as likely having a significant congenital heart malformation, a series of diagnostic and monitoring interventions is necessary. The primary diagnostic technique is a confirmatory transthoracic echocardiogram. The importance of a complete echocardiographic examination as soon as practical cannot be overstated. By the time of the echocardiogram, a complete physical examination and chest radiograph are likely to have been completed and pre- and postductal pulse oximetry probes have been placed. These evaluations may have led to a strong suspicion of CHD. Even in the setting of a convincing prenatal sonographic examination, however, the diagnosis and specific features of the anatomic abnormality must be confirmed in the nursery. With increasing experience in fetal echocardiography, false-positive results have become quite rare, typically less than 10% to 15%, if a complete examination has been possible [3]. Nonetheless, even with the best prenatal examination, diagnostic uncertainty may remain, as is frequently the case in left heart obstructive lesions. For example, the distinction between critical aortic stenosis and hypoplastic left heart syndrome (HLHS) is notoriously difficult before birth and often continues to be so afterward [4]. Other complex lesions, such as heterotaxy syndromes, may require multiple echocardiographic evaluations for complete delineation of anatomy. Even in relatively straightforward abnormalities, such as d-transposition of the great vessels, multiple studies may be required to establish the exact coronary artery anatomy. In conjunction with diagnostic echocardiography, therapeutic balloon septostomy may be performed in patients whose atrial septal defect is restrictive [5]. Although this is occasionally necessary in certain other unusual circumstances, it is most frequently performed in the setting of d-transposition with an intact ventricular septum. The resultant atrial septal defect enhances mixing and frequently greatly improves oxygen saturation, even in children whose ductal patency has been preserved with intravenous prostaglandin infusion.

In the present era, diagnostic cardiac catheterization is seldom necessary in the evaluation of a neonate with CHD, although it has been safely accomplished even in extremely small newborns [6]. A notable exception is the infant with pulmonary atresia and an intact ventricular septum whose coronary circulation is incompletely evaluated by echocardiography. Patients with pulmonary atresia and an intact ventricular septum with exceptionally small tricuspid valves and nontripartite right ventricles frequently have so-called "right ventricular–dependent coronary circulation" [7]. In such patients, there is luminal communication between the native coronary arteries and the cavity of the right ventricle, in addition to which there is proximal stenosis or even atresia of the coronary arteries. In this circumstance, significant portions of the myocardium actually receive nutrient blood flow from the right ventricle rather than antegrade through the coronary artery. Such patients would be at extreme risk if the right ventricle were to be decompressed by means of a valvotomy, and even in the absence of decompression, such patients are at high risk for lethal coronary ischemia. Cardiac transplantation may be chosen for such patients as opposed to single-ventricle palliation [7].

With the cardiac diagnosis firmly established and the infant stabilized, a secondary series of examinations and evaluations is appropriate. These include a survey of external morphology with particular attention to recognizable stigmata of various syndromes, which may be present in as many as 3% to 4% of children with congenital heart malformations [8]. The characteristic facies of Down's syndrome and webbed neck seen in Turner's syndrome are two well-known phenotypes that can be detected in the nursery. Other physical findings suggestive of more unusual syndromes include low-set ears and microcephaly. The examination must be complete and exclude abnormalities of the esophagus and airway, such as are classically seen in VATER (vertebral anomalies, anal atresia, tracheal and esophageal anomalies, and renal agenesis) syndrome, as well as evaluating the lower digestive tract. Such abnormalities, if undetected before the cardiac operation, may significantly complicate intraoperative management (eg, attempts to perform transesophageal echocardiography would be unsuccessful and dangerous in esophageal atresia). Standard chest radiography, beyond its value for assessing cardiopulmonary status as well as visceral situs, is useful in identifying bony abnormalities of the thorax, including hemivertebrae and ribcage malformations. Sequelae of a difficult delivery, such as clavicle fractures, are also identifiable on the chest radiograph.

The value of "routine" laboratory testing, including complete blood cell counts, evaluation of clotting parameters, and standard assays of electrolytes and renal function indices, should not be underestimated. An arterial blood gas assessment should also be a part of the laboratory evaluation of the neonate with CHD. Assay of liver function and bilirubin level should also be a part of the laboratory survey of the child with CHD, although both assessments are likely to be more informative on the second or third day of life than initially.

In addition to traditional methods of physical examination, radiography, echocardiography, and routine laboratory evaluation, genetic studies have come to assume increasing importance in the complete assessment of the neonate with CHD [9–11]. Standard chromosomal analysis should be performed to detect the well-known aneuploidies, including trisomy 13 (Patau's syndrome), trisomy 18 (Edward's syndrome), trisomy 21 (Down syndrome), and monosomy 45,X (Turner's syndrome) [9]. Fluorescent in situ hybridization (FISH) studies should also be performed to detect certain chromosomal deletions, such as the 22qll deletion variously known as DiGeorge syndrome or velocardiofacial syndrome. Identification of this latter defect is particularly important because of the potential for significant hypocalcemia related to congenital hypoparathyroidism as well as potential late implications with regard to immune function and neuropsychiatric abnormalities.

Preoperative management

With the diagnosis established and the medical condition stabilized, the next goal of care in the preoperative neonate with CHD is the maintenance of stability and optimization of physiology. The first requirement for the accomplishment of these goals is full physiologic monitoring. At a minimum, this mandates routine electrocardiography, pulse oximetry, hemodynamic monitoring (continuous arterial and central venous pressure monitoring if possible), and hourly assessment of total fluid administration and loss. These measures should be supplemented by appropriately frequent laboratory testing. Abnormal values on intake assessment should be followed up with repeat studies as appropriate to confirm adequacy of resuscitation and recovery of organ function. In patients requiring mechanical ventilation, continuous in-line measurement of end-tidal carbon dioxide may help to limit the number of arterial blood gas assessments, but this indicator should be regarded as supplemental information to rather than a replacement for formal blood gas analysis [12].

A relatively recent addition to the monitoring armamentarium is the use of multisite near-infrared spectroscopy (NIRS) [13]. This modality involves reflectance oximetry using a paired emitter and detector of infrared light in the region of the spectrum appropriate for saturated and desaturated hemoglobin. In effect, the monitor provides an estimate of the relative saturation of venous blood in a particular region of the body. Although initially designed for assessment of the adequacy of perfusion of the adult cerebral cortex, there is increasing experience with its use for assessing the adequacy of perfusion in infants and children in the operative and postoperative settings. We have recently extended this use to optimize preoperative management as well. It is important to stress several cautions with regard to this technology, however. There is the obvious limitation that its use is not approved by the US Food and Drug Administration (FDA) in children for the indications previously mentioned. In addition, there are certain technical limitations that reduce the certainty about which specific region is being sampled (ie, sampling depth) as well as a remarkable paucity of information about the correctness of the absolute values returned by the oximeter. At best, NIRS assessment should be only part of a comprehensive evaluation of the adequacy of cardiac output, combined with physical findings and urine output as well as with other traditional assessments. It is probably most valuable as a trend indicator. The fact that the monitor may be used to simultaneously assess two anatomic sites also serves as a helpful reminder that systemic cardiac output may be heterogeneously distributed and that adequacy of oxygen delivery in one area does not automatically indicate adequacy of oxygen delivery throughout.

Regardless of the extent and complexity of monitoring elected, the underlying theme of labile physiology must be borne in mind by those caring for the preoperative neonate with CHD. In particular, the well-known dynamism of the pulmonary vascular resistance must be constantly considered. It is to be anticipated that the pulmonary vascular resistance is going to fall over time, albeit at an unpredictable rate, with potentially devastating consequences for the systemic vascular bed in those lesions in which an unrestricted left-to-right shunt is possible. The phrase "pulmonary overcirculation" is frequently used to describe the consequence of a falling pulmonary resistance, but use of this phrase is unfortunate in that it may distract from the "systemic undercirculation" that may accompany its appearance. Inordinate focus on the lungs may lead clinicians to overlook the impact on the mesenteric, renal, and cerebral circulations. The priority must be ensuring adequacy of systemic perfusion. This may require the provision of exogenous carbon dioxide to the ventilatory circuit or the provision of subatmospheric concentrations of oxygen to alter the balance of pulmonary and systemic flow in a favorable way. It may also require the use of catecholamine infusions, such as dopamine or even epinephrine, to increase the total cardiac output rather than simply relying on restoration of appropriate distribution of that output, however. The means chosen to preserve or restore systemic circulatory adequacy is less important than that it be done.

In addition to the ongoing technologic monitoring previously described and the liberal use of laboratory data to monitor the preoperative infant, the utility of serial physical examination must be emphasized. For example, no single monitoring technique or group of techniques has been shown to eliminate the need for serial physical examinations in the early detection of necrotizing enterocolitis (NEC). The association of NEC with structural cardiovascular abnormalities is well known [14] and should stimulate an enhanced intensity of surveillance for its detection (and prevention) in clinicians caring for neonates with CHD. Likewise, skilled thoracic auscultation may detect early changes, such as major pulmonary atelectasis or endotracheal tube malposition or obstruction, that may be life threatening for a fragile cardiac neonate in extreme cases.

In addition to thoracic and abdominal organ system assessment and care, the central nervous system must be carefully considered in children with structural heart disease. There is a well-known association of significant spontaneous intracranial hemorrhage in premature neonates with patent ductus arteriosus with which neonatologists are all too familiar. The presence and severity of such abnormalities should be sonographically defined in all premature babies with patent ductus arteriosus, because this may alter the decision about when and whether to seek surgical closure or to persist with medical therapy. Even in term infants with structural heart disease, there is increasing evidence of more subtle central nervous system abnormalities, including periventricular leukomalacia, and other structural malformations, which are not likely helped by the abnormal physiology (eg, cyanosis, low diastolic blood pressure) inherent in many cardiac abnormalities [15]. Given the well-established risks of central nervous system injury and morbidity historically attributed to open-heart surgery in neonates, it is not unreasonable maintain a low threshold for preoperative CT or MRI. This is particularly true if there has been any significant abnormality in the complete neonatal neurologic examination that should be included in the intake and on-going assessment of preoperative cardiac babies. Such neuroimaging evaluations should also be considered in babies whose delivery was unusually difficult or who presented with major circulatory compromise.

Beyond monitoring and surveillance for problems, the preoperative care of the cardiac neonate should also involve as much nutritional support as can be safely provided. As with any other patient population, the nutritional route of first choice is enteral, preferably with full oral feedings supplemented by tube feedings as needed. This ideal means is seldom possible in neonates with complex heart disease or significant prematurity, however. Enteral feeding is contraindicated in the youngest and smallest infants as well as in those with umbilical artery catheters because of the risk of NEC. Oral feeding is obviously ruled out in those children requiring mechanical ventilation, and even consistent provision of full enteric support by nasoenteric feedings may prove difficult in this group. Full parenteral nutrition is therefore the only option in a significant percentage of children awaiting heart surgery, and, as with every other part of the care of these children, meticulous attention must be paid to the details. For example, the relative proportion of chloride and base must be carefully attended to so as to prevent or remedy the significant acid base abnormalities that are easily iatrogenically induced.

While children await surgery, the threat of infection must also be carefully considered. The fully monitored preoperative neonate on mechanical ventilation represents an extraordinarily vulnerable target for the numerous, and increasingly virulent, microorganisms that populate the modern hospital. Virtually all the monitoring and support modalities previously mentioned, although invaluable, also are invasive, and thus breach normal infection barriers. Recognition of this fact mandates scrupulous sterile technique in the manipulation of vascular catheters and lines, endotracheal tubes, and urinary catheters. As with all other patient populations, rigidly observed hand washing techniques must be followed before each patient contact, and this must be stressed to parents as well. In addition to prevention and prophylaxis, infection surveillance and aggressive institution of appropriately targeted antimicrobial therapy, when appropriate, are familiar concepts in the neonatal intensive care unit. The cardiac neonate with a worrisome clinical picture should undergo the "3-day rule out" or full sepsis workup used in other populations of neonates. In fact, given the increased potential for endovascular infection inherent in structural heart disease and provoked by indwelling vascular catheters, a case may be made for cardiac patients requiring the most aggressive antimicrobial approach.

The risks inherent in the placement of central venous or arterial catheters in neonates with congenital heart lesions are not only infectious, however [16]. There is also significant risk of catheter-induced thrombosis. Such thrombosis may induce local or regional problems, such as limb ischemia or swelling, but also may result in thromboembolism that may be neurologically devastating. Each catheter site has its own unique set of potential complications, including portal vein thrombosis, renal vein thrombosis, renal artery or aortic thrombosis, and ileofemoral venous or arterial thrombosis. Perforation of a central vein or cardiac chamber is a well-described risk of indwelling catheters, as is endothelial injury with late vascular obstruction or stenosis. The latter complication is particularly of concern when hypertonic hyperalimentation solutions are infused through a central venous catheter, the tip of which is near or in a pulmonary vein, because this has been reported to cause unilateral pulmonary vein stenosis and pulmonary hypertension [17].

Postoperative phase

In most cardiac units, the postoperative care for neonates undergoing open-heart surgery or complicated closed procedures is delivered in a pediatric intensive care unit or cardiac care unit. With the change in location and addition of new caregivers, there is the potential for loss of valuable insight into the particular features of a particular patient, such as the history of prior vascular access. Knowledge of the status of ongoing genetic or other evaluations is also a frequent casualty of interunit transfers. There is also the potential for disruption in the relationship of the family with the health care team if one of the previous members (the neonatologist) is no longer seen to be involved. For all these reasons, it is desirable for the involvement and input of the neonatologist to continue after surgery, even if the location of the patient has changed.

Specific lesions

Transposition of the great arteries (TGA) is among the most commonly encountered structural heart lesions presenting in the neonatal period, perhaps representing as much as 5% to 10% of CHD [18,19]. Most neonates with TGA are well grown and free from extracardiac or chromosomal anomalies, although a search for such abnormalities should be undertaken as with all children with CHD. The simple form of TGA, that is to say without a significant ventricular septal defect, represents approximately 75% of TGA patients and results in parallel circulation with the potential for extremely severe cyanosis unless there is significant mixing at the level of the ductus arteriosus and atrial septum. If the diagnosis is suspected based on prenatal imaging or postnatal cyanosis, prostaglandin infusion should be initiated while the diagnosis is confirmed by echocardiography, with particular attention paid to the coronary artery anatomy. The echocardiographic examination and clinical picture can then predict the need for a balloon atrial septostomy, which can be performed during the initial echocardiographic assessment if the atrial septal defect appears inadequate. In general, our preference is to err on the side of performance of a septostomy unless the atrial septal defect is truly large [20]. Thereafter, the neonate is generally quite stable and can be fully assessed during preparation for surgical repair, the so-called "arterial switch" operation. Preoperative management of the child then depends on institutional preference. Some units elect to discontinue prostaglandin infusion, extubate, and begin oral feedings. In other centers, or depending on the operative schedule, the child may be left intubated and prepared for early surgery. Surgery should be performed electively before hospital discharge and is typically performed in the first 2 weeks of life, although a one-stage arterial switch operation has been successfully accomplished in neonates up to 60 days of age in the setting of delayed presentation [21]. Infants older than 2 months of age should be carefully evaluated for significant left ventricular deconditioning and considered for a preliminary pulmonary artery banding and shunting procedure to "prepare" the left ventricle for systemic vascular resistance. In the group of children with TGA and large ventricular septal defects, the timing of surgery is much more elective and may be accomplished at a time of convenience for the family, so long as the defect remains nonrestrictive. In most units, in part because of parent anxiety more than physiologic considerations, the surgery for TGA with ventricular septal defects is accomplished, as in simple TGA, in the first few weeks of life.

Truncus arteriosus is a relatively uncommon congenital malformation representing approximately 2% of congenital cardiac anomalies [18,19], and because of the complete mixing nature of the lesion, which produces little cyanosis, it may be undetected for the first few days or week of life. As the pulmonary vascular resistance falls, however, classic symptoms of heart failure ensue, including tachypnea, diaphoresis, poor feeding, and consequent poor weight gain, typically manifest by 2 weeks of age. Echocardiography is diagnostic and allows definition of the spatial arrangement of the origins of the pulmonary arteries, the nature of the truncal valve anatomy and function, and the detection of aortic arch interruption, which is present in 10% to 20% of truncus arteriosus patients. Once the diagnosis is made, surgery should be electively scheduled, because there is no advantage (indeed, some disadvantage) to deferring surgery in the futile hopes of weight gain. During the preoperative interval, other anatomic and genetic abnormalities should be sought, with particular attention to detecting the 22q11 deletion, which is present in a large proportion of children with truncus arteriosus. The importance of this deletion includes its potential implications for hypocalcemia and immunodeficiency as well as for developmental and psychologic problems. Because of the potential for graft-versus-host disease in patients with immunodeficiency related to the 22q11 deletion, patients with this diagnosis should only receive irradiated blood products.

Total anomalous pulmonary venous return (TAPVR) is relatively rare, representing approximately 2% of CHD [18,19]; however, in its obstructed form, it represents one of the few pediatric cardiac surgical emergencies. The term *obstructed* refers to relative narrowing of the pathway for blood to pass from the lungs to the right atrium. It is most common in the infracardiac type of TAPVR, less common in the supracardiac type, and rare in the cardiac variant. In the case of obstruction, prostaglandin infusion may allow for increased systemic perfusion by enhancing right-to-left shunting through a previously restrictive ductus arteriosus. With or without prostaglandin, however, infants with obstructed TAPVR should be taken directly to surgery for repair. In infants presenting in extremis, a period of preoperative or postoperative extracorporeal membrane oxygenation may be necessary. If there is no obstruction in the venous pathway, the mode of presentation should be that of a left-to-right shunt, with the size of the shunt being determined by the size of the atrial septal defect. In general, the diagnosis of TAPVR should lead to prompt referral for surgical correction, with the urgency of the surgery being proportional to the severity of symptoms. During the preoperative phase, unobstructed patients should undergo complete evaluation, although most patients with uncomplicated TAPVR do not have other cardiac or extracardiac anomalies.

Tetralogy of Fallot is among the most common of the cyanotic congenital heart lesions, occurring at approximately the same frequency as TGA [18,19]. The classic presentation is that of the development of cyanosis with ductal closure, which defines ductal dependence, on the basis of severe right ventricular outflow tract obstruction or even complete pulmonary atresia. As with TGA, suspicion of the diagnosis mandates the institution of prostaglandin therapy while diagnostic echocardiography is arranged. If the obstruction to the right ventricular outflow tract is less severe, the cyanosis may be minimal or mild after ductal closure. Neonates with ductal-dependent tetralogy require surgical intervention before discharge from the hospital. Such intervention has increasingly taken the form of complete repair (closure of ventricular septal defect and relief of right ventricular outflow tract obstruction using cardiopulmonary bypass) [22], although certain anatomic or clinical circumstances, or institutional preference, may indicate a preliminary, palliative, systemic-to-pulmonary shunt procedure. In ductal-dependent infants awaiting surgery or those who do not require a neonatal operation, a complete genetic and physical evaluation is mandatory because of the frequent association of tetralogy with chromosomal abnormalities (eg, trisomy 21); 22q11 deletions; or multisystem malformation, such as the CHARGE (coloboma, heart defects, atresia choanae, retardation of growth and development, genitourinary problems, and ear abnormalities) syndrome or VACTERL (vertebral anomalies, anal atresia, cardiac abnormalities, tracheoesophageal fistula, renal agenesis, and limb defects)/VATER syndrome. A special subset of tetralogy patients is the 5% with complete absence of pulmonary valve tissue. These patients typically have giant central pulmonary arterial dilation with secondary compression and malacia of the central airways, which may severely compromise respiratory status. If the airway obstruction is severe, these children require urgent operation in the newborn period, with surgical plication of the enlarged arteries, placement of a competent pulmonary valve, and possibly transposition of the pulmonary artery bifurcation anterior to the aorta (the Lecompte maneuver) [23] to minimize airway compression. In the preoperative setting, neonates with tetralogy and an absent pulmonary valve may be most effectively ventilated in the prone position to minimize anterior compression on the airway; in extreme circumstances, they may require preoperative extra-corporeal membrane oxygenation.

Another right heart obstructive lesion, pulmonary atresia with an intact ventricular septum, accounts for approximately 3% of CHD [7,18,19], and like severe tetralogy, is a cyanotic ductal-dependent anomaly. Symptoms appear with ductal closure, mandating the institution of prostaglandin therapy. Echocardiographic evaluation can confirm the diagnosis and allow a preliminary management plan with regard to the potential for a biventricular or univentricular reconstructive strategy. As with many congenital cardiac anomalies, the diagnosis of pulmonary atresia with an intact ventricular septum represents a spectrum of morphologies, ranging from near-complete right heart hypoplasia on one end to near-normal right heart anatomy with only an imperforate pulmonary valve at the more favorable end of the spectrum. Included in the more severe group are those patients with right ventricular–dependent coronary circulation described in a previous section. These infants are typically quite stable while awaiting initial surgery or, in some cases, interventional catheterization-based pulmonary valvotomy. Occasionally, however, a balloon atrial septostomy may be advisable, particularly in those infants who proceed down a single-ventricle pathway.

An interrupted aortic arch represents approximately 1% to 2% of CHD and is virtually always associated with an outlet type ventricular septal defect [18,19]. In the absence of prenatal diagnosis, the neonate is typically asymptomatic until ductal closure begins, after which the consequences of progressive lower body hypoperfusion predominate: anuria, metabolic acidosis, and intestinal and hepatic ischemia. The findings of the physical examination and pulse oximetry depend on the origin of the subclavian arteries (there is frequently an aberrant origin of the right subclavian artery from the distal descending aorta). In all cases in which ductal-dependent perfusion of the distal aorta is suspected, the initiation of prostaglandin therapy is mandatory. Echocardiography is then performed and is diagnostic of an interrupted aortic arch as well as providing intracardiac and great vessel origination details. Particular attention must be paid by the echocardiographer to the left ventricular outflow tract region as well as to other left heart structures so as to identify the suitability for two-ventricle repair. Before surgery, the importance of allowing complete metabolic recovery in this lesion, along with other left heart and aortic obstructive lesions, cannot be overemphasized. The consequences of visceral ischemia, beyond end organ injury reflected in abnormalities indicated by abnormal serum chemistry values, may also include bacteremia as a consequence of an injured gut mucosal barrier, and a period of prophylactic antibiotic therapy is wise after a delayed diagnosis of an interrupted aortic arch or similar lesions. During the recovery phase in the preoperative period, a 22q11 deletion should be identified if present for the reasons previously discussed.

As with an interrupted aortic arch, in the absence of a prenatal diagnosis or suspicion, neonates with significant coarctation of the aorta are typically asymptomatic until ductal closure, which occurs only after discharge from the hospital in many instances. Such patients may present in profound shock; however, with careful resuscitation, they may undergo an urgent operation with excellent outcomes [24]. If the diagnosis is suspected, the baby should be observed in the hospital until ductal closure, which, in effect, forces the infant to become ill to prove that he or she has CHD. In such circumstances, serial echocardiography and careful physical assessments are absolutely mandatory. In the event that a coarctation is "unmasked" by the trial of observation, prostaglandin should be restarted and elective surgery scheduled. Frequently associated cardiac anomalies, such as a bicuspid aortic valve and ventricular septal defect, must be sought in conjunction with the coarctation. Approaches to a ventricular septal defect depend on its perceived size and potential for spontaneous closure. The variety of options may range from simple observation to combined coarctation repair and pulmonary banding, or even closure of the defect in conjunction with coarctation repair (which may be accomplished through two incisions or as a one-stage operation via a median sternotomy) [25]. Associated syndromes, such as Turner's syndrome, Noonan's syndrome, and von Recklinghausen disease, should be considered in the neonate with coarctation, as should now rare congenital rubella.

HLHS is a surprisingly common diagnosis, accounting for approximately 8% of children diagnosed with structural heart disease in the first year of life [18,19]. Although it is now frequently identified or suspected prenatally, undiagnosed HLHS presents in a similar way to an interrupted aortic arch or severe coarctation of the aorta with ductal closure. As with other ductal-dependent lesions, prostaglandin therapy is mandatory. A major difference to be borne in mind between HLHS and coarctation or an interrupted aortic arch is the fact that HLHS patients have limited circulatory reserve as a consequence of having only a single ventricle. As neonates with HLHS await first-stage palliative surgery (Sano procedure or classic Norwood operation) or transplantation (in some centers), hypervigilance is necessary to prevent the potential hemodynamic deterioration seen with pulmonary overcirculation secondary to falling pulmonary resistance. This is a group of patients in whom full monitoring is mandatory and in which our group has found the previously described NIRS probes to be particularly helpful. Although children with HLHS are said to be rarely troubled with extracardiac anomalies, a systematic review [26] contradicts this impression and mandates full preoperative noncardiac assessment.

Although HLHS is the most common congenital cardiac malformation with a functionally single ventricle, there are numerous other cardiac anomalies with "single-ventricle physiology." The anomalies share the unifying trait of ultimately requiring a Fontan operation but differ widely with regard to details like ventricular morphology (left or right ventricle) and atrioventricular valve anatomy (eg, double-inlet ventricle, atrioventricular canal, mitral or tricuspid stenosis or atresia) as well as the numerous other details of segmental anatomy and chamber and great vessel orientation. Although all these specific details are of incredible importance in the planning of palliative reconstruction, two questions assume particular importance during the neonatal period. Is there systemic obstruction (at the aortic, ventricular, mitral, or atrial level)? Is there a reliable (nonductal) source of (and unobstructed egress for) pulmonary blood flow? If both questions cannot be answered affirmatively, an appropriately tailored surgical procedure must address the problem(s). After the anatomic details of the particular malformation have been clearly delineated for a child with a functional single ventricle, preoperative care is customized to the relevant physiology, including prostaglandin for ductal-dependent anatomy or strategies to address pulmonary overcirculation if present. Known associations with identifiable cardiac malformations, such as the heterotaxy syndromes (with predictable risks of asplenia and intestinal malrotation), must provoke a thorough chromosomal, genetic, and physical survey for such anomalies.

The last lesion to be discussed separately in this article is isolated patent ductus arteriosus in the premature underweight neonate. The identification of a patent ductus in such a patient is a matter of routine for neonatologists. The algorithm for when to refer such a patient for surgery is often less straightforward. Unless there are specific contraindications, intravenous prostaglandin inhibitors, of which the best studied is indomethacin, represent first-line therapy, with ultimate referral for ductal ligation only after treatment failure (or even retreatment failure). Interestingly, a recent Cochrane review identified only a single randomized study comparing medical therapy with surgery [27]. This trial showed surgery to be more efficacious, albeit with a higher risk of pneumothorax [28]. The basis for the preference for medical therapy as opposed to surgical therapy thus seems to be based not on data but on the wish to avoid surgery. The low mortality and morbidity of ductal ligation with a metal clip, which is performed in the neonatal intensive care unit, is well established [29], as is the fact that indomethacin is least efficacious in the smallest and youngest infants. It might be suggested that a prospective randomized trial be undertaken in premature infants with very low birth weight (<800 g) comparing primary ductal ligation with primary medical therapy. Apart from such a study, earlier consideration of surgical ligation in these infants seems reasonable, particularly in the youngest and sickest, because under present management schemes, they are often not referred for surgery until after a major complication, typically intraventricular hemorrhage or intestinal perforation, has ensued.

Summary

In this article, we have reviewed some of the specific points in the continuum of care of the neonate with CHD wherein communication between the neonatologist, cardiac surgeon, and cardiologist is of particular benefit to the patient, the patient's family, and, for that matter, the health care team. (It is hard to conceive of an aspect of medical care that is not enhanced by better communication within the health care team.) We have also highlighted some specific considerations relevant to particular congenital cardiac malformations. Lastly, we would like to emphasize that the involvement of the neonatologist and the cardiologist should not end when the patient enters the operating room but should continue after the operation, particularly as regards the nonsurgical aspects of the patient's care.

References

[1] Mohan UR, Kleinman CS, Kern JH. Fetal echocardiography and its evolving impact 1992 to 2002. Am J Cardiol 2005;96(1):134–6.

[2] Yates RS. The influence of prenatal diagnosis on postnatal outcome in patients with structural congenital heart disease. Prenat Diagn 2004;24(13):1143–9.

[3] DeVore GR. The role of fetal echocardiography in genetic sonography. Semin Perinatol 2003; 27(2):160–72.

[4] Corno AF. Borderline left ventricle. Eur J Cardiothorac Surg 2005;27(1):67–73.

[5] Zellers TM, Dixon K, Moake L, et al. Bedside balloon atrial septostomy is safe, efficacious, and cost-effective compared with septostomy performed in the cardiac catheterization laboratory. Am J Cardiol 2002;89(5):613–5.

[6] McMahon CJ, Price JF, Salerno JC, et al. Cardiac catheterisation in infants weighing less than 2500 grams. Cardiol Young 2003;13(2):117–22.

[7] Bichell DP. Evaluation and management of pulmonary atresia with intact ventricular septum. Curr Opin Cardiol 1999;14(1):60–6.

[8] Pajkrt E, Weisz B, Firth HV, et al. Fetal cardiac anomalies and genetic syndromes. Prenat Diagn 2004;24(13):1104–15.

[9] Wimalasundera RC, Gardiner HM. Congenital heart disease and aneuploidy. Prenat Diagn 2004;24(13):1116–22.

[10] Gelb BD. Recent advances in the understanding of genetic causes of congenital heart defects. Front Biosci 2000;5:D321–33.

[11] Prasad C, Chudley AE. Genetics and cardiac anomalies: the heart of the matter. Indian J Pediatr 2002;69(4):321–32.

[12] Wu CH, Chou HC, Hsieh WS, et al. Good estimation of arterial carbon dioxide by end-tidal carbon dioxide monitoring in the neonatal intensive care unit. Pediatr Pulmonol 2003;35(4): 292–5.

[13] Nagdyman N, Fleck T, Barth S, et al. Relation of cerebral tissue oxygenation index to central venous oxygen saturation in children. Intensive Care Med 2004;30(3):468–71.

[14] Ostlie DJ, Spilde TL, St. Peter SD, et al. Necrotizing enterocolitis in full-term infants. J Pediatr Surg 2003;38(7):1039–42.

[15] Wernovsky G, Shillingford AJ, Gaynor JW. Central nervous system outcomes in children with complex congenital heart disease. Curr Opin Cardiol 2005;20(2):94–9.

[16] Hermansen MC, Hermansen MG. Intravascular catheter complications in the neonatal intensive care unit. Clin Perinatol 2005;32(1):141–56.

[17] Jaillard SM, Godart FR, Rakza T, et al. Acquired pulmonary vein stenosis as a cause of life-threatening pulmonary hypertension. Ann Thorac Surg 2003;75(1):275–7.

[18] Ferencz C, Rubin JD, Loffredo CA, et al. The epidemiology of congenital heart disease, the Baltimore-Washington Infant Study (1981–1989). In: Perspectives in pediatric cardiology, vol.4. Mount Kisco, NY: Futura Publishing Company; 1993.

[19] Fyler DC. Report of the 1980 New England Regional Infant Cardiac Program. Pediatrics 1980;65(Suppl):375–461.

[20] Chantepie A, Schleich JM, Gournay V, et al. Preoperative mortality in transposition of the great vessels. Arch Pediatr 2000;7(1):34–9.

[21] Duncan BW, Poirier NC, Mee RB, et al. Selective timing for the arterial switch operation. Ann Thorac Surg 2004;77(5):1691–6 [discussion: 1697].

[22] Kolcz J, Pizarro C. Neonatal repair of tetralogy of Fallot results in improved pulmonary

artery development without increased need for reintervention. Eur J Cardiothorac Surg 2005; 28:394–9.

[23] Hraska V. Repair of tetralogy of Fallot with absent pulmonary valve using a new approach. Semin Thorac Cardiovasc Surg Pediatr Card Surg Annu 2005;8:132–4.

[24] Fesseha AK, Eidem BW, Dibardino DJ, et al. Neonates with aortic coarctation and cardiogenic shock: presentation and outcomes. Ann Thorac Surg 2005;79(5):1650–5.

[25] Kostelka M, Walther T, Geerdts I, et al. Primary repair for aortic arch obstruction associated with ventricular septal defect. Ann Thorac Surg 2004;78(6):1989–93 [discussion: 1993].

[26] Natowicz M, Chatten J, Clancy R, et al. Genetic disorders and major extracardiac anomalies associated with the hypoplastic left heart syndrome. Pediatrics 1988;82(5):698–706.

[27] Malviya M, Ohlsson A, Shah S. Surgical versus medical treatment with cyclooxygenase inhibitors for symptomatic patent ductus arteriosus in preterm infants. Cochrane Database Syst Rev 2003;3:CD003951.

[28] Gersony WM, Peckham GJ, Ellison RC, et al. Effects of indomethacin in premature infants with patent ductus arteriosus: results of a national collaborative study. J Pediatr 1983;102(6): 895–906.

[29] Little DC, Pratt TC, Blalock SE, et al. Patent ductus arteriosus in micropreemies and full-term infants: the relative merits of surgical ligation versus indomethacin treatment. J Pediatr Surg 2003;38(3):492–6.

ELSEVIER
SAUNDERS

CLINICS IN
PERINATOLOGY

Clin Perinatol 32 (2005) 963–978

DiGeorge Syndrome: New Insights

Elizabeth Goldmuntz, MD

Division of Cardiology, The Children's Hospital of Philadelphia,
University of Pennsylvania School of Medicine, Abramson Research Center 702A,
3615 Civic Center Boulevard, Philadelphia, PA 19104–4318, USA

DiGeorge syndrome was first described in 1968 as a rare developmental field defect affecting structures derived from the third and fourth embryonic pharyngeal arches [1,2]. Characteristic features included distinct facial features, hypoplasia or aplasia of the thymus, hypoplasia or aplasia of the parathyroid glands, and conotruncal cardiac defects. Infants presented with hypocalcemia, immunodeficiency, and severe heart defects, which, at the time, were often incompatible with life. The syndrome was observed to be etiologically heterogeneous, occurring in the context of maternal diabetes or alcohol use and in conjunction with a variety of chromosomal abnormalities. Studies subsequently demonstrated that approximately 10% to 20% of patients with the DiGeorge phenotype had a chromosomal alteration resulting in the loss of the proximal long arm of chromosome 22. Further molecular analysis demonstrated that nearly 90% of patients with the clinical features of DiGeorge syndrome had a microdeletion of a section of chromosome 22, called a 22q11 deletion [3–5].

Two patient populations that shared common features with DiGeorge syndrome, namely, velocardiofacial (or Shprintzen's) and conotruncal anomaly face (CTAF) syndromes, had also been described. Velocardiofacial syndrome was characterized in 1978 by typical facial features, a cleft palate, learning disabilities, and specific congenital heart defects [6]. CTAF syndrome was originally described in Japan in 1976 and was defined by conotruncal cardiac defects, hypernasal speech, mild mental retardation, neonatal tetany, thymic aplasia or hypoplasia, and facial dysmorphia [7]. As of 1993, molecular investigations had identified chromosome 22q11 deletions in 80% to 90% of patients with velocardiofacial or CTAF syndrome [8–11]. Thus, three clinical

This work was supported by grant P50 HL74731 from the National Institutes of Health.
E-mail address: goldmuntz@email.chop.edu

0095-5108/05/$ – see front matter © 2005 Elsevier Inc. All rights reserved.

syndromes—DiGeorge, velocardiofacial, and CTAF—were found to share a common genetic cause in most cases, namely, a chromosome 22q11 deletion. These studies defined the most common deletion syndrome currently known, namely, the 22q11 deletion syndrome, estimated to occur in approximately 1 in 4000 to 6000 live births [12].

Clinical characteristics of the 22q11 deletion syndrome

The clinical phenotype of the 22q11 deletion syndrome is highly variable among related and unrelated individuals. Most patients have a subset of the most common features. The presentation can be subtle and difficult to identify or more severe and easily recognized at birth. Approximately 6% to 10% of cases are familial; frequently, one of the parents is only recognized to carry the 22q11 deletion after a more severely affected child is diagnosed. The most common features are listed in Box 1 and are described briefly here.

Congenital heart disease

Hospital-based studies estimate that approximately 75% to 80% of patients with a 22q11 deletion have congenital heart disease [13,14]. These studies may overestimate the true frequency with which cardiac defects are seen in the deleted population, given that children and adults without significant heart disease may escape diagnosis in the current era. As noted, many parents only learn of their own deletion status on the delivery of a child with congenital heart disease who is diagnosed with a 22q11 deletion. A recent report identified two families

---

Box 1. Common features of the 22q11 deletion syndrome

Congenital heart disease
Immunodeficiency
Hypocalcemia
Palate anomalies
Velopharyngeal dysfunction and other speech disorders
Feeding disorders and growth retardation
Otorhinolaryngologic issues
Dysmorphic facies
Renal anomalies
Skeletal anomalies
Cognitive or learning disabilities
Behavioral or psychiatric disorders

transmitting a 22q11 deletion over three generations, where the deletion was only identified with the delivery of children with heart defects [15].

Regardless, congenital heart defects are a common finding in the 22q11 deletion syndrome. The most common cardiac defects include a subset of cono-truncal defects (tetralogy of Fallot, interrupted aortic arch, and truncus arteriosus) and perimembranous ventricular septal defects (Table 1) [13,14]. Aortic arch anomalies, including a cervical aortic arch, double aortic arch, and right-sided aortic arch, and an abnormal origin of the subclavian arteries (aberrant and isolated subclavian arteries) are also common findings (unpublished data). Aortic arch anomalies can be identified in conjunction with intracardiac defects or in isolation. Although conotruncal, septal, and aortic arch anomalies are by far the most common cardiac findings, a 22q11 deletion has been identified in patients with a variety of congenital heart defects, including patients with hypoplastic left heart syndrome, heterotaxy syndrome, valvar pulmonary stenosis, and a bicuspid aortic valve.

Immunodeficiency

Nearly 80% of patients with a 22q11 deletion have demonstrable abnormalities of their immune system [13,16–18]. Most commonly, they have mild to moderate decrements in T-cell numbers because of thymic hypoplasia with preserved T-cell function. Only rare cases (<0.5%) have complete absence of T cells and require an immediate thymic transplant. Humoral deficits, including IgA deficiency, have also been identified in approximately 10% of the population. As a result, patients with a 22q11 deletion commonly experience prolonged viral infections with frequent bacterial superinfections of the upper and lower respiratory tracts. Even those with normal T-cell numbers have frequent

Table 1
Cardiac defects in the 22q11 deletion syndrome

Cardiac diagnosis	Percentage of total (%)
Normal	21
Tetralogy of Fallot	23
Interrupted aortic arch	15
Ventricular septal defect[a]	15
Truncus arteriosus	9
Isolated aortic arch anomalies	5
Atrial septal defects	2
Other	10

[a] Perimembranous, malalignment, or conoseptal hypoplasia types of ventricular septal defects.
Data from McDonald-McGinn DM, LaRossa D, Goldmuntz E, et al. The 22q11.2 deletion: screening, diagnostic workup, and outcome of results; report on 181 patients. Genet Test 1997;1(2):99–108; and Ryan AK, Goodship JA, Wilson DI, et al. Spectrum of clinical features associated with interstitial chromosome 22q11 deletions: a European collaborative study. J Med Genet 1997;34(10):798–804.

infections, suggesting that other factors contribute to the risk of infection. Graft-versus-host disease has historically been of significant concern in these patients, given their history of immunodeficiency and exposure to blood products. In fact, this complication is quite rare and most likely to occur in those with the most severe T-cell deficiency. In contrast, studies have recently demonstrated that adults with a 22q11 deletion continue to have frequent infections and have an increased risk of developing a range of autoimmune diseases.

Hypocalcemia and other endocrinologic disorders

Hypoplasia or aplasia of the parathyroid glands results in hypoparathyroidism in a significant subset of patients. Reports vary but estimate that 49% to 60% of neonates with a 22q11 deletion experience transient hypocalcemia [14]. Recent cross-sectional studies suggest that hypoparathyroidism occurs in 13% to 69% of patients outside the neonatal period [19,20]. Reports have clearly documented cases in which hypoparathyroidism recurred or occurred for the first time in later decades of life and may even be the first presenting symptom indicative of the 22q11 deletion syndrome [21,22]. Other endocrinologic abnormalities have been reported in the deleted population, including growth hormone deficiency and thyroid disease [14,23].

Palate anomalies

Anomalies of the palate are a common problem resulting in significant morbidity for these patients. In our center's experience, only 19% of patients with a 22q11 deletion escaped such problems and had normal palate architecture and function. Approximately 44% of patients had a cleft palate, of which a few had an overt cleft of the soft (13%) or soft and hard (13%) palates or a bilateral cleft lip and palate (2%), whereas most had a submucous cleft palate (72%) [24,25]. Careful examination of the palate is required, including identification of a bifid uvula, which can indicate the presence of a submucous cleft in the palate.

In addition to cleft palate, nearly 80% of patients have velopharyngeal insufficiency defined by incomplete closure of the velopharyngeal valve during speech (Fig. 1). This disorder is manifest as hypernasal speech, nasal air emission, and compensatory articulation disorders. Velopharyngeal insufficiency can only be diagnosed with the emergence of speech, which is almost uniformly delayed.

The pathogenesis of velopharyngeal insufficiency is multifactorial. Velopharyngeal disproportion whereby the palate is too short relative to the depth of the pharynx has been observed in this patient population. Neurologic or muscular velopharyngeal hypotonia may also be present. Adenoid hypoplasia is commonly observed in patients with a 22q11 deletion and can contribute to velopharyngeal insufficiency. In fact, adenoidectomy should be avoided in patients with a 22q11 deletion in most cases, because this procedure may secondarily increase the

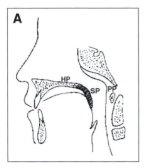
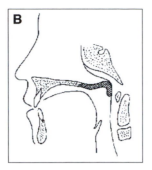
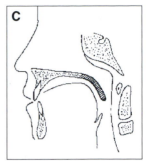

Fig. 1. Velopharyngeal function in normal individuals and patients with velopharyngeal dysfunction. The velopharynx is pictured at rest (*A*), during normal phonation (*B*), and during phonation in a patient with velopharyngeal dysfunction (*C*). Note that in the patient with velopharyngeal dysfunction, the soft palate fails to move juxtaposed to the posterior pharynx and therefore allows the escape of air during phonation. HP, hard palate; PP, posterior pharynx; SP, soft palate. (Courtesy of Richard Kirschner, MD, Philadelphia, PA.)

likelihood of velopharyngeal dysfunction. The presence of an overt or submucous cleft palate also contributes to velopharyngeal insufficiency.

Speech and language disabilities

Infants with a 22q11 deletion almost uniformly experience delayed emergence of speech [26,27]. When speech emerges, most demonstrate hypernasality (64%–84%) and articulation disorders (62%–77%). The latter may result from compensatory mechanisms in the presence of velopharyngeal dysfunction or motor speech disorders. Some also have voice disorders, including hoarseness and reduced vocal volume. The speech disorders can be of such severity that some families resort to sign language to improve communication, although this approach is controversial.

Feeding disorders

Feeding disorders are a common problem and daily challenge for the patient with a 22q11 deletion and his or her family [13,24,28]. Nearly 70% of patients are estimated to have nasopharyngeal reflux, characterized by reflux of liquids out of the nose because of insufficient closure of the velopharynx during swallowing. A hallmark sign of the infant with a 22q11 deletion, this symptom resolves without intervention during the toddler years and does not predict hypernasality of speech.

In addition, patients with a 22q11 deletion are commonly diagnosed with gastroesophageal reflux, esophageal dysmotility, and constipation, all of which compound their feeding disorders. Gastric tubes are used occasionally to supplement caloric intake.

Otorhinolaryngologic problems

Patients with a 22q11 deletion frequently have otolaryngologic disorders ranging from acquired to congenital anomalies [29]. Chronic otitis media and sinusitis are common problems, given their propensity to frequent infections. Reported congenital anomalies include laryngeal web, tracheomalacia, laryngomalacia, and tracheal compression or distortion from vascular rings. One series reported the triad of the 22q11 deletion with a laryngeal web and vascular rings in numerous patients [30]. Thus, any patient diagnosed with a 22q11 deletion treated for one of these two malformations who continues to have significant respiratory symptoms should be evaluated for concurrent anomalies.

Facial features

Typical facial dysmorphia may include hooded eyelids, auricular anomalies (eg, squared off or overfolded helices, protuberant ears, preauricular tags or pits, attached lobes, small ears), a prominent nasal root (more commonly seen in older children), a bulbous nasal tip with hypoplastic nasal alae, a small mouth, micrognathia, a short forehead, and some midfacial flattening (Fig. 2). These features can be particularly difficult to recognize in the neonate and often become more apparent in the toddler or school-aged child.

Additional anomalies

Renal anomalies, including abnormalities of the urinary tract (31%), renal agenesis, or multidysplastic kidneys (10%), have been described [13,14]. Skeletal anomalies involving the extremities, vertebral bodies (including butterfly vertebra), ribs, and cranium have been observed as well [13,14]. Growth retar-

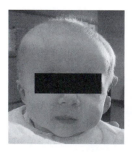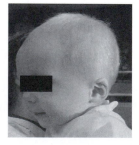

Fig. 2. Facial dysmorphia of a child diagnosed with a 22q11 deletion. This child demonstrates some of the typical facial features of the 22q11 deletion syndrome, including a short broad forehead, thick overfolded helices, small attached ear lobes, a bulbous nasal tip, a small mouth, and micrognathia. (Courtesy of Elaine Zackai, MD, Philadelphia, PA and Donna McDonald-McGinn, MS, Philadelphia, PA.)

dation is also well described and may result from a combination of issues described previously.

Neurocognitive and behavioral and/or psychiatric disorders

Most patients with a 22q11 deletion demonstrate below average full-scale IQ scores [26,31–33]. In particular, our center has reported that approximately 13% have average, 23% have low average, and 31% have borderline IQ scores, whereas 26% have scores consistent with mild mental retardation. A few have moderate (7%) or severe (< 1%) mental retardation. Many centers have reported higher verbal than performance IQ, implying that these patients' ability to process and use verbal information is better than their ability in perceptual processing and organization. Although some have described this difference as a "nonverbal learning disability," that term is likely misleading, because other areas of the verbal and language domains are areas of weakness. Relative strengths and weaknesses can be described (Table 2), although these must be interpreted with caution, because even the "strengths" often fall below normal levels of performance. Particular deficits in visual-spatial skills have been identified and may partially explain the observed impairment in mathematic abilities [34,35]. Consequently, a survey in our center found that 15% of children were in a regular classroom with no additional services, whereas 55% were in a regular class with special education services and 30% of school-aged children were in a special education classroom full time. Although this hospital-based survey may be biased toward more severely affected individuals, it nonetheless demonstrates that most affected children experience learning disabilities and require additional educational support services.

A wide range of behavioral and psychiatric disorders is commonly observed in this patient population [35]. A recent survey of our population has documented a 14% incidence of autistic spectrum disorders. These are first diagnosed in the toddler and preschool years, with impairment in social interaction, impairments in verbal and nonverbal communication, and restricted and repetitive patterns of behavior [36]. Attention deficit and hyperactivity disorders occur with increased frequency as compared with the general population. A number of children are diagnosed with anxiety disorders, depression, somatization, or social withdrawal (19% collectively) or with obsessive-compulsive disorder (5%). Multiple retrospective studies have identified a markedly increased frequency of schizophrenia

Table 2
Relative "strengths" and "weaknesses" of cognitive function

Strengths	Weaknesses
Rote verbal learning and memory	Complex verbal memory (stories)
Word reading/phonics	Reading comprehension
Initial auditory attention	Visual perception
Simple focused attention	Visual memory
Reading and spelling measured by standardized tests	Visual-spatial information processing
	Cognitive flexibility and executive function

among adolescents and adults with the 22q11 deletion syndrome and estimate that 25% to 30% of deletion-bearing children develop schizophrenia or schizo-affective disorders as adults [37–40].

Neuroimaging studies have identified structural abnormalities, which affect the white matter to a greater extent than the gray matter, in the patient population with a 22q11 deletion. In particular, several volumetric MRI studies report a reduction in white matter volume, particularly in the parietal regions of the brain [41]. Further study revealed reduced white matter anisotropy in regions of the brain that correlate with observed neurocognitive deficits [42].

It should be noted that the neurocognitive, developmental, behavioral, and psychiatric disorders described here represent an integral component of the 22q11 deletion syndrome and are not merely a secondary consequence of congenital heart disease or surgery. These findings have been described in those patients with a 22q11 deletion in the absence of cardiac defects. Further study to examine the interplay between the deletion syndrome and cardiac defects is warranted, but the deficits must not solely be attributed to the presence of congenital heart disease and must be anticipated as an important feature of the deletion syndrome itself. The neurocognitive and psychiatric profile of the 22q11 deletion syndrome is an active area of research. Novel neuroimaging techniques promise to corre-late structure with function and to provide increased understanding of the mecha-nism underlying these profound difficulties. This research may provide insight into new management for patients with, and perhaps without, a 22q11 deletion.

Diagnosis and management of the patient with a 22q11 deletion

Identifying the patient with a 22q11 deletion

Identifying the patient with a 22q11 deletion early in life is important, given the numerous associated medical problems and developmental challenges. Early diagnosis not only permits premorbid evaluation and intervention for medical issues but allows for appropriate family counseling about the syndrome and testing for risk of recurrence. Approximately 6% to 10% of cases are familial, implying that one of the parents, usually with mild symptoms, may unknowingly carry a 22q11 deletion. The parent carrying a 22q11 deletion has a 50% chance of transmitting the deletion to each offspring. Reports highlight cases in which the diagnosis of a 22q11 deletion is only made on the delivery of a severely affected newborn, only to find that multiple siblings or even generations carry the same diagnosis when examined "retrospectively" [15]. These studies highlight the marked clinical variability associated with a 22q11 deletion and the challenge of diagnosing the deletion-bearing person with a more subtle presentation.

Identifying the newborn or infant with a 22q11 deletion can be particularly challenging. The facial features can be subtle; palate anomalies most commonly are not overt; and the neurocognitive, developmental, and speech disorders that characterize the 22q11 deletion syndrome are not apparent. Therefore, in the newborn or infant, noteworthy signs include hypocalcemia, nasopharyngeal reflux, facial features (if apparent, the ears and nose can be particularly informative), absent thymus (although this can be seen in many nondeleted newborns under stress), and congenital heart disease. Numerous studies have demonstrated that a significant proportion of newborns or infants with specific types of congenital heart disease have a 22q11 deletion. As such, the newborn or infant presenting with cardiovascular disease offers the opportunity for early identification of the deletion-bearing patient.

A significant proportion of newborns with tetralogy of Fallot, truncus arteriosus, or an interrupted aortic arch are found to have a 22q11 deletion on testing (Table 3) [43]. In addition, patients with a perimembranous ventricular septal defect or isolated aortic arch anomaly are frequently found to have a 22q11 deletion as well [44,45]. For each of these diagnoses, the presence of an aortic arch anomaly (cervical, double, or right sided), abnormal origin of one of the subclavian arteries, or discontinuous branch pulmonary arteries markedly increases the likelihood that that patient carries a 22q11 deletion. In contrast, patients with d-transposition of the great arteries or a double-outlet right ventricle are rarely found to have a 22q11 deletion.

Therefore, we currently recommend that all newborns or infants with tetralogy of Fallot, truncus arteriosus, an interrupted aortic arch, or isolated aortic arch anomalies undergo testing for a 22q11 deletion (Box 2). Those with a perimembranous ventricular septal defect and aortic arch anomaly are at high risk (45%) and warrant testing as well [45]. Those with an isolated perimembranous ventricular septal defect should be strongly considered and evaluated carefully for concurrent symptoms but are less commonly found to carry a 22q11 deletion (3%). Any patient with congenital heart disease of a different variety with other signs of the 22q11 deletion syndrome should be tested as well. Similar testing strategies for the fetus diagnosed with these specific types of cardiac defects or additional features of the 22q11 syndrome are recommended.

Table 3
22q11 deletion frequency in congenital heart defects

Cardiac defect	Frequency (%)[a]
Tetralogy of Fallot	16
Truncus arteriosus	35
Interrupted aortic arch	50
Ventricular septal defect[b]	10
With aortic arch anomaly	40
With normal aortic arch	3
Isolated aortic arch anomaly	24
Double-outlet right ventricle	<5
Transposition of the great arteries	<1

[a] Frequencies increase in the face of concurrent aortic arch anomalies, such as right-sided or cervical locations, double aortic arch, or abnormal branching patterns.

[b] Perimembranous, malalignment, or conoseptal hypoplasia ventricular septal defects.

Data from Refs. [43–45].

Box 2. Current recommendations for 22q11 deletion testing

1. Any fetus, newborn, or infant with the following:
   Tetralogy of Fallot
   Truncus arteriosus
   Interrupted aortic arch
   Isolated aortic arch anomalies
   Perimembranous ventricular septal defect with concurrent
     aortic arch anomaly
2. Consider testing a child with a perimembranous ventricular
   septal defect in conjunction with any other feature of the
   22q11 deletion syndrome.
3. Test any fetus, newborn, infant, or child with other types
   of congenital heart disease in conjunction with other features
   of the 22q11 deletion syndrome.
4. Test any older child or adult with one of the high-risk lesions
   and any other feature of the 22q11 deletion syndrome if he or
   she has not already been evaluated.

Testing for a 22q11 deletion is now routinely clinically available in most cytogenetics laboratories. The test requires a small sample of whole blood (before a transfusion is given), and it takes, on average, 1 week to obtain a result. The deletion itself is identified by fluorescence *in situ* hybridization (FISH) (Fig. 3).

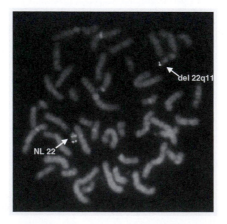

Fig. 3. FISH of metaphase chromosomes with fluorescently labeled probes to detect a deletion of chromosome 22q11. Note the signal for the green control probe at the distal end of both homologues of chromosome 22. Note the presence of the red signal for the test probe on one homologue of chromosome 22 (NL 22) and the absence of the test probe on the other homologue (del 22q11), implying a deletion of that locus on one chromosome. (Courtesy of Beverly Emanuel, PhD, Philadelphia, PA.)

Clinical evaluation of the deleted patient

The diagnosis of a 22q11 deletion in a patient should prompt evaluation of multiple systems or referral to appropriate subspecialists to offer premorbid diagnosis and early intervention (Table 4). Additional services and consultations are obviously tailored to individual patient needs. Three particular evaluations are described briefly here.

Cardiology

The patient with known congenital heart disease should be carefully examined for associated aortic arch anomalies if they are not already clearly defined, because nearly 50% of patients with the 22q11 deletion syndrome are found to have an aortic arch anomaly (unpublished data). Particular attention should be paid to identify those with an isolated or absent subclavian artery as opposed to assuming an aberrant subclavian artery when abnormal branching patterns are suspected. Suprasternal frontal imaging on echocardiography for aortic arch sidedness and a branching pattern is important to perform. If the echocardiogram is equivocal, cardiac MRI has been proven instrumental to diagnose and detail aortic arch anatomy (Fig. 4) [46]. Identification of a vascular ring is important before surgical intervention for a concurrent intracardiac defect to allow for simultaneous ligation of the vascular ring.

If the patient with a 22q11 deletion has not been evaluated for a cardiac defect, referral to a cardiologist for complete evaluation is warranted, particularly in the presence of respiratory or airway symptoms. The evaluation should include a complete history for respiratory and airway symptoms as well as an echocardiogram or cardiac MRI even when the results of the physical examination are normal. In our case series, approximately 34% (10 of 29) of patients diagnosed with a 22q11 deletion after 6 months of age (when critical congenital heart defects would have already manifested themselves) were found to have an aortic arch anomaly, of which nearly one third (3 of 10 patients) had a vascu-

Table 4
Evaluation of the patient newly diagnosed with a 22q11 deletion

Testing/referrals for all patients	Testing/referrals commonly needed
Cardiology consultation	Feeding evaluation
Immunology consultation	Gastroenterology consultation
Palate evaluation (plastic surgery or ORL)	Skeletal films
Calcium level	Endocrine evaluation
Renal ultrasound	Psychiatric evaluation
Developmental evaluation	
Speech evaluation	
Genetics consultation	
Parental testing for 22q11 deletion	

Abbreviation: ORL, otorhinolaryngology.

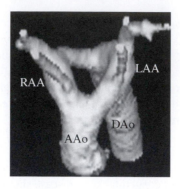

Fig. 4. MRI of a patient with a double aortic arch. This shaded-surface display of a double aortic arch was acquired by MRI on a child with airway symptoms by injection of gadolinium (magnetic contrast agent). This three-dimensional reconstruction was created from the maximum intensity projection image with removal of all structures other than the double aortic arch system. This three-dimensional reconstruction can be rotated in any fashion to acquire any view needed to display the salient anatomy. This image illustrates why a double aortic arch is called a vascular ring, because it encircles the trachea and esophagus (not pictured). AAo, ascending aorta, DAo, descending aorta, LAA, left aortic arch; RAA, right aortic arch. (Courtesy of Mark Fogel, MD, Philadelphia, PA.)

lar ring compressing the trachea and most likely contributing to respiratory symptoms [44].

Immunology

On diagnosis, the infant with a 22q11 deletion should be tested for T-cell markers to identify those with severe immunodeficiency in need of a thymic transplant. Families should also be apprised of the risk of infection. In our center, live vaccines are not given in the first year of life, at which point, repeat testing for T-cell numbers, immunoglobulin levels, and diphtheria and tetanus titers should be performed. If there are functional antibodies and the CD8 count exceeds 250 cells per cubic meter, all immunizations, including live vaccines, are permitted. If the patient fails these tests, live vaccines should continue to be postponed and repeat testing performed. Studies have shown that live vaccines are ultimately well tolerated in most cases [47]. If the patient is diagnosed with the 22q11 deletion syndrome at a later age beyond infancy, immunologic testing need only be performed in those children with frequent infections or particular concerns. Long-term follow-up with an immunologist may not be required except to assist with frequent infections or to evaluate for autoimmune disorders.

Palate and speech evaluation

On diagnosis of the 22q11 deletion syndrome, the palate should be examined for the presence of an overt or submucosal cleft. Speech and language therapy should begin early between 1 and 2 years of life. Annual evaluations for perceptual evidence of velopharyngeal insufficiency should be performed as speech emerges, and, when suspected, the diagnosis should be confirmed by imaging studies, such as nasendoscopy or multiview videofluoroscopy. If there is clinically significant velopharyngeal insufficiency, pharyngoplasty is undertaken at approximately 5 years of age.

Molecular considerations

As noted, most patients with the clinical diagnosis of DiGeorge, velocardiofacial, or CTAF syndrome share a common genetic cause, namely, a deletion of chromosome 22 on the long arm (q) at band 11, or a 22q11 deletion. The deletion most commonly (87%) encompasses 3 megabytes (Mb) of DNA from one of the two copies of chromosome 22 [5]. Approximately 30 to 40 genes map to the deleted region, such that the patient is left with only one rather than two copies of each of the deleted genes and is said to be haploinsufficient at that locus [48]. This deletion presumably decreases the amount or dosage of the gene product, which presumably leads to the multitude of observed malformations. Some patients have been found to have smaller or uniquely placed deletions of the same region, but studies found that the variable deletion size or location did not account for the observed clinical variability. Thus, there does not seem to be a genotype–phenotype correlation when the size of the deletion is considered. Instead, other genetic variants or environmental factors probably account for the notable clinical variability observed in the 22q11 deletion syndrome.

Over many years, investigators identified approximately 30 genes that map into the region to determine whether deletion of a single gene or multiple genes results in the observed phenotype. Elegant experiments in a mouse model in several laboratories demonstrated that *TBX1*, a T-box transcription factor, was an excellent candidate gene for the disorder [49–51]. Subsequent studies in human beings, where mutations of *TBX1* were identified in rare patients with the CTAF syndrome but without a 22q11 deletion, support this hypothesis [52]. Many questions remain as to whether other genes in the region contribute to the phenotype, however.

Molecular studies have also tried to determine why this chromosome so commonly experiences a deletion at this locus. Experiments have demonstrated that there are chromosome-specific, low-copy, repeat segments throughout the locus of the deleted segment, which probably allow for misalignment during meiosis and consequent duplication and deletion [53].

Summary

In conclusion, molecular analysis of a presumably rare developmental disorder led to the discovery of the most common deletion syndrome known to date, namely, the 22q11 deletion syndrome. The syndrome is characterized in part by congenital heart disease, immunodeficiency, hypocalcemia, palate anomalies, speech and feeding disorders, and facial dysmorphia as well as neurocognitive, behavioral, and psychiatric disorders. A significant proportion of infants with specific types of congenital heart defects have been found to have the 22q11 deletion syndrome and warrant early diagnosis to provide optimal anticipatory medical care and family counseling. Preliminary studies indicate that deletion status may also have an impact on clinical outcome, further emphasizing the need to identify the deletion-bearing patient for counseling and clinical purposes [54]. Routine testing of a subset of newborns and infants with cardiac disease should be considered, given the marked variability of clinical features associated with the deletion syndrome. Of note, a small number of infants with the clinical appearance of DiGeorge syndrome do not have a 22q11 deletion and should be evaluated for other etiologies, including different chromosomal abnormalities or maternal environmental factors. Additional research should continue to lend insight into the neurocognitive features of this syndrome, with potential applicability to a broader population. Investigations on the impact of genotype on clinical outcome should also serve to improve our clinical management of these infants.

Acknowledgments

The critical review of this manuscript by Kathleen Sullivan, MD, Richard Kirschner, MD, Marsha Gerdes, PhD, and Donna McDonald-McGinn, MS, is gratefully acknowledged.

References

[1] Kirkpatrick Jr JA, DiGeorge AM. Congenital absence of the thymus. Am J Roentgenol Radium Ther Nucl Med 1968;103(1):32–7.

[2] Conley ME, Beckwith JB, Mancer JF, et al. The spectrum of the DiGeorge syndrome. J Pediatr 1979;94(6):883–90.

[3] Scambler PJ, Carey AH, Wyse RK, et al. Microdeletions within 22q11 associated with sporadic and familial DiGeorge syndrome. Genomics 1991;10(1):201–6.

[4] Driscoll DA, Budarf ML, Emanuel BS. A genetic etiology for DiGeorge syndrome: consistent deletions and microdeletions of 22q11. Am J Hum Genet 1992;50(5):924–33.

[5] Emanuel BS, Budarf ML, Scambler PJ. The genetic basis of conotruncal cardiac defects: the chromosome 22q11.2 deletion. In: Harvey RP, Rosenthal N, editors. Heart development. Toronto: Academic Press; 1999. p. 463–78.

[6] Shprintzen RJ, Goldberg RB, Lewin ML, et al. A new syndrome involving cleft palate, cardiac anomalies, typical facies, and learning disabilities: velo-cardio-facial syndrome. Cleft Palate J 1978;15(1):56–62.

[7] Kinouchi A, Mori K, Ando M, et al. Facial appearance of patients with conotruncal abnormalities. Pediatr Jpn 1976;17:84.

[8] Driscoll DA, Spinner NB, Budarf ML, et al. Deletions and microdeletions of 22q11.2 in velo-cardio-facial syndrome. Am J Med Genet 1992;44(2):261–8.

[9] Kelly D, Goldberg R, Wilson D, et al. Confirmation that the velo-cardio-facial syndrome is associated with haplo-insufficiency of genes at chromosome 22q11. Am J Med Genet 1993; 45(3):308–12.

[10] Burn J, Takao A, Wilson D, et al. Conotruncal anomaly face syndrome is associated with a deletion within chromosome 22q11. J Med Genet 1993;30(10):822–4.

[11] Matsuoka R, Takao A, Kimura M, et al. Confirmation that the conotruncal anomaly face syndrome is associated with a deletion within 22q11.2. Am J Med Genet 1994;53(3):285–9.

[12] Botto LD, May K, Fernhoff PM, et al. A population-based study of the 22q11.2 deletion: phenotype, incidence, and contribution to major birth defects in the population. Pediatrics 2003;112(1 Pt 1):101–7.

[13] McDonald-McGinn DM, LaRossa D, Goldmuntz E, et al. The 22q11.2 deletion: screening, diagnostic workup, and outcome of results; report on 181 patients. Genet Test 1997;1(2):99–108.

[14] Ryan AK, Goodship JA, Wilson DI, et al. Spectrum of clinical features associated with interstitial chromosome 22q11 deletions: a European collaborative study. J Med Genet 1997;34(10): 798–804.

[15] Shooner KA, Rope AF, Hopkin RJ, et al. Genetic analyses in two extended families with deletion 22q11 syndrome: importance of extracardiac manifestations. J Pediatr 2005;146(3):382–7.

[16] Sullivan KE, Jawad AF, Randall P, et al. Lack of correlation between impaired T cell production, immunodeficiency, and other phenotypic features in chromosome 22q11.2 deletion syndromes. Clin Immunol Immunopathol 1998;86(2):141–6.

[17] Jawad AF, McDonald-McGinn DM, Zackai E, et al. Immunologic features of chromosome 22q11.2 deletion syndrome (DiGeorge syndrome/velocardiofacial syndrome). J Pediatr 2001; 139(5):715–23.

[18] Sullivan KE. The clinical, immunological, and molecular spectrum of chromosome 22q11.2 deletion syndrome and DiGeorge syndrome. Curr Opin Allergy Clin Immunol 2004;4(6):505–12.

[19] Brauner R, Le Harivel de Gonneville A, Kindermans C, et al. Parathyroid function and growth in 22q11.2 deletion syndrome. J Pediatr 2003;142(5):504–8.

[20] Taylor SC, Morris G, Wilson D, et al. Hypoparathyroidism and 22q11 deletion syndrome. Arch Dis Child 2003;88(6):520–2.

[21] Scire G, Dallapiccola B, Iannetti P, et al. Hypoparathyroidism as the major manifestation in two patients with 22q11 deletions. Am J Med Genet 1994;52(4):478–82.

[22] Greig F, Paul E, DiMartino-Nardi J, et al. Transient congenital hypoparathyroidism: resolution and recurrence in chromosome 22q11 deletion. J Pediatr 1996;128(4):563–7.

[23] Weinzimer SA, McDonald-McGinn DM, Driscoll DA, et al. Growth hormone deficiency in patients with 22q11.2 deletion: expanding the phenotype. Pediatrics 1998;101(5):929–32.

[24] McDonald-McGinn DM, Kirschner R, Goldmuntz E, et al. The Philadelphia story: the 22q11.2 deletion: report on 250 patients. Genet Couns 1999;10(1):11–24.

[25] Kirschner RE. Palatal anomalies in 22q11.2 deletion syndrome. Cambridge, UK: Cambridge University Press; 2005.

[26] Gerdes M, Solot C, Wang PP, et al. Cognitive and behavior profile of preschool children with chromosome 22q11.2 deletion. Am J Med Genet 1999;85(2):127–33.

[27] Solot CB, Gerdes M, Kirschner RE, et al. Communication issues in 22q11.2 deletion syndrome: children at risk. Genet Med 2001;3(1):67–71.

[28] Eicher PS, McDonald-McGinn DM, Fox CA, et al. Dysphagia in children with a 22q11.2 deletion: unusual pattern found on modified barium swallow. J Pediatr 2000;137(2):158–64.

[29] Dyce O, McDonald-McGinn D, Kirschner RE, et al. Otolaryngologic manifestations of the 22q11.2 deletion syndrome. Arch Otolaryngol Head Neck Surg 2002;128(12):1408–12.

[30] McElhinney DB, Jacobs I, McDonald-McGinn DM, et al. Chromosomal and cardiovascular anomalies associated with congenital laryngeal web. Int J Pediatr Otorhinolaryngol 2002;66(1): 23–7.

[31] Moss EM, Batshaw ML, Solot CB, et al. Psychoeducational profile of the 22q11.2 microdeletion: a complex pattern. J Pediatr 1999;134(2):193–8.

[32] Swillen A, Vogels A, Devriendt K, et al. Chromosome 22q11 deletion syndrome: update and review of the clinical features, cognitive-behavioral spectrum, and psychiatric complications. Am J Med Genet 2000;97(2):128–35.

[33] Gerdes M, Solot C, Wang PP, et al. Taking advantage of early diagnosis: preschool children with the 22q11.2 deletion. Genet Med 2001;3(1):40–4.

[34] Bearden CE, Woodin MF, Wang PP, et al. The neurocognitive phenotype of the 22q11.2 deletion syndrome: selective deficit in visual-spatial memory. J Clin Exp Neuropsychol 2001;23(4): 447–64.

[35] Simon TJ, Bearden CE, Moss EM, et al. Cognitive development in VCFS. Prog Pediatr Cardiol 2002;15:109–17.

[36] Fine SE, Weissman A, Gerdes M, et al. Autism spectrum disorders and symptoms in children with molecularly confirmed 22q11.2 deletion syndrome. J Autism Dev Disord 2005;35(4):70.

[37] Shprintzen RJ, Goldberg R, Golding-Kushner KJ, et al. Late-onset psychosis in the velo-cardio-facial syndrome. Am J Med Genet 1992;42(1):141–2.

[38] Bassett AS, Hodgkinson K, Chow EW, et al. 22q11 deletion syndrome in adults with schizophrenia. Am J Med Genet 1998;81(4):328–37.

[39] Murphy KC, Jones LA, Owen MJ. High rates of schizophrenia in adults with velo-cardio-facial syndrome. Arch Gen Psychiatry 1999;56(10):940–5.

[40] Bassett AS, Chow EW, Abdel Malik P, et al. The schizophrenia phenotype in 22q11 deletion syndrome. Am J Psychiatry 2003;160(9):1580–6.

[41] Eliez S, Blasey CM, Schmitt EJ, et al. Velocardiofacial syndrome: are structural changes in the temporal and mesial temporal regions related to schizophrenia? Am J Psychiatry 2001;158(3): 447–53.

[42] Barnea-Goraly N, Menon V, Krasnow B, et al. Investigation of white matter structure in velocardiofacial syndrome: a diffusion tensor imaging study. Am J Psychiatry 2003;160(10): 1863–9.

[43] Goldmuntz E, Clark BJ, Mitchell LE, et al. Frequency of 22q11 deletions in patients with conotruncal defects. J Am Coll Cardiol 1998;32(2):492–8.

[44] McElhinney DB, Clark III BJ, Weinberg PM, et al. Association of chromosome 22q11 deletion with isolated anomalies of aortic arch laterality and branching. J Am Coll Cardiol 2001; 37(8):2114–9.

[45] McElhinney DB, Driscoll DA, Levin ER, et al. Chromosome 22q11 deletion in patients with ventricular septal defect: frequency and associated cardiovascular anomalies. Pediatrics 2003; 112(6 Pt 1):e472–6.

[46] Johnson TR, Goldmuntz E, McDonald-McGinn DM, et al. Cardiac magnetic resonance imaging for accurate diagnosis of aortic arch anomalies in patients with 22q11.2 deletion. Am J Cardiol, in press.

[47] Perez EE, Bokszczanin A, McDonald-McGinn D, et al. Safety of live viral vaccines in patients with chromosome 22q11.2 deletion syndrome (DiGeorge syndrome/velocardiofacial syndrome). Pediatrics 2003;112(4):e325–7.

[48] Scambler PJ. The 22q11 deletion syndromes. Hum Mol Genet 2000;9(16):2421–6.

[49] Baldini A. DiGeorge syndrome: the use of model organisms to dissect complex genetics. Hum Mol Genet 2002;11(20):2363–9.

[50] Yamagishi H, Srivastava D. Unraveling the genetic and developmental mysteries of 22q11 deletion syndrome. Trends Mol Med 2003;9(9):383–9.

[51] Baldini A. Dissecting contiguous gene defects: TBX1. Curr Opin Genet Dev 2005;15(3):279–84.

[52] Yagi H, Furutani Y, Hamada H, et al. Role of TBX1 in human del22q11.2 syndrome. Lancet 2003;362(9393):1366–73.

[53] Shaikh TH, Kurahashi H, Emanuel BS. Evolutionarily conserved low copy repeats (LCRs) in 22q11 mediate deletions, duplications, translocations, and genomic instability: an update and literature review. Genet Med 2001;3(1):6–13.

[54] Mahle WT, Crisalli J, Coleman K, et al. Deletion of chromosome 22q11.2 and outcome in patients with pulmonary atresia and ventricular septal defect. Ann Thorac Surg 2003;76(2): 567–71.

Clin Perinatol 32 (2005) 979–997

Cardiovascular Drugs for the Newborn

Robert M. Ward, MD[a],*, Ralph A. Lugo, PharmD[b]

[a]University of Utah, Division of Neonatology, 50 North Medical Drive, Salt Lake City, UT 84132, USA
[b]College of Pharmacy, University of Utah, 30 South 2000 East, Room 267,
Salt Lake City, UT 84112-5820, USA

Antiarrhythmics

Antiarrhythmic drugs are classified according to their mechanisms of action, such as effects on ion channels, duration of repolarization, and receptor interaction (Table 1) [1–3]. Such classification systems help with understanding the effects of individual antiarrhythmic drugs and selection of drugs for specific arrhythmias. Drugs and their metabolites, however, may interact with multiple ion channels and one or more antiarrhythmic mechanisms [2,4]. Drugs within a given class may differ in effectiveness for a given arrhythmia. Dosages for drugs used frequently for resuscitation of newborns are listed (Table 2) [5,6]. Whenever possible, arrhythmias should be treated by drugs indicated for the specific type of arrhythmia.

Supraventricular tachycardia

In neonates, the most frequent arrhythmia that needs treatment is supraventricular tachycardia (SVT) [7]. In general, SVT occurs from either aberrant conduction pathways or abnormal automaticity within a discrete atrial focus [7]. Reentrant mechanisms are the most common causes of SVT in neonates and usually involve retrograde conduction via accessory conduction pathways from the ventricle to the atrium, producing premature atrial depolarization, designated as orthodromic reciprocating tachycardia (ORT). A variant of ORT arises from a posterior accessory conducting pathway that causes a slower, but incessant form

Supported in part by NICHD 1 U10 HD 045986-01.
* Corresponding author.
E-mail address: Robert.Ward@hsc.utah.edu (R.M. Ward).

0095-5108/05/$ – see front matter © 2005 Elsevier Inc. All rights reserved.
doi:10.1016/j.clp.2005.09.013

Table 1
Antiarrhythmic drugs by mechanism of action

Class	Action/Structure	Drugs
IA	Sodium ± potassium channel blockade Phase 0 dV/dt slowed Conduction slowed (prolonged PR, QRS, and QT) Repolarization usually delayed Anticholinergic	Quinidine Procainamide Dysopyramide
IB	Sodium channel blockade Phase 0 dV/dt minimal change Repolarization usually shortened (QT shortened) Fibrillation thresholds elevated	Lidocaine Mexilitine Moricizine
IC	Sodium channel blockade Phase 0 dV/dt markedly slowed Repolarization minimally changed PR and QRS markedly prolonged	Flecainide Propafenone
II	Beta-adenergic blockade, variable selectivity	Propranolol Atenolol Esmolol
III	Repolarization and action potential prolonged	Amiodarone Sotalol
IV	Calcium channel blockade	Verapamil
V	Digitalis glycosides	Digoxin Ouabain
VI	Purinergic agonists	Adenosine

Abbreviations: dt, change in time; dV, change in voltage.
Data from Grant AO. Mechanisms of action of antiarrhythmic drugs: from ion channel blockage to arrhythmia termination. Pacing Clin Electrophysiol 1997;20:432–44; and Perry JC. Pharmacologic therapy of arrhythmias. In: Deal B, Wolff G, Gelband H, editors. Current concepts in diagnosis and management of arrhythmias in infants and children. Armonk (NY): Futura Publishing Co.; 1998. p. 267–305.

of SVT—permanent junctional reciprocating tachycardia, which left untreated causes cardiomyopathy and congestive heart failure (CHF). In the Wolff-Parkinson-White syndrome (WPW), the accessory conduction pathway can be identified during sinus rhythm from early depolarization that creates a shoulder (delta wave) on the R wave and a shortened PR interval [7]. Almost 50% of reentrant SVT in infants does not show preexcitation overtly during sinus rhythm. When the depolarization returns from the ventricle through the atrioventricular node to cause SVT, a wide, complex tachycardia results.

Nonreentrant SVT is rare in infancy and difficult to treat pharmacologically. SVT caused by a nonsinus node focus of abnormal automaticity is designated automatic atrial tachycardia (AAT) [4]. AAT is distinguished from sinus tachycardia because the heart rate may gradually increase or decrease. The P-wave morphology during AAT differs from that during sinus rhythm and the PR interval of conducted beats may lengthen rather than shorten as the heart rate increases. SVT may also arise from a site of abnormal automaticity within or near the atrioventricular (AV) node, designated junctional ectopic tachycardia [4], which is also difficult to treat [8,9].

Table 2
Drugs for newborn resuscitation

Drug and formulation	Final concentration	Dose (amount/kg)	Dose (mL/kg)
Adenosine 6 mg/2 mL	3 mg/mL	Start: 50 µg/kg rapid IV push, followed by flush of IV catheter; if no response within 0.5–2 min, increase dose by 50 µg/kg and repeat until conversion of SVT or AV block, to maximum single dose of 250–500 µg/kg	Dilute 0.5 ml with 2.5 ml saline, infuse 0.1mL/kg IV for every 50 µg/kg dose
Atropine 10.0%	0.1 mg/mL	IV dosage: 0.01–0.02 mg/kg (minimum dose 0.1 mg); may repeat in 10 min to maximum of 0.04 mg/kg; IT dosage: 0.02–0.04 mg/kg	0.1–0.2 mL/kg IV 0.2–0.4 mL/kg IT
Bicarbonate 0.05 mEq/mL	0.5 mEq/mL	1–2 mEq/kg; treat measured metabolic acidosis; avoid 1.0 mEq/mL formulation in newborns; maintain ventilation	1–2 mL/kg IV
Calcium gluconate 10%	100 mg/mL (9.3 mg Ca++/mL)	60 mg/kg infused slowly; stop infusion for symptomatic bradycardia; repeat as needed for clinical effect; extravasation causes tissue necrosis	0.6 mL/kg IV
Calcium chloride 10%	100 mg/mL (27 mg Ca++/mL)	20 mg/kg infused slowly; stop infusion for symptomatic bradycardia; repeat as needed for clinical effect; extravasation causes tissue necrosis	0.2 mL/kg IV
Direct current defibrillation		1 Watt-sec/kg; increase by 1 Watt-sec/kg if unsuccessful	
Epinephrine 1:10,000	0.1 mg/mL	0.01–0.03 mg/kg IV or IO 0.1 mg/kg IT	0.1–0.3 mL/kg IV, IO 1.0 mL/kg IT
Glucose 10%	100 mg/mL	200–500 mg/kg	2–5 mL/kg IV
Lidocaine 2%	20 mg/mL	0.5–1.0 mg/kg; repeat every 5–10 min to maximum of 3 mg/kg	Dilute 0.5 mL + 9.5 mL D5W Infuse: 0.5–1.0 mL/kg IV, IT
Naloxone 0.4 mg/mL	0.4 mg/mL	0.1 mg/kg; dose may be repeated to maintain opiate reversal. This dose is indicated for acute opiate intoxication. Titration to effect with lower initial doses (0.01 mg/kg or 10 µg/kg) should be considered for respiratory depression during pain management. WARNING: May induce acute withdrawal in opioid dependent patients.	0.25 mL/kg IV, IM
Procainamide 100 mg/mL	100 mg/mL	3–6 mg/kg over 5 min, repeat to a titrated maximum of 15 mg/kg loading dose, infuse slowly with myocardial dysfunction	Dilute 1 mL + 9 mL D5W Infuse: 0.3–0.6 mL/kg IV

With use of endotracheal tube, dose should be diluted in saline or tube flushed with saline after dose.
Abbreviations: D5W, 5% dextrose in water; IM, intramuscular; IO, intraosseous; IT, intratracheal; IV, intravenous.
Data from references [5,6,14].

Treatment of SVT may be required in two situations: acute termination of a symptomatic tachycardia and chronic suppression of recurrent SVT. Vagal maneuvers, such as stimulation of the diving reflex through ice applied to the face, are still frequently used for the acute termination of SVT, although bilateral carotid massage or pressure on the eyes should be avoided. Synchronized electrocardioversion terminates SVT in about 50% of cases, but it is more successful if P waves are not present [10].

Adenosine has been used in the acute treatment of SVT, with moderate success. Adenosine slows spontaneous heart rate, prolongs the PR interval, and decreases the slope of phase 4 repolarization through activation of A_1-purinoceptors coupled to sarcolemmal potassium channels. Electroconversion is rarely required for conversion of infantile onset SVT since the introduction of adenosine [11]. Adenosine has a 9-second half-life and must be administered by rapid intravenous (IV) push to be effective. Adenosine slows the heart rate within seconds of administration; however, its short half-life limits its usefulness to the acute treatment of SVT. The initial dose of adenosine is 50 to150 mcg/kg. The dose may be increased by 50 mcg/kg every minute to a maximum of 250 to 500 mcg/kg [2,12,13]. Theophylline is a competitive antagonist of adenosine [14], and thus higher adenosine dosages may be required in infants treated with theophylline [15]. Adverse effects of adenosine include bronchoconstriction, wheezing, and hypotension caused by vasodilatation [16].

Procainamide is a class 1A drug that blocks sodium and potassium channels and may be used to treat SVT that is unresponsive to adenosine [2]. Rapid infusion of procainamide may precipitate hypotension, and chronic treatment produces a systemic lupus erythematosus-type syndrome with antinuclear antibodies present in 50% to 90% of patients [2,16]. High serum concentrations of procainamide may depress myocardial contractility and predispose the patient to CHF [2]. More than 50% of procainamide is excreted unchanged in the urine, whereas the rest of a dose is metabolized by N-acetyltransferase in the liver to N-acetylprocainamide (NAPA), an active metabolite that acts through a different (class III) antiarrhythmic mechanism [2]. Adults may be phenotyped as fast or slow acetylators [17]; however, infants between birth and 2 months of age are uniformly slow acetylators because of immaturity of the enzyme system [18]. NAPA and procainamide accumulate with renal insufficiency. Procainamide levels of 4 to 8 mcg/mL are generally effective for control of arrhythmias. Procainamide and NAPA levels need to be followed periodically.

Lidocaine, a class 1B antiarrhythmic, and its metabolites primarily block the fast inward sodium channel [2,16]. Its effects are much greater on the conducting system and the ventricular muscle than on the atrium. Drugs known to decrease hepatic blood flow, such as cimetidine, will decrease hepatic clearance of lidocaine. Plasma concentrations should be maintained between 2 and 5 μg/mL. Concentrations exceeding 6 μg/mL may produce seizures or respiratory arrest [2,16].

Chronic treatment of SVT is not needed in every patient. If the frequency of SVT is rare, not associated with cardiovascular compromise, and is easily terminated with vagal maneuvers, chronic treatment may not be required [4]. The presence of WPW, however, is a significant predictor of SVT recurrence after discontinuing medications [19]. Digoxin treatment of WPW is controversial, because it has been associated with sudden death in 1% to 5% of these patients [4,20]. In another series of patients who had SVT, digoxin treatment was successful in 65% regardless of whether patients showed preexcitation [11]. A review of patients treated for SVT at Texas Children's Hospital revealed no difference in the success rate for treatment of SVT with digitalis among patients who had and who did not have WPW [10].

Propranolol is frequently used to treat neonates who have SVT in situations when digoxin is contraindicated because of the presence of WPW [2]. Following oral or enteral administration, propranolol is cleared largely through first-pass extraction by the liver. It is metabolized extensively to an active metabolite, 4-hydroxypropranolol [21]. With multiple doses, hepatic extraction decreases, more drug reaches the systemic circulation, and plasma concentrations vary widely at steady-state. If administered IV, the dose of propranolol must be reduced at least tenfold because it bypasses hepatic extraction and produces a dose- and concentration-related decrease in heart rate and cardiac contractility. Propranolol is used most frequently to treat supraventricular and ventricular arrhythmias and sinus tachycardia related to hypermetabolic states such as thyrotoxicosis [16]. Data on dosing, kinetics, and efficacy for other beta-adrenergic blocking drugs in neonates, such as atenolol, nadolol, sotalol, and esmolol, are limited.

Verapamil has been used for treatment of SVT with moderate success, but its use in neonates and infants less than 12 months of age has been discouraged [2,22]. Because of its negative inotropic activity and ability to decrease sinus function, verapamil should not be used with beta-adrenergic blocking drugs in infants and children [16].

Amiodarone is a benzofuran compound that was approved as a 'last resort' drug for refractory, life-threatening arrhythmias [23]. During the last few years, much more information has accumulated about its efficacy and its toxicity. Amiodarone illustrates the limitations of a classification system for antiarrhythmics. It inhibits the fast sodium channel and the slow calcium channel, has non-competitive antisympathetic effects, and modulates thyroid function [24]. Amiodarone has a low negative inotropic effect and therefore may be the preferred antiarrhythmic treatment for infants and children who have depressed myocardial function caused by incessant tachycardias or perioperative tachycardias following surgery for congenital heart disease [34]. Acutely, amiodarone slows AV node conduction with little effect on the rate corrected QT interval (QTc), whereas during chronic therapy, it lengthens QTc and prolongs the refractory period [26]. Although reports are limited in neonates, the following adverse effects have been observed after amiodarone treatment of infants and children: photosensitivity [25,26], corneal deposits [26], gray skin color [26], abnormal liver function tests [26], hypothyroidism [25,26], hyperthyroidism [25,26], accelerated bone maturation [25], delayed longitudinal growth [25], excess weight gain [25], headaches [25], pulmonary infiltrates [27], and sleep disturbances [26]. Amiodarone may increase the concentration of several drugs, such as digoxin, quinidine, procainamide, and phenytoin, by decreasing clearance and volume of distribution. Decreased clearance of warfarin by amiodarone may precipitate hemorrhage. Overall, the frequency of adverse effects is greater in adults than in children and greater in older children than in infants.

In infants and children, the treatment of refractory and serious arrhythmias with amiodarone has been successful with limited acute toxicity. In a multicenter trial, Perry reported [28] a 93% rate of improvement with the use of amiodarone for life-threatening arrhythmias in 40 patients from eight centers. Arrhythmias in pediatric patients who have been treated successfully with amiodarone include: multifocal atrial tachycardia (chaotic atrial tachycardia) [29,30], ventricular tachycardia (caused by intracardiac tumor) [31], and refractory SVT [32,33]. In a study by Burri and colleagues [34], IV amiodarone was reported to be safe and effective therapy for life-threatening incessant tachycardias in infants. Twenty-three hemodynamically unstable infants (median age 8 days) who had life-threatening tachycardias (17 supraventricular, 6 ventricular) were treated with IV amiodarone, 5 mg/kg over 1 hour followed by 5 µg/kg/min with stepwise increase to 25 µg/kg/min [34]. Amiodarone was effective in 83% of infants. Median time to arrhythmia control was 24 hours, and the median maintenance dose was 15 µg/kg/min (range 5–26 µg/kg/min). Adverse effects, sinus bradycardia in two patients and hypotension in one infant, were not significant and resolved after dose reduction. Choreoathetotic movements and elevated liver enzymes occurred in two patients.

Dosages of amiodarone have varied widely between studies. Initial treatment with amiodarone begins with a loading dose of 5–7 mg/kg followed by an infusion of 7.5 to 15 mg/kg/d [26,28] for 9 to 10 days [35]. Larger dosages were required for infants less than 1 year of age in one study [26]. Oral monotherapy has been successful [26,36]. In a study by Etheridge and colleagues [36], 44 of 50 neonates and infants (1.0 ± 1.5 months) who had difficult-to-control tachycardias were successfully treated with oral amiodarone using a 7- to 10-day load at either 10 or 20 (higher dose for more difficult-to-control tachyarrhythmias) mg/kg/d in two divided doses. Twenty-five patients also required oral propranolol (2 mg/kg/d) for sustained or symptomatic episodes of tachycardia. Rhythm control was achieved in all patients. Infants were discharged on maintenance amiodarone doses of 5 to 10 mg/kg/d (mean dose 7 ± 2 mg/kg/d) and drugs were discontinued as tolerated. Sixty-eight percent of patients remained free of arrhythmias at 1 year, despite discontinuation of propranolol and amiodarone. No significant side effects occurred. The prolonged loading time likely relates to amiodarone's extremely long half-life, which is estimated to exceed 50 days in adults [23]. Plasma concentrations of amiodarone are kept between 0.8 and 2.0 mg/L in adults [26]; however there is no clear relationship between the concentrations of amiodarone or its metabolite desethylamiodarone and toxicity or efficacy [37,38].

Fetuses that have arrhythmias may be treated with amiodarone, however newly born infants should be evaluated for potential adverse effects. Neonatal hyperthyroidism and hypothyroidism with or without a goiter have been observed after fetal exposure to amiodarone [39–42].

Antihypertensives

The relationship among blood pressure, gestational age, birth weight and postconceptional age was defined by Zubrow and colleagues [43] in 695 neonates studied over a period of 3 months. Based on these data, hypertension in term and preterm infants may be identified if blood pressure exceeds the upper limit of the 95% confidence interval for infants of similar gestational or postconceptual age and size [44]. Drug treatement for hypertension should start with a single drug from one of the following classes: angiotensin converting enzyme (ACE) inhibitors, angiotensin-receptor antagonists, beta-receptor antagonists, calcium channel blockers, or diuretics [45].

For severe hyptertension in the neonate, a continuous intravenous infusion is advantageous, because the dose of medication may be titrated and blood pressure may be kept within narrow parameters, thus minimizing the fluctuations observed with intermittent dosing. Antihypertensive agents that have been used in neonates or infants by continuous infusion include esmolol [46], nitroprusside, and nicardipine [47,48]. Small studies have found that intravenous nicardipine may be effective in treating hypertensive neonates [47,48]. Milou and colleagues [47] administered 0.5 µg/kg/min of nicardipine (maximum 0.74 ± 0.41 µg/kg/min) to 20 neonates (15 preterm) for 14.6 ± 11.6 days. Blood pressure significantly decreased after 3, 6, 12, 24, and 48 hours of nicardipine treatment without hypotension. Gouyon and colleagues [48] treated 8 preterm infants who had systemic hypertension with either 0.5 µg/kg/min (2 infants) or 1.7 µg/kg/min (6 infants) for 15.9 ± 10.3 days. Systolic blood pressure decreased significantly without hypotension or other side effects after 12 and 24 hours of nicardipine treatment ($-17 \pm 17\%$ and $-21 \pm 10\%$, respectively) and diastolic blood pressure decreased after 24 hours of treatment ($-22 \pm 16\%$).

Hypertensive emergencies are uncommon in neonates, but can be treated with sodium nitroprusside if renal function is normal or with diazoxide if renal function is inadequate [45]. As observed in older patients, thiocyanate and cyanide may accumulate during sodium nitroprusside treatment; and hyperglycemia may occur with diazoxide infusions.

Mild-to-moderate hypertension may be treated with intermittently administered intravenous agents, such as hydralazine, labetalol, and enalaprilat [49], although enalaprilat should be used with great caution because of the potential for significant and prolonged hypotension [44]. Oral antihypertensives may be used in infants who have mild-to-moderate hypertension or in patients being transitioned from intravenous therapy.

Angiotensin-converting enzyme inhibitors (eg, captopril) have a special role in the treatment of neonatal renovascular hypertension caused by elevated serum levels of renin and angiotensin [50]. Aortic catheters may be associated with microemboli to the kidneys and increased secretion by the kidneys of renin and angiotensin. Although captopril may be a relatively specific treatment for this etiology of renovascular hypertension in neonates, dosage adjustments are difficult because a liquid dosage form is not commercially available. An extemporaneously compounded dosage form containing ascorbate has been shown to be stable for 14 days at room temperature [51]. To avoid hypotension and acute renal insufficiency [52], the dose of captopril in neonates should be initiated at 0.01 mg/kg, rather than the earlier recommendations of 0.1 to 0.3 mg/kg dose; and doses should be increased daily if hypertension persists. Captopril may also be useful for afterload reduction in the treatment of chronic CHF in newborns [53]. Other oral agents that have been used include the vasodilators hydralazine and minoxidil, and the calcium channel blocker isradipine [44]. Isradipine can be compounded into a suspension, and its successful and safe use has been reported in infants and children [44,54]. The use of isradipine suspension allows infants and young children to be treated as readily as older children.

Inotropes

Although inotropy refers specifically to myocardial contractility, inotropic drugs not only improve cardiac contractility, but also may increase heart rate and alter vascular tone [55,56]. The inotropic drug should be selected according to its specific pharmacologic properties and the specific cardiovascular abnormality to be corrected. Despite frequent administration of inotropes to newborns, they have received limited study in this population.

Cardiac output is determined by preload, afterload, and contractility; and it is the product of stroke volume and heart rate. Shock occurs when cardiac output and oxygen delivery are inadequate to meet tissue demands. Inotropic drug treatment for the failing heart must balance increasing myocardial oxygen consumption from increased work against the increase in cardiac output that provides more oxygenated blood through the coronary circulation to the myocardium. Disproportionate increases in myocardial wall stiffness from increased contractility and increased afterload may impede coronary flow and worsen myocardial ischemia. Conversely, excess peripheral vasodilation may reduce systemic blood pressure to a level where there is too little pressure to maintain adequate coronary flow during diastole.

Specific receptor interactions, cardiovascular effects, and controlled clinical trials of inotropic drugs in newborns should guide their clinical use (Table 3) [56–58]. Dosages for drugs used frequently in newborn resuscitation are indicated in Table 2. All inotropes should be dosed to effect. Prolonged infusion of catecholamines has been shown to down-regulate receptors with resultant tachyphylaxis.

Isoproterenol is a direct-acting, potent, pure beta-adrenergic agonist whose usefulness is limited by tachycardia and peripheral vasodilation, which may steal perfusion away from more vital organs and produce myocardial ischemia [59]. Isoproterenol is most effective for increasing heart rate, such as in the treatment of complete heart block.

Epinephrine stimulates all adrenergic receptors directly, but its vascular effects vary among organs, with beta$_2$ vasodilation usually exceeding beta$_1$ vasoconstriction so that peripheral vascular resistance decreases [56]. The effects of

Table 3
Relative cardiovascular receptor interactions of inotropes and the associated effects

Cardiovascular receptor interactions and effects

Catecholamine	α_1 Vasoconstriction; ⇑ Cardiac contractility	α_2 Vasoconstriction; ⇓ Norepinephrine release	β_1 ⇑ Contractility, ⇑ Conduction velocity	β_2 Vasodilation, bronchodilation	Dopamine, D_1 Renal, mesenteric & coronary vasodilation	Indirect Release of endogenous norepinephrine
Dobutamine	1+	0	3+	1+	0	0
Dopamine	0 to 3+	1+	2+ to 3+	2+	3+	1+
Epinephrine	2+	2+	3+	3+	0	0
Isoproterenol	0	0	3+	3+	0	0

0 = lowest to 3+ = highest interaction.

Data from Zaritsky A, Chernow B. Use of catecholamines in pediatrics. J Pediatr 1984;105:341–50; and Hoffman BB, Hoffman BB, Taylor P. Neurotransmission. Catecholamines, sympathomimetic drugs, and adrenergic receptor antagonists. In: Hardman JG, Limbird LE, Gilman AG, editors. Goodman & Gilman's the pharmacological basis of therapeutics. 10th edition. New York: McGraw-Hill; 2001. p. 215–68.

epinephrine infusions of 0.05 to 2.6 mcg/kg/min were described in 31 hypotensive newborns of 23 to 30 weeks gestation who had not responded to treatment with three 10 to 15 mL/kg infusions of crystalloid and dopamine infused at 15 mcg/kg/min [60]. Epinephrine normalized blood pressure in all, increased heart rate an average of 10 beats/min, and improved urine output in 5 of 6 patients who had oliguria; but it worsened the base deficit an average of 3 mEq/L. No controlled trials have compared epinephrine to dopamine or dobutamine as the intitial treatment of hypotensive premature newborns.

Dopamine, the immediate precursor of norepinephrine, is unique among inotropes because it dilates renal, coronary, and mesenteric vascular beds of adults at low doses through activation of the D_1-dopaminergic receptors [56]. Dopamine exerts some of its effects through release of endogenous norepinephrine, which may become depleted during prolonged infusions [56]. Dopamine does not cross the blood-brain barrier, so there is no interaction with central nervous system dopamine receptors. Extravasation of dopamine may cause severe ischemic tissue damage, which may be treated by local infiltration of diluted phentolamine [61].

The dose–response relationship of dopamine in regards to raising blood pressure in neonates seems to begin at 2 mcg/kg/min [62]; however, the upper limit of dopamine's dose response in neonates has not been defined. At high concentrations, dopamine's alpha$_1$ receptor activity is reported to cause vasoconstriction in all circulations [55]. Studies of renal vascular resistance in newborn animals receiving 32 to 50 μg/kg/minute of dopamine have not detected this effect [63,64]. Similarly high-dose (30–50 μg/kg/min) infusions in oliguric, hypotensive, near-term newborns improved urine output and increased heart rate, suggesting that the alpha$_1$ vasoconstrictor effects that are expected at high dosages may not predominate and may not decrease renal perfusion in all newborns [65].

The regional blood-flow effects of dopamine have been studied in premature newborns using Doppler measures of blood-flow velocity to derive a pulsatility index (PI), which provides indirect evidence of vascular tone. The greater the degree of initial vasoconstriction in the renal arteries, the greater the degree of dopamine-induced vasodilation as measured by a decrease in PI [66]. Whereas dopamine did not change flow in the cerebral or mesenteric arteries, aortic blood pressure increased without changing aortic PI, suggesting peripheral vasoconstriction as the mechanism. A related study of dopamine in 18 hypotensive preterm newborns who had patent ductus arteriosus estimated pulmonary and systemic blood pressures after dopamine treatment using Doppler blood flow velocities [67]. In this study, pulmonary/systemic artery mean blood pressure ratio decreased or remained the same in 9 patients and increased in 9 others. In 2 patients who had lower baseline pulmonary artery blood pressure, the increase in pulmonary artery pressure was sufficient to reverse ductal flow and create a right-to-left shunt. For the 9 neonates whose mean pulmonary artery pressure/mean systemic blood pressure (mPAP/mSBP) increased, the increase was similar in magnitude to the decrease in the other 9 (+17% versus −19%). This unpredictability of pulmonary artery response implies that dopamine needs to be used carefully and with frequent reevaluation of its effects.

Dobutamine is the product of directed structural manipulation of dopamine and isoproterenol to produce hydroxyphenyl-isobutyl-dopamine (dobutamine), an inotrope designed to increase contractility without significant tachycardia or vasodilation [68]. Initially, dobutamine was thought to possess balanced vascular alpha$_1$ and beta$_2$ activities. Later study demonstrated that dobutamine exists in two enantiomorphic forms, each with different receptor activities [69]. The (−) isomer is a potent alpha$_1$-agonist that increases cardiac contractility, whereas the (+) isomer is a potent alpha$_2$-antagonist. The (+) isomer is several-fold more potent for beta receptors than the (−) isomer. Overall, dobutamine is more selective for beta$_1$ than for beta$_2$ receptors. With infusions at less than 20 μg/kg/min, dobutamine increases cardiac output and contractility with minimal changes in peripheral resistance and modest increases in heart rate [56]. In neonates, dosages of 5 and 7.5 μg /kg/min increased cardiac output without changing heart rate or blood pressure [70]. The lack of vasoconstriction may limit dobutamine's usefulness in patients who have severe hypotension, but may be useful in patients who have cardiogenic failure in whom cardiac function may worsen with increased afterload.

The effectiveness of dopamine and dobutamine to raise blood pressure has been studied in hypotensive, premature newborns who had respiratory distress syndrome [71–74]. In this specific group of neonates who do not have asphyxia or sepsis, dopamine is more effective than dobutamine for treatment of hypotension unresponsive to volume expansion, likely related to the peripheral vasodilating effects of dobutamine and the vasoconstricting effects of dopamine. The effects of dobutamine and dopamine on systemic blood pressure and flow were compared using SVC blood flow velocity [74]. Although dopamine raised blood pressure to a greater degree, dobutamine increased SVC blood-flow velocity more than dopamine, consistent with lowering systemic vascular resistance while increasing cardiac output.

Inamrinone and milrinone

Phosphodiesterase inhibitors represent a new class of inotropic drugs for newborns, although they have been used extensively since the 1980s to treat adults and older children, especially following cardiac surgery [75,76]. These drugs increase cardiac output through a combination of increased contractility and decreased afterload without receptor interactions. In contrast to catecholamines that increase intracellular cyclic AMP through activation of adenyl cyclase, these newer bipyridine compounds increase cyclic AMP by inhibition of the cyclic nucleotide phosphodiesterase.

The first of these drugs studied, approved, and used to treat neonates was amrinone, which has since been renamed inamrinone to prevent drug name confusion with amiodarone [77–81]. Rapid redistribution of inamrinone after cardiac surgery creates complex pharmacokinetics. Neonates have a smaller distribution volume and lower clearance of inamrinone than infants, despite equal rates of N-acetylation, leading to a half-life of 10.7 hours versus 6.1 hours for infants [82].

In infants, inamrinone increases cardiac index more than nitroprusside alone, likely caused by the combination of increased cardiac contractility and vasodilation [78]. The use of inamrinone has been limited because of potential for developing reversible thrombocytopenia in 20% [76] to 44% of patients [83]. The latter study found that thrombocytopenia correlated with the area under the concentration time curve of N-acetylamrinone, but not that of inamrinone [83].

Milrinone represents the next generation of bipyridine phosphodiesterase inhibitor to be marketed in the United States. In an open-labeled study of 10 neonates who had low cardiac output after cardiac surgery, milrinone treatment (50 µg/kg loading dose followed by 0.50 µg/kg/min for 30 minutes) increased heart rate, decreased average atrial pressures, decreased systemic and pulmonary arterial pressures, and increased cardiac index in 9 of 10 patients [84] while decreasing systemic and pulmonary vascular resistances. Hoffman studied 238 infants greater than 35 weeks postconceptual age undergoing cardiac surgery [75]. In this study, high-dose milrinone (75 µg/kg over 60 minutes followed by 0.75 µg/kg/min for 35 hours) was superior to low-dose milrinone (25 µg/kg over 60 minutes followed by 0.25 µg/kg/min for 35 hours) and to placebo for prevention of low cardiac output state (9.6% in high dose, 17.7% in low dose, and 26.7% in placebo) [75]. As with inamrinone, milrinone has a lower clearance in infants than in children and has been associated with the development of thrombocytopenia [85]. Before adopting widespread treatment of premature neonates with milrinone, the kinetics and cardiovascular effects must be studied in this population. Maturation of responses by the heart and vasculature might occur at different rates and predispose to excessive vasodilatation and hypotension. The phosphodiesterase inhibitors, however, may provide an important new treatment for low cardiac output in neonates that avoids adrenergic receptor down-regulation, and depletion of endogenous catecholamines.

Digoxin

Digoxin remains a useful drug for the chronic treatment of CHF. The efficacy of digitalis for the treatment of CHF varies according to myocardial dynamics [86]. In a study of 21 infants who had CHF caused by ventricular septal defects, digoxin improved 12 by clinical evaluation, but only 6 by echocardiographic measurements [87]. The half-life of digoxin averages 35 hours (range 17–52 hours) in term newborns and 57 hours (range 38–88 hours) in premature neonates who had birth weights greater than 1150 grams [88]. This difference in half-life likely reflects differences in renal function between term and preterm neonates [89] and suggests that premature neonates require a smaller digoxin maintenance dose [90]. Digoxin toxicity, like efficacy, is not defined by a specific concentration, but by signs and symptoms, such as emesis, arrhythmias, or conduction abnormalities, for example complete heart block [91]. Various drugs may increase digoxin concentrations, such as antibiotics that reduce inactivation by gut flora [92], spironolactone that reduces its clearance [93], and amiodarone that may either reduce the clearance or increase the bioavailability of digoxin [23]. Life-threatening arrhythmias resulting from excessive digitalis concentrations may be treated successfully with antidigoxin Fab antibody fragments [94].

Older assays for therapeutic monitoring of digoxin cross-reacted with an endogenous molecule, digoxin-like immunoreactive substance (DLIS), which was increased in the circulation of preterm newborns, pregnant women, and patients who have renal failure [95,96]. This cross-reactivity with the newer assays has been eliminated, and the circulating DLIS has been identified as ouabain [97].

Pulmonary vasodilators

Because the pulmonary vasculature of many neonates is in parallel with the systemic vasculature, through patency of the ductus arteriosus and foramen ovale, an effective pulmonary vasodilator must dilate the pulmonary vasculature more than the systemic vasculature [98]. Endothelium-derived relaxing factor was shown to be involved in control of the perinatal pulmonary circulation as it dilates after birth [99,100]. It was shown to have the same properties as nitric oxide (NO) [101]. NO dilates pulmonary arteries selectively through release of cyclic guanosine monophosphate (cGMP) [102,103]. Infants who have persistent pulmonary hypertension of the newborn (PPHN) have lower circulating cGMP, likely because of inadequate NO production needed to dilate the pulmonary vasculature after birth [104]. The selectivity of NO for the pulmonary vasculature derives from its administration by inhalation and inactivation by binding to hemoglobin as soon as it enters the blood stream. This same binding, however, may induce methemoglobinemia at higher doses of NO [105]. NO is a highly reactive compound whose dose must be carefully monitored to avoid potentially severe or even lethal toxicity [102].

Improved oxygenation and a reduced need for extracorporeal membrane oxygenation (ECMO), have been demonstrated in randomized, controlled trials of NO treatment of near-term neonates who have respiratory failure [106–110]. A metaanalysis of 12 controlled trials found that NO improves oxygenation in about 50% of treated patients and significantly reduces the need for ECMO. No improvement in outcome was demonstrated for infants who had diaphragmatic hernia. Although NO has been used to treat a variety of disorders [111], when respiratory failure is accompanied by pulmonary disease and severe infiltrates, NO treatment is less successful, possibly because inhalational delivery does not reach the pulmonary vasculature [112]. Dose–response studies indicate that neonates achieve maximum improvement in oxygenation at 20 ppm [113] to 40 ppm [114–116]. Prolonged treatment longer than 10 days has been associated with pulmonary toxicity demonstrated by detection of nitrotyrosine [117]. Platelet function has been reduced during NO treatment of adults, likely through increased cGMP, and may represent a risk for neonates [118]. In the critically-ill neonatal population treated with NO, long-term outcome should be evaluated in comparison with control, comparably sick infants not exposed to NO. From a randomized, controlled study of NO treatment in 248 neonates, evaluation at

1 year showed no increase in mortality, reactive airway disease, chronic lung disease, or developmental delay in the NO-treated group [119].

Although NO was approved for the near-term neonate who has pulmonary hypertension, preterm neonates of less than 32 weeks gestation have been treated with NO [120]. A group of 70 infants born at 23 to 31 weeks gestation who had hypoxic respiratory failure defined by alveolar-arterial oxygen gradient (AaO2) less than 22 mmHg were randomized to treatment with 5 ppm NO or no treatment, and pulmonary blood flow velocity was measured by Doppler. NO treatment increased pulmonary blood flow and significantly improved oxygenation with a 71% increase in AaO2.

Several other drugs have been used for treatment of PPHN, including to-lazoline, PGE_1, PGI_2, PGD_2, acetylcholine, isoproterenol, chlorpromazine, nitroprusside, and sildenafil [121]. None of these drugs have proven to be selective for the pulmonary vasculature. Although tolazoline has been reported to improve oxygenation in approximately 60% of patients, high mortality persisted, and adverse effects occurred at an unacceptably high rate [122]. Improvement in oxygenation was recently reported in 72% of 43 extremely low birth weight (ELBW) neonates whose birth weight was less than 750 grams who were treated with slow bolus tolazoline infusions of 0.5 to 2.0 mg/kg [123]. Inappropriately high prolonged infusion doses of tolazoline, used without the guidance of kinetic studies, may have contributed to the high rate of adverse effects associated with tolazoline treatment [122]. Despite this recent report of efficacy of tolazoline in ELBW neonates, it has been removed from production.

Investigations of the mechanisms through which NO controls neonatal pulmonary vascular tone and the mechanisms that control NO production in the pulmonary vasculature point to potential new alternatives for treatment of PPHN [100,102]. Inhibition of phosphodiesterase 5 increases cGMP and dilates pulmonary arteries. Despite hopes that sildenafil, a phosphodiesterase 5 inhibitor, would be a specific pulmonary vasodilator, a small randomized study in infants following cardiac surgery found that sildenafil reduced systemic and pulmonary vascular resistance and worsened oxygenation and the aAO2 gradient [124]. Studies of prostacyclin administered via the airway have shown promise in a small number of neonates who have PPHN, but controlled studies are needed to evaluate the efficacy of this prostanoid [125,126]. For now, inhaled NO remains the only selective pulmonary vasodilator in neonates. Alternate drug treatment may still be successful at improving pulmonary perfusion in patients who have PPHN, but their effectiveness must be confirmed in appropriate controlled trials.

References

[1] Grant AO. Mechanisms of action of antiarrhythmic drugs: from ion channel blockage to arrhythmia termination. Pacing Clin Electrophysiol 1997;20(2 Pt 2):432–44.

[2] Perry JC. Pharmacologic therapy of arrhythmias. In: Deal BJ, Wolff G, Gelband H, editors. Current concepts in diagnosis and management of arrhythmias in infants and children. Armonk, (NY): Futura Publishing Co., Inc.; 1998. p. 267–305.

[3] Vaughan Williams EM. Classification of antiarrhythmic drugs. In: Sandoe E, Flensted-Jensen E, Olsen EH, editors. Symposium on cardiac arrhythmias. Denmark: Astra; 1970. p. 449–501.

[4] Young M-L, Deal BJ, Wolff GS. Supraventricular tachycardia—electrophysiologic evaluation and treatment. In: Deal BJ, Wolff G, Gelband H, editors. Current concepts in diagnosis and management of arrhythmias in infants and children. Armonk (NY): Futura Publishing Co., Inc; 1998. p. 145–79.

[5] Roberts RJ. Drug therapy in infants. pharmacologic principles and clinical experience. Philadelphia: WB Saunders Company; 1984.

[6] American Academy of Pediatrics Committee on Drugs. Drugs for pediatric emergencies. Pediatrics 1998;10:e13.

[7] Deal BJ. Supraventricular tachycardia mechanisms and natural history. In: Deal BJ, Wolff G, Gelband H, editors. Current concepts in diagnosis and management of arrhythmias in infants and children. Armonk (NY): Futura Publishing Co., Inc.; 1998. p. 117–43.

[8] Cilliers AM, du Plessis JP, Clur SA, et al. Junctional ectopic tachycardia in six paediatric patients. Heart 1997;78(4):413–5.

[9] Garson Jr A, Gillette PC. Junctional ectopic tachycardia in children: electrocardiography, electrophysiology and pharmacologic response. Am J Cardiol 1979;44(2):298–302.

[10] Ludomirsky A, Garson Jr A. Supraventricular tachycardia. In: Gillette PC, Garson Jr A, editors. Pediatric arrhythmias: electrophysiology and pacing. Philadelphia: WB Saunders; 1990. p. 380–426.

[11] Pfammatter JP, Stocker FP. Re-entrant supraventricular tachycardia in infancy: current role of prophylactic digoxin treatment. Eur J Pediatr 1998;157(2):101–6.

[12] Luedtke SA, Kuhn RJ, McCaffrey FM. Pharmacologic management of supraventricular tachycardias in children. Part 2: atrial flutter, atrial fibrillation, and junctional and atrial ectopic tachycardia. Ann Pharmacother 1997;31(11):1347–59.

[13] Paret G, Steinmetz D, Kuint J, et al. Adenosine for the treatment of paroxysmal supraventricular tachycardia in full-term and preterm newborn infants. Am J Perinatol 1996;13(6):343–6.

[14] Smits P, Lenders JW, Thien T. Caffeine and theophylline attenuate adenosine-induced vaso-dilation in humans. Clin Pharmacol Ther 1990;48(4):410–8.

[15] Berul CI. Higher adenosine dosage required for supraventricular tachycardia in infants treated with theophylline. Clin Pediatr (Phila) 1993;32(3):167–8.

[16] Moak JP. Pharmacology and electrophysiology of antiarrhythmic drugs. In: Gillette PC, Garson Jr A, editors. Pediatric arrhythmias: electrophysiology and pacing. Philadelphia: WB Saunders; 1990. p. 37–115.

[17] Reidenberg MM, Drayer DE, Levy M, et al. Polymorphic acetylation procainamide in man. Clin Pharmacol Ther 1975;17(6):722–30.

[18] Leeder JS, Kearns GL. Pharmacogenetics in pediatrics. Implications for practice. Pediatr Clin North Am 1997;44(1):55–77.

[19] Lemler MS, Schaffer MS. Neonatal supraventricular tachycardia: predictors of successful treatment withdrawal. Am Heart J 1997;133(1):130–1.

[20] Byrum CJ, Wahl RA, Behrendt DM, et al. Ventricular fibrillation associated with use of digitalis in a newborn infant with Wolff-Parkinson-White syndrome. J Pediatr 1982;101(3):400–3.

[21] Nies AS, Shand DG. Clinical pharmacology of propranolol. Circulation 1975;52(1):6–15.

[22] Epstein ML, Kiel EA, Victorica BE. Cardiac decompensation following verapamil therapy in infants with supraventricular tachycardia. Pediatrics 1985;75(4):737–40.

[23] Mason JW. Amiodarone. N Engl J Med 1987;316(8):455–66.

[24] Kodama I, Kamiya K, Toyama J. Cellular electropharmacology of amiodarone. Cardiovasc Res 1997;35(1):13–29.

[25] Ardura J, Hermoso F, Bermejo J. Effect on growth of children with cardiac dysrhythmias treated with amiodarone. Pediatr Cardiol 1988;9(1):33–6.

[26] Keeton BR, Bucknall CA, Curry PV, et al. Use of amiodarone in childhood. Br J Clin Pract Suppl 1986;44:115–20.

[27] Daniels CJ, Schutte DA, Hammond S, et al. Acute pulmonary toxicity in an infant from intravenous amiodarone. Am J Cardiol 1997;80(8):1113–6.

[28] Perry JC, Fenrich AL, Hulse JE, et al. Pediatric use of intravenous amiodarone: efficacy and safety in critically ill patients from a multicenter protocol. J Am Coll Cardiol 1996;27(5): 1246–50.

[29] Dodo H, Gow RM, Hamilton RM, et al. Chaotic atrial rhythm in children. Am Heart J 1995; 129(5):990–5.

[30] Fish FA, Mehta AV, Johns JA. Characteristics and management of chaotic atrial tachycardia of infancy. Am J Cardiol 1996;78(9):1052–5.

[31] Bouillon T, Schiffmann H, Bartmus D, et al. Amiodarone in a newborn with ventricular tachycardia and an intracardiac tumor: adjusting the dose according to an individualized dosing regimen. Pediatr Cardiol 1996;17(2):112–4.

[32] Chen RP, Ignaszewski AP, Robertson MA. Successful treatment of supraventricular tachycardia-induced cardiomyopathy with amiodarone: case report and review of literature. Can J Cardiol 1995;11(10):918–22.

[33] Rosenberg EM, Elbl F, Solinger RE, et al. Neonatal refractory supraventricular tachycardia: successful treatment with amiodarone. South Med J 1988;81(4):539–40.

[34] Burri S, Hug MI, Bauersfeld U. Efficacy and safety of intravenous amiodarone for incessant tachycardias in infants. Eur J Pediatr 2003;162(12):880–4.

[35] Fenrich Jr AL, Perry JC, Friedman RA. Flecainide and amiodarone: combined therapy for refractory tachyarrhythmias in infancy. J Am Coll Cardiol 1995;25(5):1195–8.

[36] Etheridge SP, Craig JE, Compton SJ. Amiodarone is safe and highly effective therapy for supraventricular tachycardia in infants. Am Heart J 2001;141(1):105–10.

[37] Kannan R, Yabek SM, Garson Jr A, et al. Amiodarone efficacy in a young population: relationship to serum amiodarone and desethylamiodarone levels. Am Heart J 1987;114(2): 283–7.

[38] Vrobel TR, Miller PE, Mostow ND, et al. A general overview of amiodarone toxicity: its prevention, detection, and management. Prog Cardiovasc Dis 1989;31(6):393–426.

[39] De Wolf D, De Schepper J, Verhaaren H, et al. Congenital hypothyroid goiter and amiodarone. Acta Paediatr Scand 1988;77(4):616–8.

[40] Laurent M, Betremieux P, Biron Y, et al. Neonatal hypothyroidism after treatment by amiodarone during pregnancy. Am J Cardiol 1987;60(10):942.

[41] Magee LA, Downar E, Sermer M, et al. Pregnancy outcome after gestational exposure to amiodarone in Canada. Am J Obstet Gynecol 1995;172(4 Pt 1):1307–11.

[42] Tubman R, Jenkins J, Lim J. Neonatal hyperthyroxinaemia associated with maternal amiodarone therapy: case report. Ir J Med Sci 1988;157(7):243.

[43] Zubrow AB, Hulman S, Kushner H, et al. Determinants of blood pressure in infants admitted to neonatal intensive care units: a prospective multicenter study. Philadelphia Neonatal Blood Pressure Study Group. J Perinatol 1995;15(6):470–9.

[44] Flynn JT. Neonatal hypertension: diagnosis and management. Pediatr Nephrol 2000;14(4): 332–41.

[45] National High Blood Pressure Education Program Working Group on High Blood Pressure in Children and Adolescents. The fourth report on the diagnosis, evaluation, and treatment of high blood pressure in children and adolescents. Pediatrics 2004;114:555–76.

[46] Wiest DB, Garner SS, Uber WE, et al. Esmolol for the management of pediatric hypertension after cardiac operations. J Thorac Cardiovasc Surg 1998;115(4):890–7.

[47] Milou C, Debuche-Benouachkou V, Semama DS, et al. Intravenous nicardipine as a first-line antihypertensive drug in neonates. Intensive Care Med 2000;26(7):956–8.

[48] Gouyon JB, Geneste B, Semama DS, et al. Intravenous nicardipine in hypertensive preterm infants. Arch Dis Child Fetal Neonatal Ed 1997;76(2):F126–7.

[49] Wells TG, Bunchman TE, Kearns GL. Treatment of neonatal hypertension with enalaprilat. J Pediatr 1990;117(4):664–7.

[50] Bauer SB, Feldman SM, Gellis SS, et al. Neonatal hypertension. a complication of umbilical–artery catheterization. N Engl J Med 1975;293(20):1032–3.

[51] Nahata MC, Morosco RS, Hipple TF. Stability of captopril in three liquid dosage forms. Am J Hosp Pharm 1994;51(1):95–6.

[52] O'Dea RF, Mirkin BL, Alward CT, et al. Treatment of neonatal hypertension with captopril. J Pediatr 1988;113(2):403–6.

[53] Romankiewicz JA, Brogden RN, Heel RC, et al. Captopril: an update review of its pharmacological properties and therapeutic efficacy in congestive heart failure. Drugs 1983;25(1):6–40.

[54] Strauser LM, Groshong T, Tobias JD. Initial experience with isradipine for the treatment of hypertension in children. South Med J 2000;93(3):287–93.

[55] Driscoll DJ. Use of inotropic and chronotropic agents in neonates. Clin Perinatol 1987;14(4):931–49.

[56] Hoffman BB. Catecholamines, sympathomimetic drugs, and adrenergic receptor antagonists. In: Hardman JG, Limbird LE, Gilman AG, editors. Goodman & Gilman's the pharmacological basis of therapeutics. 10th edition. New York: McGraw-Hill; 2001. p. 215–68.

[57] Zaritsky A, Chernow B. Use of catecholamines in pediatrics. J Pediatr 1984;105(3):341–50.

[58] Hoffman BB, Taylor P. Neurotransmission: The autonomic and somatic motor nervous systems. In: Hardman JG, Limbird LE, Gilman AG, editors. Goodman and Gilman's the pharmacological basis of therapeutics. 10th edition. New York: McGraw Hill; 2001. p. 115–53.

[59] Rude RE, Bush LR, Izquierdo C, et al. Effects of inotropic and chronotropic stimuli on acute myocardial ischemic injury. III. Influence of basal heart rate. Am J Cardiol 1984;53(11):1688–94.

[60] Heckmann M, Trotter A, Pohlandt F, et al. Epinephrine treatment of hypotension in very low birthweight infants. Acta Paediatr 2002;91(5):566–70.

[61] Siwy BK, Sadove AM. Acute management of dopamine infiltration injury with Regitine. Plast Reconstr Surg 1987;80(4):610–2.

[62] Seri I, Tulassay T, Kiszel J, et al. Cardiovascular response to dopamine in hypotensive preterm neonates with severe hyaline membrane disease. Eur J Pediatr 1984;142(1):3–9.

[63] Driscoll DJ, Gillette PC, Lewis RM, et al. Comparative hemodynamic effects of isoproterenol, dopamine, and dobutamine in the newborn dog. Pediatr Res 1979;13(9):1006–9.

[64] Fiser DH, Fewell JE, Hill DE, et al. Cardiovascular and renal effects of dopamine and dobutamine in healthy, conscious piglets. Crit Care Med 1988;16(4):340–5.

[65] Perez CA, Reimer JM, Schreiber MD, et al. Effect of high-dose dopamine on urine output in newborn infants. Crit Care Med 1986;14(12):1045–9.

[66] Seri I, Abbasi S, Wood DC, et al. Regional hemodynamic effects of dopamine in the sick preterm neonate. J Pediatr 1998;133(6):728–34.

[67] Liet JM, Boscher C, Gras-Leguen C, et al. Dopamine effects on pulmonary artery pressure in hypotensive preterm infants with patent ductus arteriosus. J Pediatr 2002;140(3):373–5.

[68] Tuttle RR, Mills J. Dobutamine: development of a new catecholamine to selectively increase cardiac contractility. Circ Res 1975;36(1):185–96.

[69] Ruffolo Jr RR, Yaden EL. Vascular effects of the stereoisomers of dobutamine. J Pharmacol Exp Ther 1983;224(1):46–50.

[70] Martinez AM, Padbury JF, Thio S. Dobutamine pharmacokinetics and cardiovascular responses in critically ill neonates. Pediatrics 1992;89(1):47–51.

[71] Roze JC, Tohier C, Maingueneau C, et al. Response to dobutamine and dopamine in the hypotensive very preterm infant. Arch Dis Child 1993;69(1 Spec No):59–63.

[72] Greenough A, Emery EF. Randomized trial comparing dopamine and dobutamine in preterm infants. Eur J Pediatr 1993;152(11):925–7.

[73] Klarr JM, Faix RG, Pryce CJ, et al. Randomized, blind trial of dopamine versus dobutamine for treatment of hypotension in preterm infants with respiratory distress syndrome. J Pediatr 1994;125(1):117–22.

[74] Osborn D, Evans N, Kluckow M. Randomized trial of dobutamine versus dopamine in preterm infants with low systemic blood flow. J Pediatr 2002;140(2):183–91.

[75] Hoffman TM, Wernovsky G, Atz AM, et al. Efficacy and safety of milrinone in preventing low cardiac output syndrome in infants and children after corrective surgery for congenital heart disease. Circulation 2003;107(7):996–1002.

[76] Ward A, Brogden RN, Heel RC, et al. Amrinone. a preliminary review of its pharmacological properties and therapeutic use. Drugs 1983;26(6):468–502.

[77] Williams GD, Sorensen GK, Oakes R, et al. Amrinone loading during cardiopulmonary bypass in neonates, infants, and children. J Cardiothorac Vasc Anesth 1995;9(3):278–82.

[78] Bailey JM, Miller BE, Kanter KR, et al. A comparison of the hemodynamic effects of amrinone and sodium nitroprusside in infants after cardiac surgery. Anesth Analg 1997;84(2):294–8.

[79] Laitinen P, Happonen JM, Sairanen H, et al. Amrinone versus dopamine-nitroglycerin after reconstructive surgery for complete atrioventricular septal defect. J Cardiothorac Vasc Anesth 1997;11(7):870–4.

[80] Laitinen P, Happonen JM, Sairanen H, et al. Amrinone versus dopamine and nitroglycerin in neonates after arterial switch operation for transposition of the great arteries. J Cardiothorac Vasc Anesth 1999;13(2):186–90.

[81] Levy JH, Bailey JM. Phosphodiesterase inhibitors: the inotropes of choice for the new millennium? J Cardiothorac Vasc Anesth 2000;14(4):365–6.

[82] Laitinen P, Ahonen J, Olkkola KT, et al. Pharmacokinetics of amrinone in neonates and infants. J Cardiothorac Vasc Anesth 2000;14(4):378–82.

[83] Ross MP, Allen-Webb EM, Pappas JB, et al. Amrinone-associated thrombocytopenia: pharmacokinetic analysis. Clin Pharmacol Ther 1993;53(6):661–7.

[84] Chang AC, Atz AM, Wernovsky G, et al. Milrinone: systemic and pulmonary hemodynamic effects in neonates after cardiac surgery. Crit Care Med 1995;23(11):1907–14.

[85] Ramamoorthy C, Anderson GD, Williams GD, et al. Pharmacokinetics and side effects of milrinone in infants and children after open heart surgery. Anesth Analg 1998;86(2):283–9.

[86] Smith TW. Digitalis: mechanisms of action and clinical use. N Engl J Med 1988;318(6):358–65.

[87] Berman Jr W, Yabek SM, Dillon T, et al. Effects of digoxin in infants with congested circulatory state due to a ventricular septal defect. N Engl J Med 1983;308(7):363–6.

[88] Lang D, von Bernuth G. Serum concentration and serum half-life of digoxin in premature and mature newborns. Pediatrics 1977;59(6):902–6.

[89] Steiness E. Renal tubular secretion of digoxin. Circulation 1974;50(1):103–7.

[90] Hastreiter AR, van der Horst RL, Voda C, et al. Maintenance digoxin dosage and steady-state plasma concentration in infants and children. J Pediatr 1985;107(1):140–6.

[91] Ingelfinger JA, Goldman P. The serum digitalis concentration—does it diagnose digitalis toxicity? N Engl J Med 1976;294(16):867–70.

[92] Lindenbaum J, Rund DG, Butler Jr VP, et al. Inactivation of digoxin by the gut flora: reversal by antibiotic therapy. N Engl J Med 1981;305(14):789–94.

[93] Waldorff S, Andersen JD, Heeboll-Nielsen N, et al. Spironolactone-induced changes in digoxin kinetics. Clin Pharmacol Ther 1978;24(2):162–7.

[94] Smith TW, Butler Jr VP, Haber E, et al. Treatment of life-threatening digitalis intoxication with digoxin-specific Fab antibody fragments: experience in 26 cases. N Engl J Med 1982;307(22):1357–62.

[95] Seccombe DW, Pudek MR, Whitfield MF, et al. Perinatal changes in a digoxin-like immuno-reactive substance. Pediatr Res 1984;18(11):1097–9.

[96] Valdes Jr R. Endogenous digoxin-immunoactive factor in human subjects. Fed Proc 1985;44(12):2800–5.

[97] Mathews WR, DuCharme DW, Hamlyn JM, et al. Mass spectral characterization of an endogenous digitalis-like factor from human plasma. Hypertension 1991;17(6 Pt 2):930–5.

[98] Ward RM. Persistent pulmonary hypertension. In: Nelson NM, editor. Current therapy in neonatal-perinatal medicine-2. Toronto: BC Decker; 1990. p. 331–8.

[99] Abman SH, Chatfield BA, Hall SL, et al. Role of endothelium-derived relaxing factor during transition of pulmonary circulation at birth. Am J Physiol 1990;259(6 Pt 2):H1921–7.

[100] Shaul PW. Ontogeny of nitric oxide in the pulmonary vasculature. Semin Perinatol 1997;21(5):381–92.

[101] Palmer RM, Ferrige AG, Moncada S. Nitric oxide release accounts for the biological activity of endothelium-derived relaxing factor. Nature 1987;327(6122):524–6.

[102] McAndrew J, Patel RP, Jo H, et al. The interplay of nitric oxide and peroxynitrite with signal transduction pathways: implications for disease. Semin Perinatol 1997;21(5):351–66.

[103] Steinhorn RH, Morin 3rd FC, Fineman JR. Models of persistent pulmonary hypertension of

the newborn (PPHN) and the role of cyclic guanosine monophosphate (GMP) in pulmonary vasorelaxation. Semin Perinatol 1997;21(5):393–408.

[104] Christou H, Adatia I, Van Marter LJ, et al. Effect of inhaled nitric oxide on endothelin-1 and cyclic guanosine 5'-monophosphate plasma concentrations in newborn infants with persistent pulmonary hypertension. J Pediatr 1997;130(4):603–11.

[105] Nakajima W, Ishida A, Arai H, et al. Methaemoglobinaemia after inhalation of nitric oxide in infant with pulmonary hypertension. Lancet 1997;350(9083):1002–3.

[106] Finer NN, Barrington KJ. Nitric oxide in respiratory failure in the newborn infant. Semin Perinatol 1997;21(5):426–40.

[107] Kinsella JP, Truog WE, Walsh WF, et al. Randomized, multicenter trial of inhaled nitric oxide and high-frequency oscillatory ventilation in severe, persistent pulmonary hypertension of the newborn. J Pediatr 1997;131(1 Pt 1):55–62.

[108] Roberts Jr JD, Fineman JR, Morin III FC, et al. Inhaled nitric oxide and persistent pulmonary hypertension of the newborn. The Inhaled Nitric Oxide Study Group. N Engl J Med 1997; 336(9):605–10.

[109] Cornfield DN, Maynard RC, deRegnier RA, et al. Randomized, controlled trial of low-dose inhaled nitric oxide in the treatment of term and near-term infants with respiratory failure and pulmonary hypertension. Pediatrics 1999;104(5 Pt 1):1089–94.

[110] Finer NN, Barrington KJ. Nitric oxide for respiratory failure in infants born at or near term. Cochrane Database Syst Rev 2001;4:CD000399.

[111] Nelin LD, Hoffman GM. The use of inhaled nitric oxide in a wide variety of clinical problems. Pediatr Clin N Am 1998;45(3):531–48.

[112] Day RW, Lynch JM, White KS, et al. Acute response to inhaled nitric oxide in newborns with respiratory failure and pulmonary hypertension. Pediatrics 1996;98(4 Pt 1):698–705.

[113] Demirakca S, Dotsch J, Knothe C, et al. Inhaled nitric oxide in neonatal and pediatric acute respiratory distress syndrome: dose response, prolonged inhalation, and weaning. Crit Care Med 1996;24(11):1913–9.

[114] Lonnqvist PA. Inhaled nitric oxide in newborn and paediatric patients with pulmonary hypertension and moderate to severe impaired oxygenation: effects of doses of 3–100 parts per million. Intensive Care Med 1997;23(7):773–9.

[115] Nakagawa TA, Morris A, Gomez RJ, et al. Dose response to inhaled nitric oxide in pediatric patients with pulmonary hypertension and acute respiratory distress syndrome. J Pediatr 1997; 131(1 Pt 1):63–9.

[116] Tworetzky W, Bristow J, Moore P, et al. Inhaled nitric oxide in neonates with persistent pulmonary hypertension. Lancet 2001;357(9250):118–20.

[117] Hallman M, Bry K, Turbow R, et al. Pulmonary toxicity associated with nitric oxide in term infants with severe respiratory failure. J Pediatr 1998;132(5):827–9.

[118] Cheung PY, Salas E, Schulz R, et al. Nitric oxide and platelet function: implications for neonatology. Semin Perinatol 1997;21(5):409–17.

[119] Clark RH, Huckaby JL, Kueser TJ, et al. Low-dose nitric oxide therapy for persistent pulmonary hypertension: 1-year follow-up. J Perinatol 2003;23(4):300–3.

[120] Desandes R, Desandes E, Droulle P, et al. Inhaled nitric oxide improves oxygenation in very premature infants with low pulmonary blood flow. Acta Paediatr 2004;93(1):66–9.

[121] Kulik TJ, Lock JE. Pulmonary vasodilator therapy in persistent pulmonary hypertension of the newborn. Clin Perinatol 1984;11(3):693–701.

[122] Ward RM. Pharmacology of tolazoline. Clin Perinatol 1984;11(3):703–13.

[123] Nuntnarumit P, Korones SB, Yang W, et al. Efficacy and safety of tolazoline for treatment of severe hypoxemia in extremely preterm infants. Pediatrics 2002;109(5):852–6.

[124] Stocker C, Penny DJ, Brizard CP, et al. Intravenous sildenafil and inhaled nitric oxide: a randomised trial in infants after cardiac surgery. Intensive Care Med 2003;29(11):1996–2003.

[125] Ehlen M, Wiebe B. Iloprost in persistent pulmonary hypertension of the newborn. Cardiol Young 2003;13(4):361–3.

[126] Kelly LK, Porta NF, Goodman DM, et al. Inhaled prostacyclin for term infants with persistent pulmonary hypertension refractory to inhaled nitric oxide. J Pediatr 2002;141(6):830–2.

ELSEVIER
SAUNDERS

CLINICS IN
PERINATOLOGY

Clin Perinatol 32 (2005) 999–1015

Management of Low Birth Weight Infants with Congenital Heart Disease

Anne Ades, MD[a,*], Beth Ann Johnson, MD, MA[b],
Stuart Berger, MD[b,c]

[a]Division of Neonatology, Children's Hospital of Philadelphia, 2nd Floor Main Building,
34th and Civic Center Boulevard, Philadelphia, PA 19104, USA
[b]Herma Heart Center, Children's Hospital of Wisconsin, 9000 West Wisconsin Avenue, Milwaukee,
WI 53226, USA
[c]Medical College of Wisconsin, Milwaukee, WI, USA

Low birth weight (LBW), defined as birth weight less than 2500 g, occurs in approximately 8% of births [1]. Congenital heart disease (CHD) is also quite common, with a prevalence of 4 in 1000 live births [2]. Infants may be of LBW because of prematurity or being small for gestational age (SGA). Several studies have revealed a higher incidence of LBW, SGA, and/or prematurity for many cardiac lesions [3–5]. Studies also have reported an incidence of 13% to 20% of associated congenital anomalies or genetic syndromes in infants with CHD [4–6]. Many congenital syndromes and chromosomal anomalies are associated with poor intrauterine growth. Thus, it is not surprising that up to 30% of infants who are of LBW and have CHD have associated extracardiac anomalies, syndromes, or chromosomal anomalies [7,8].

Infants who are of LBW and have CHD have a higher risk of mortality than infants with CHD who are not of LBW. This increased risk is most likely multifactorial, related to the underlying etiology of the LBW and technical issues related to the absolute size of the neonate. Management of this high-risk group of patients must take into account the pathophysiology of the CHD, the pathophysiology attributable to prematurity, intrauterine growth restriction, or the associated anomalies or syndromes as well as the absolute size of the neonate.

---

* Corresponding author.
E-mail address: ades@email.chop.edu (A. Ades).

0095-5108/05/$ – see front matter © 2005 Elsevier Inc. All rights reserved.
doi:10.1016/j.clp.2005.09.001   *perinatology.theclinics.com*

These factors also have an impact on surgical management in terms of the timing of surgery, the approach taken, and the procedure performed.

Pathophysiology associated with prematurity and intrauterine growth restriction

It is clear that even without CHD, infants who are premature or SGA have higher morbidity and mortality than those who are not. Prematurity is associated with organ immaturity, which predisposes infants to diseases, such as respiratory distress syndrome (RDS), chronic lung disease (CLD), necrotizing enterocolitis (NEC), infection, renal failure, intraventricular hemorrhage (IVH), periventricular leukomalacia, and retinopathy of prematurity (ROP). Term and preterm infants who are SGA are at higher risk of adverse outcomes, usually because of the underlying etiology of the SGA and intrauterine growth restriction. The etiology of being SGA is diverse, with fetal, maternal, and placental causes. Many of these etiologies have fetal hypoxia, abnormal fetal vascular flow patterns, or poor fetal nutrition as the end result, however. The in utero response and adaptations to these insults can become problematic after birth and affect many organ systems.

Pulmonary

Premature infants are at high risk of developing RDS because of surfactant deficiency. CLD is the end result of a variety of insults to the lungs, including lung immaturity, surfactant deficiency, oxygen toxicity, infection, poor nutrition, and mechanical ventilation. The incidence of RDS and CLD is as high as 50% and 23%, respectively, in very low birth weight (VLBW) infants (501–1500 g) [9]. The incidence of RDS and CLD increases significantly with decreasing gestational age and birth weight. The influence of being SGA on the incidence of RDS is unclear, with some studies reporting a higher incidence compared with counterparts matched for gestational age but of appropriate weight for gestational age and others studies showing no difference [10–12]. Most studies have found an increased risk of CLD in preterm infants who are SGA, however [11–13].

Pre- and postoperative management of the infant with CHD can be more difficult with accompanying lung disease. The guiding principle of managing patients with CHD who have ductal-dependent lesions is to ensure adequate systemic blood flow to avoid end-organ ischemia while maintaining adequate pulmonary blood flow to prevent severe hypoxemia at the same time. Changes in pulmonary compliance can affect pulmonary blood flow. Therefore, trying to maintain balanced pulmonary and systemic circulations may be difficult in premature infants with RDS and changes in pulmonary compliance attributable to surfactant therapy, resolving RDS, and evolving CLD. Surfactant is still the standard therapy for premature infants with RDS whether or not they have CHD. In some infants with abnormal chest radiographs and oxygenation on the basis of

CHD, such as may be seen in total anomalous pulmonary venous return and hypoplastic left heart syndrome (HLHS) with an intact atrial septum, the diagnosis of RDS may be unclear, however. This makes it difficult to determine whether interventions like repeated doses of surfactant are appropriate. In addition, although repeat surfactant doses are given routinely to preterm infants with an ongoing need for mechanical ventilation and supplemental oxygen, there is concern that with a large left-to-right shunt through a patent ductus arteriosus, pulmonary hemorrhage may occur with surfactant treatment. Presumably, infants with ductal-dependent lesions are also at risk of this complication, especially those who are dependent on the ductus arteriosus for pulmonary blood flow. Thus, the severity of the lung disease and benefit from surfactant therapy need to be weighed against the risks of treatment.

Several studies have shown evidence of surfactant dysfunction in infants and children undergoing cardiopulmonary bypass [14,15]. In addition, there is evidence that premature infants are at risk for surfactant dysfunction, even after the initial RDS has resolved [16]. Thus, secondary surfactant dysfunction may complicate the postoperative course in preterm and term infants with CHD. There are no reports in the literature on changes in outcome with postoperative administration of surfactant, however, and the postoperative infant may be less tolerant to the potential side effects of endotracheal tube obstruction, sinus bradycardia, and desaturation associated with the administration of surfactant.

The now common use of permissive hypercapnia in premature infants may be less desirable in an infant with CHD. Higher $PaCO_2$ levels may induce pulmonary vasoconstriction, and the accompanying lower pH may be detrimental to cardiac function. Nevertheless, there is reasonable evidence that hypocapnia puts preterm infants at higher risk for periventricular leukomalacia [17], cerebral palsy [18], and CLD [19]. Thus, attempts to maintain $PaCO_2$ levels at greater than 35 mm Hg before and after surgery may be beneficial in this subset of patients with CHD. The upper desirable limit for $PaCO_2$ and lower limit for pH depend on the type of heart disease and the severity of lung disease to balance the benefits and risks associated with permissive hypercapnia, especially given that permissive hypercapnia has thus far only been shown to improve CLD in a subgroup of infants with a birth weight of 501 to 750 g [20].

In general, the desired oxygen saturation levels to avoid pulmonary overcirculation in ductal-dependent lesions and those obtainable in cyanotic heart lesions are close to those now used for goal saturations in premature infants with RDS to minimize oxygen toxicity. In other cardiac lesions, maintaining this lower saturation goal should not be harmful, and saturation goals based on gestational age should be used per unit policy. Supplemental oxygen should be used as needed to maintain desired saturations in the face of lung disease if the cardiac physiology (ie, adequate pulmonary blood flow) and ventilatory support are otherwise optimal.

The need for prolonged support with mechanical ventilation attributable to lung disease also may make pre- and postoperative management more difficult and increase subsequent morbidity. There is a fine balance needed with positive pressure ventilation in maintaining appropriate lung inflation without adversely affecting right heart afterload. The current mode of ventilating postoperative cardiac patients typically uses high tidal volumes, low rates, and variable amounts of positive end-expiratory pressure (PEEP) depending on the expected post-operative physiology. Although this strategy minimizes effects on right heart afterload, these higher tidal volumes place immature lungs at high risk for ventilator-induced lung injury and subsequent CLD. A strategy of using more moderate settings immediately postoperatively and rapidly adjusting to the more traditional mode of ventilating premature infants with tidal volumes of 4 to 7 mL/kg and a higher rate, after the hemodynamic effects of surgery are improving, may be appropriate. In addition, many premature infants with RDS or evolving CLD need high PEEP on the ventilator or nasal continuous positive airway pressure (CPAP) to help stabilize the highly compliant chest wall. The added chest wall instability after a sternotomy may be ameliorated with the use of PEEP and CPAP. PEEP and CPAP are also useful to help prevent atelectasis and maintain functional residual capacity, but high levels of PEEP and CPAP can increase pulmonary vascular resistance and impede systemic venous return to the heart, particularly if the higher levels result in lung overdistention. Thus, it might be prudent to increase PEEP slowly so as to maintain the fine line of preventing atelectasis while preserving low pulmonary vascular resistance and adequate venous return.

Also, if complicated by increases in pulmonary vascular resistance, CLD could make staging to Fontan circulation more difficult, because patients with Fontan physiology are dependent on low pulmonary vascular resistance for pulmonary blood flow. There are no studies published yet on the influence of RDS or CLD on outcome in infants with CHD or on the influence of CHD on the incidence of RDS or CLD. One study did report that CLD was associated with late mortality in a population of patients operated on for CHD at a weight of less than 2500 g, however [21].

Cardiac

The myocardium of premature neonates is less compliant than that of term neonates or adults. This stiffness may confer a limited ability to increase cardiac output in response to a volume load and to respond to increases in afterload that may be seen after cardiopulmonary bypass. The inability to respond appropriately to volume overload could lead to impaired systemic blood flow in the face of a large left-to-right shunt associated with some forms of CHD. In addition, the neonatal myocardium is more sensitive to changes in calcium and relies more on glucose metabolism (compared with fat) than that of older patients. Thus, premature and SGA infants may be more at risk for myocardial dysfunction given their decreased stores of calcium, inadequate glycogen stores, and impaired gluconeogenesis. Monitoring these infants closely for hypoglycemia and hypo-calcemia is critical not only for the potential adverse cardiac effects but because of the other complications associated with hypoglycemia and hypocalcemia.

CHD itself with the associated abnormal cardiac physiology may prevent or alter some of the normal postnatal development of the heart. The fact that the newborn heart is more resistant to ischemia may temper some of the risks associated with surgery, however.

Hypotension is frequently seen in premature infants. Although hypotension can be caused by hypovolemia, hypotension in the preterm neonate is commonly attributable to myocardial dysfunction or altered peripheral vasoregulation. The first-line treatment for hypotension usually is volume administration; however, given the limitations of the immature myocardium to respond to volume as discussed previously, boluses should be limited to 10 to 20 mL/kg in the absence of known hypovolemia. Dopamine is frequently used after volume resuscitation and has been shown to be effective in preterm infants for improving blood pressure. The adverse effects of tachycardia and increased afterload with dopamine at higher doses may be detrimental, however, especially in the postoperative patient. Hydrocortisone is also used more frequently now in "pressor-resistant" hypotension or capillary leak syndromes, which are common in cardiac and premature infants. The effects of hydrocortisone on the developing premature brain are unclear; however, given the evidence associating dexamethasone with adverse neurodevelopmental outcomes and concerns of intestinal damage with steroid use, caution should be used with any steroid administration in premature patients.

Gastrointestinal

NEC is the most concerning disease of the gastrointestinal tract of premature infants given the profound deleterious effects on morbidity and mortality in those infants who develop NEC. The etiology of NEC is multifactorial, but hyperosmolar feeds, ischemia, infection, and immature gut host defenses have all been proposed as factors in the development of NEC in the preterm population. Again, as with RDS and CLD, the evidence for increased risk of NEC in SGA infants is unclear [10–13,22]. Several studies have documented abnormal mesenteric or umbilical artery flow in SGA and growth-restricted infants [23,24], however, which has been shown to be associated with an increased incidence of NEC [25,26]. Several studies have documented an increased risk of NEC in preterm and term patients with CHD [7,27,28]. In a population of preterm and term infants with CHD, factors associated with a higher risk for NEC included left-sided obstructive lesions, prematurity, prostaglandin doses greater than 0.05 μg/kg/min, and episodes of poor systemic perfusion [28]. Another study also showed a higher risk of NEC in infants who were premature with CHD compared with a control group of premature infants without CHD and again reported patients with left-sided obstructive lesions to be most at risk [7]. In both of these studies, most of the cases of NEC occurred before surgery. Given this increased risk of NEC, feedings are usually established and advanced slowly when they are able to be started before surgery or when they are started after surgery in preterm and severely growth-restricted patients. The ensuing inability to provide adequate enteral nutrition in these infants makes them dependent on central venous access for parenteral nutrition. Prolonged central venous access, however, increases the risk of line-associated infection as well as venous thrombosis. If concerns of NEC arise in these infants, particularly in those with left-sided obstructive lesions or those with larger ductal run-off, earlier correction of the heart defect may be indicated to prevent further bowel ischemia.

Renal

Preterm infants are at risk for disruption of fluid and electrolyte homeostasis because of renal glomerular and tubular immaturity. Extremely preterm infants are also at risk for dehydration because of increased insensible losses, particularly transepidermal water loss. Placement in a humidified isolette is important to prevent water loss and to maintain a thermoneutral environment. The immature tubular function leads to bicarbonate and sodium losses, thus requiring replacement to maintain normal sodium balance and avoid acidemia. Testing urine pH in these patients, in the face of acidemia, may be useful to clarify if all that is needed is replacement of renal losses of bicarbonate versus further investigation of other causes of acidemia, such as ischemia or hypoxia on the basis of the CHD. Frequent monitoring and close attention are needed to maintain adequate fluid and electrolyte balance, especially in the face of diuretic administration.

Premature infants are at higher risk for renal insufficiency than term infants because they have more immature kidneys functionally and anatomically. The kidneys of premature infants have even lower glomerular filtration rates, higher vascular resistance, and more impaired concentrating and diluting ability than those of term infants. The insults of poor systemic flow associated with some forms of CHD, cardiopulmonary bypass, and exposure to potentially nephrotoxic medications may further impair renal function. Thus, careful medication dosing and monitoring of levels, when appropriate, based on weight, postconceptional age, and renal function are important.

Brain

The immature germinal matrix of premature infants along with the physiologic instability of the perinatal period puts them at high risk for IVH. Most cases of IVH occur in the first 72 hours after birth, and most patients who develop severe IVH are younger than 30 weeks of gestational age and weigh less than 1000 g at birth. Given the heparinization, dilution of clotting factors, ischemia if circulatory arrest is used, postoperative thrombocytopenia, and ensuing hemodynamic instability that occur with cardiopulmonary bypass, one would predict that premature infants undergoing surgery for CHD would be at higher risk for developing IVH. Surprisingly, Dees and colleagues [7] showed a lower incidence of severe IVH in premature infants with CHD (mean weight of 1852 g, median gestational age of 33 weeks) compared with a similar gestational age group of premature infants without CHD (mean weight of 1533 g, median gestational age of 32 weeks). Other studies of LBW infants operated on for CHD also do not report significant incidences of IVH. In these studies, however, the LBW populations are diverse, with some milder forms of CHD not needing cardiopulmonary bypass for repair included; in general, the mean weight and gestational age are high and intracranial imaging is not routinely used. One study that routinely performed head ultrasound before and after surgery found no neurologic complications after surgery; however, the mean birth weight was 2190 g, and most of the patients were born at greater than 33 weeks of gestation [29]. In the most premature infants with CHD, it might be reasonable to delay the operative repair beyond the first few days of life, because that is the period of highest risk for the development of IVH. If moderate or severe IVH is present, delaying surgery if possible may help to prevent extension. The potential deleterious effects of unrepaired CHD should also be taken into consideration when deciding on the timing for surgery, however. In addition, treating thrombocytopenia and coagulation defects in the immediate postoperative period may be more important in preterm infants compared with term infants.

Premature infants and infants with CHD (before and after surgery) are also at high risk of periventricular leukomalacia and other neurologic morbidity, including worsened long-term neurodevelopmental outcomes. It is unknown at this time if the combination of prematurity and CHD increases the incidence of these adverse neurologic outcomes.

Retinopathy of prematurity

ROP is a disease found primarily in preterm infants less than 32 weeks of gestational age. Several factors have been implicated as increasing the risk of ROP, including white race, worse severity of illness, lower birth weight, and decreasing gestational age. In addition, patients exposed to oxygen and episodes of hyperoxia are at high risk for the development of ROP, especially if they are also premature. It might be expected that infants with cyanotic CHD would be less likely to develop ROP because they are rarely exposed to supplemental oxygen and usually do not achieve high PaO_2 levels. Only one study has attempted to evaluate this hypothesis [30]. This particular study identified six patients who were preterm, had cyanotic CHD, and met criteria to be evaluated for ROP. Of these six patients, three were diagnosed with ROP. It seems reasonable that infants with CHD should be screened as per unit policy or the American Academy of Pediatrics guidelines based on gestational age and birth weight, especially given that there is some evidence that hypoxic episodes may also be a risk factor for ROP [31,32]. Again, there are conflicting reports about the effect of SGA on the risk for ROP [11–13,22].

Diagnostic and therapeutic considerations

Echocardiography

Echocardiography is now routinely used to diagnose CHD, perhaps more so in LBW infants given the risks associated with cardiac catheterization. Although echocardiography is a less invasive procedure than catheterization, it can be associated with adverse effects, especially in premature infants. It is not infrequent that these infants experience bradycardic and desaturation episodes with the pressure of the probe on the chest. Sedation and increased ventilator support may be necessary to allow the study to be completed for full anatomic definition without these detrimental effects. In addition, the gel for the echocardiography probes and the need to have the isolette windows open may induce hypothermia in patients with lower gestational ages and birth weights. It is thus important that someone, other than the sonographer, is at the bedside monitoring the infant to observe for these adverse events and to intervene if needed.

Echocardiography is usually an extremely accurate modality in diagnosing CHD. In LBW infants, several factors, such as intolerance to the procedure requiring aborting the echocardiogram before completion, more difficult windows given the small size of the patient, pulmonary hypertension, lung disease, or use of high-frequency ventilation, may limit the accuracy of the study. One study showed that the incidence of major errors in diagnosing CHD by echocardiography was higher (5.2% versus 1.9%) in LBW infants compared with non-LBW controls matched for diagnosis [33].

Cardiac catheterization

Despite the utility of echocardiography, cardiac catheterization is still needed in some cases, especially for diseases of the great arteries, defining pulmonary blood flow, and performing interventions. Catheterization can be helpful in delineating anatomy if the echocardiogram is unclear and can better evaluate pulmonary blood supply and the presence of aortopulmonary collaterals in the tetralogy of Fallot with pulmonary atresia. Also, catheterization may be used in patients with pulmonary atresia with an intact ventricular septum to determine the appropriate surgical procedure (ie, outflow patch versus shunt depending on the presence of coronary stenoses in addition to the sinusoids) or in transposition of the great arteries if the coronary anatomy is not adequately visualized on echocardiography. Catheterizations are frequently used therapeutically for the indications listed in Table 1. They are usually performed through the umbilical or femoral vessels in neonates, and in the case of balloon atrial septostomies, such interventions can be done at the bedside in the intensive care unit with echocardiographic guidance. Given the sedation needed and risks of cardiovascular and respiratory instability, mechanical ventilation is frequently instituted electively before the procedure begins.

Table 1
Common neonatal cardiac catheterization interventions

Intervention	Lesions
Balloon valvuloplasty	Pulmonary stenosis
	Aortic stenosis
Atrial septostomy/septoplasty	Transposition of the great arteries
	Hypoplastic left heart syndrome with intact/restrictive atrial septum
Stent placement	Patent ductus arteriosus stenting
Laser, wire, or radiofrequency-assisted valve perforation	Membranous atresia of the pulmonary valve
Coil embolization	Aortopulmonary collaterals
	Arteriovenous malformation
	Pulmonary sequestration

Successful cardiac catheterization has been reported in an infant weighing 700 g who underwent a balloon pulmonary valvuloplasty [34]. Although mortality is infrequent, complications may occur in 10% to 20% of infants overall. These complications include vascular perforations, bleeding, arrhythmias, respiratory instability, and thromboses. Few studies have evaluated the risk of catheterization in LBW infants. One study did reveal a higher incidence of complications in infants weighing 5 kg or less compared with those weighing greater than 5 kg but did not find a difference when comparing those weighing 2.5 kg or less with those weighing between 2.5 and 5 kg [35]. Other studies have reported on complications of cardiac catheterization in the LBW population, with an incidence of approximately 10% for major complications [8,34].

Operative strategies

Several different approaches have been used for the surgical repair of LBW infants with CHD. These include delaying surgery; performing less complex palliative procedures initially, followed by a reparative procedure; and performing operations in a manner and time as if these patients were of higher birth weight and gestational age.

Delaying surgery

The principle behind delaying cardiac surgery in LBW infants is to achieve weight gain to alleviate the technical issues related to size and to avoid initial neonatal physiologic instability, especially in the more premature neonates. Several problems may arise from the delay in surgery, however, including (1) difficulty in achieving good weight gain, (2) prolonged need for central venous access, (3) prolonged volume overload in defects with excess pulmonary blood flow (Box 1), (4) prolonged need for prostaglandin administration in ductal-dependent lesions (see Box 1), and (5) prolonged hypoxemia.

Box 1. Physiology in newborn congenital heart disease

Diseases that typically have increased pulmonary blood flow
    Ventricular septal defect
    Truncus arteriosus
    Transposition of the great arteries
    Complete atrioventricular canal
    Patent ductus arteriosus
    Aortopulmonary window
    Single-ventricle lesions (with open ductus arteriosus)
Diseases with ductal-dependent systemic blood flow
    Aortic stenosis
    Aortic coarctation
    Interrupted aortic arch
    HLHS
Diseases with ductal-dependent pulmonary blood flow
    Severe forms of tetralogy of Fallot
    Pulmonary atresia with intact ventricular septum
    Severe pulmonary stenosis (especially in association with
        other complex CHD)
    Some forms of tricuspid atresia
    Some forms of heterotaxy

Premature infants commonly have postnatal failure of weight gain, which is only exacerbated by associated heart disease, especially if the heart defect causes excessive pulmonary blood flow and subsequent congestive heart failure. Strategies to enhance weight gain include fortification of feeds up to as high as 126 J/oz. Fortification of feeds may increase the risk for NEC by providing hyperosmolar feeds to the immature gut, however. Also, if fluid restriction is desired in those infants at risk for congestive heart failure and excessive pulmonary blood flow, even maximal fortification may not provide adequate calories for successful weight gain. Another strategy is to give supplemental parenteral hyperalimentation; this, however, puts these infants at increased risk of infections and venous thrombosis with the necessary use of central venous lines to provide nutritionally replete hyperalimentation. Another problem of parenteral nutrition is hyperalimentation-associated liver disease, which is already more common in SGA infants [36] and may further complicate operative repairs if severe enough to affect liver synthetic function with subsequent coagulation defects.

Delaying surgery also increases exposure of infants with ductal-dependent heart disease to prostaglandin E_1. Morbidities associated with prostaglandin E_1 can be significant and include apnea (at times requiring intubation), fever, hypotension, seizures, complications related to the need for venous access, gastric outlet obstruction attributable to gastric foveolar hyperplasia, and cortical hyperostosis (reversible) with prolonged use.

Another disadvantage to delaying surgery is a longer exposure to abnormal physiology. Patients with lesions at risk for increased pulmonary blood flow (see Box 1) or pulmonary venous engorgement (total anomalous pulmonary venous return) have decreased pulmonary compliance, which may render them more difficult to extubate and thus increase ventilator days and risk for CLD. The increased pulmonary blood flow may increase the likelihood of progression to CLD as seen in premature infants with persistent patent ductus arteriosus [37]. Furthermore, in treating excessive pulmonary blood flow and heart failure, diuretics are frequently required, with subsequent risk for electrolyte abnormalities and a longer term risk of nephrocalcinosis if loop diuretics are used. The prolonged exposure to decreased systemic flow and hypoxemia seen in some CHD could affect developing organs, such as the brain, kidneys, heart, and intestine, by exposing them to episodes of ischemia and hypoxia.

Only one study has evaluated the mortality associated with delaying surgery in LBW infants [8]. This study retrospectively evaluated 100 LBW patients with CHD from 1987 through 1991. Sixty-two patients had early operations (before discharge from initial hospitalization), and 26 patients had operations delayed until after initial hospitalization. Twelve patients died as a result of their heart disease without the intent to attempt intervention. The mortality rate of those who had early repairs was 19%. In those patients who survived to late repair, 18 of 20 survived the operation; however, 23% died of sepsis, NEC, or severe hypoxemia with respiratory failure while waiting for the repair. Thus, the overall mortality rate of the late group was 30%. Although this suggests that delaying repair does not improve mortality and actually may worsen mortality because of interval events, the groups were not comparable from a physiologic perspective, because patients with ductal-dependent circulations were essentially always operated on early.

Palliation versus primary repair

Another approach used to avoid some of the mortality seen in LBW infants with CHD is to perform an initial palliative procedure with reparative surgery delayed until a greater weight is achieved. Not all heart lesions are amenable to this approach. These palliative procedures include balloon atrial septostomies, systemic-to-pulmonary arterial shunts, and pulmonary artery bands. Although allowing for the discontinuation of prostaglandin E_1 in ductal-dependent lesions and attempting to decrease morbidity associated with excessive pulmonary blood flow in others, these procedures still leave the infant with abnormal physiology. In small neonates, it is difficult to select an appropriately sized shunt, particularly one allowing for growth. Shunts that are too big have excess pulmonary blood flow, but if they are too small, they cause more hypoxemia than desired and an increased risk of shunt thrombosis. Placement of a pulmonary artery band also is complicated by some of the same risks, with too much or too little pulmonary blood flow depending on the tightness of the band. Although these procedures usually can be accomplished without cardiopulmonary bypass for term infants, doing so may be more difficult in the LBW infant. In addition, these palliations add another chest entry and may thus make subsequent surgery more difficult because of postoperative changes, such as scarring and potential distortion of the anatomy.

Two retrospective studies evaluated the effect on mortality of performing a palliative repair when a reparative procedure would have been done if the patient were of greater weight. One study looked at 30 patients operated on from 1992 through 1997 who weighed less than 2000 g at the time of the operation [38]. There was no difference in mortality between those patients who had palliative procedures versus reparative procedures. Another more recent study in infants weighing less than 2500 g at the time of surgery again showed no difference in mortality between those patients who had anatomy amenable to reparative repair but were palliated and those who underwent a reparative procedure [29]. These data suggest that exposing patients to a palliative procedure in an attempt to delay reparative operations until they are of greater weight may not be beneficial.

Outcomes

Early mortality (in-hospital before discharge home)

Several centers have reported their experience with LBW infants with CHD who were operated on (Table 2). Early mortality rates in these studies ranges from 10% to 43%, with most centers reporting mortality rates from 10% to 25% [7,8,21,29,38–43]. Reported risk factors for mortality include persistent pre-operative acidosis [21,42], longer cardiopulmonary bypass and cross-clamp times [29,42], and single-ventricle hearts [21,42]. Except for the studies by Chang and coworkers [8] and Kecskes and Cartwright [40], none of these studies report on infants who died while waiting for surgery or were not considered to be candidates for surgical repair based on size or gestational age.

Weight less than 1500 g and mortality

Four studies have evaluated mortality in VLBW patients with CHD. Reddy and Hanley [44] published a report of 20 VLBW patients weighing less than 1500 g whose operative mortality rate was 10%. Survivors included a 1350-g operative weight neonate with truncus arteriosus, a 750-g operative weight patient with aortic coarctation and patent ductus arteriosus, a 1040-g patient who had repair for total anomalous pulmonary venous return, and a patient with an operative weight of 1300 g who had an arterial switch operation for transposition of the great arteries. Rossi and colleagues [38] reported on 8 patients who weighed less than 1500 g at the time of surgery, with a 25% mortality rate compared with a mortality rate of 14% for those patients weighing 1501 to 2000 g.

Table 2
Reported outcomes after cardiac surgery in low-birth-weight infants with chronic heart disease

Author	Time period	Weight inclusion	No. patients	Mortality rate (in-hospital)	Hypoplastic left heart syndrome mortality	Actuarial survival
Dees et al [7]	July 1976–May 1999	<2500 g birth weight	201 (108 operated on)	26% overall (25.4% mortality rate for open procedures, 10.4% mortality rate for closed procedures)	78% (7/9)	47% at 10 years
Pawade et al [21]	January 1979–December 1990	<2500 g at surgery	60	16.5%		
Numa et al [39]	January 1985–December 1989	<2000 g at surgery	21	43%		
Chang et al [8]	January 1987–January 1991	≤2500 g birth weight	100	30%	100% (6/6) (only one operative repair attempted)	
Kecskes and Cartwright [40]	January 1988–December 1999	≤1500 g birth weight	47 (16 operated on)	40% overall (44% mortality rate for those operated on)		
Reddy et al [41]	July 1990–December 1997	≤2500 g birth weight	102	10%		82% at 1–5 years
Beyens et al [42]	September 1990–February 1997	<2500 g at surgery	23	22%		88% at 2 years
Rossi et al [38]	January 1992–June 1997	<2000 g at surgery	30	17%	66% (2/3)	62% at 5 years
Oppido et al [29]	January 1993–August 2002	<2500 g at surgery	60	15%	28.6% (2/7)	70% at 5 years
Bové et al [43]	June 1995–January 2003	<2500 g at surgery	49	18%	0% (1/1)	

Four of the 8 patients weighing less than 1500 g had documented IVH, however, although the timing of the hemorrhage was unknown. Chang and coworkers [8] reported a 50% mortality rate in 18 patients who were of VLBW compared with 26% in infants with a birth weight of 1501 to 2500 g. Of the 9 VLBW patients who survived to surgery, however, all survived. In addition, Kecskes and Cartwright [40] documented a 40% mortality rate in VLBW infants with CHD compared with 12.5% in infants with VLBW without CHD in their institution. Only 34% (16 of 47) of the patients were operated on, and 44% of these patients died after surgery.

Hypoplastic left heart syndrome

More recent reports have evaluated the mortality of neonates with HLHS and variants, given that most of the earlier studies had few patients with single-ventricle lesions, and reported an almost 100% mortality rate in the patients who underwent surgery and were of LBW. Weinstein and coworkers [45] evaluated 67 patients who weighed less than 2500 g at the time of surgery and had a stage 1 palliation for HLHS or variant thereof from 1992 through 1997. This study included 14 patients weighing less than 2000 g and 2 weighing less than 1500 g who were operated on. The overall early mortality rate was 51%. A more recent study by Pizarro and colleagues [46] reporting on 20 LBW patients with HLHS or variants of operated on from 1998 through 2000 found an early mortality rate of 45% after a stage 1 palliation. An even more recent review (2000–2002) from the Children's Hospital of Philadelphia reports an improved mortality rate of 37% in LBW infants with HLHS or variants, however [47]. This parallels the improvement in mortality, now approaching 10%, after a stage 1 palliation in term infants with HLHS.

Postoperative morbidity

Morbidity rates range from 35% to 83% after surgery in this LBW population [29,42,43]. Reported frequent complications include cardiac arrest, arrhythmias, infections, seizures, acute renal insufficiency, pulmonary hypertensive crises, phrenic nerve palsies, and low cardiac output syndrome. These are similar to those reported after cardiac repair in all neonates and infants. The incidence of these varied widely in the literature; however, although it is reasonable to assume that morbidity is higher in this population of LBW infants with CHD, there is no evidence to support this currently.

Summary

LBW infants with CHD have a higher mortality risk and likely a higher morbidity risk than their preterm or appropriate for gestational age counterparts without CHD and term counterparts with CHD. As our understanding of the pathophysiology and treatment of the diseases associated with prematurity and growth restriction improves, the outcomes for these infants should continue to improve. In addition, as more of these infants survive and are referred for surgery, operative techniques and strategies are likely to continue to improve. At this time, there is not adequate evidence that mortality is improved by delaying surgery for weight gain or performing palliative operations initially. Currently, at the Children's Hospital of Philadelphia, patients who weigh less than 1000 g are operated on as soon as they are stabilized from their perinatal events and reparative surgeries are generally done, except in extenuating circumstances (eg, associated anomalies also requiring surgery, continued pulmonary instability thought to be mainly attributable to prematurity). Given the challenging physiology in this population, optimal management includes early referral to a tertiary or quaternary facility and a multidisciplinary team approach consisting of cardiologists, neonatologists, surgeons, nurses, perfusionists, and anesthesiologists.

References

[1] Martin JA, Kochanek KD, Strobino DM, et al. Annual summary of vital statistics-2003. Pediatrics 2005;115(3):619–34.

[2] Ferencz C, Rubin JD, McCarter RJ. Congenital heart disease: prevalence at livebirth. The Baltimore-Washington Infant Study. Am J Epidemiol 1985;121:31–6.

[3] Rosenthal GL, Wilson DP, Permutt T, et al. Birth weight and cardiovascular malformations: a population-based study. Am J Epidemiol 1991;133(12):1273–81.

[4] Kramer HH, Trampisch HJ, Rammos S, et al. Birth weight of children with congenital heart disease. Eur J Pediatr 1990;149:752–7.

[5] Levy RJ, Rosenthal A, Fyler DC, et al. Birthweight of infants with congenital heart disease. Am J Dis Child 1978;132:249–54.

[6] Ferencz C, Boughman JA, Neill CA, et al. Congenital cardiovascular malformations: questions on inheritance. J Am Coll Cardiol 1989;14(3):756–63.

[7] Dees E, Lin H, Cotton RB, et al. Outcome of preterm infants with congenital heart disease. J Pediatr 2000;137:653–9.

[8] Chang AC, Hanley FH, Lock JE, et al. Management and outcome of low birth weight neonates with congenital heart disease. J Pediatr 1994;124:461–6.

[9] Lemons JA, Bauer CR, Oh W, et al. Very low birth weight outcomes of the National Institute of Child Health and Human Development Neonatal Research Network, January 1995 through 1996. Pediatrics 2001;107(1):e1.

[10] Simchen MJ, Beiner ME, Liviathan NS, et al. Neonatal outcome in growth-restricted versus appropriately grown preterm infants. Am J Perinatol 2000;17(4):187–92.

[11] Bardin C, Zelkowitz P, Papageorgiou A. Outcomes of small-for-gestational age and appropriate-for-gestational age infants born before 27 weeks of gestation. Pediatrics 1997;100(1):e4.

[12] Regev RH, Lusky A, Dolfin T, et al. Excess mortality and morbidity among small-for-gestational-age premature infants: a population based study. J Pediatr 2003;143:186–91.

[13] Aucott SW, Donohue PK, Northington FJ. Increased morbidity in severe early intrauterine growth restriction. J Perinatol 2004;24:435–40.

[14] Paul DA, Greenspan JS, Davis DA, et al. The role of cardiopulmonary bypass and surfactant decompensation after surgery for congenital heart disease. J Thorac Cardiovasc Surg 1999; 117:1025–6.

[15] Rinker C, Jansen S, Wilnhammer C, et al. Cardiopulmonary bypass reduces pulmonary surfactant activity in infants. J Thorac Cardiovasc Surg 1999;118:237–44.

[16] Merrill JD, Ballard RA, Cnaan A, et al. Dysfunction of pulmonary surfactant in chronically ventilated premature infants. Pediatr Res 2004;56:918–26.

[17] Okumara A, Hayakawa F, Kato T, et al. Hypocarbia in preterm infants with periventricular leukomalacia: the relation between hypocarbia and mechanical ventilation. Pediatrics 2001; 107(3):469–75.

[18] Collins MP, Lorenz JM, Jetton JR, et al. Hypocapnia and other ventilation-related risk factors for cerebral palsy in low birth weight infants. Pediatr Res 2001;50(6):712–9.

[19] Kraybill EN, Runyan DK, Bose CL, et al. Risk factors for chronic lung disease in infants with birth weights of 751 to 1000 grams. J Pediatr 1989;115:115–20.

[20] Mariani G, Cifuentes J, Waldemar C. Randomized trial of permissive hypercapnia in preterm infants. Pediatrics 1999;104(5):1082–8.

[21] Pawade A, Waterson K, Laussen P, et al. Cardiopulmonary bypass in neonates weighing less than 2.5 kg: analysis of the risk factors for early and late mortality. J Card Surg 1993;8:1–8.

[22] Garite TJ, Clark R, Thorp JA. Intrauterine growth restriction increases morbidity and mortality among premature infants. Am J Obstet Gynecol 2004;191:481–7.

[23] Rhee E, Detti L, Mari G. Superior mesenteric artery flow velocity waveforms in small for gestational age fetuses. J Matern Fetal Med 1998;7:120–3.

[24] Kempley ST, Gamsu HR, Vyas S, et al. Effects of intrauterine growth retardation on postnatal visceral and cerebral flow velocity. Arch Dis Child 1991;66:1115–8.

[25] Malcolm G, Ellwood D, Devonald K, et al. Absent or reversed end diastolic flow velocity in the umbilical artery and necrotising enterocolitis. Arch Dis Child 1991;66:805–7.

[26] Bhatt AB, Tank PD, Barmade KB, et al. Abnormal Doppler flow velocimetry in the growth restricted foetus as a predictor for necrotising enterocolitis. J Postgrad Med 2002;48(3):182–5.

[27] Martinez-Tallo E, Claure N, Bancalari E. Necrotizing enterocolitis in full-term and near-term infants: risk factors. Biol Neonate 1997;71:291–8.

[28] McElhinney DB, Hedrick HL, Bush DM, et al. Necrotizing enterocolitis in neonates with congenital heart disease: risk factors and outcome. Pediatrics 2000;106:1080–7.

[29] Oppido G, Napoleone CP, Formigari R, et al. Outcome of cardiac surgery in low birth weight premature infants. Eur J Cardiothorac Surg 2004;24:44–53.

[30] Johns KJ, Johns JA, Feman SS, et al. Retinopathy of prematurity in infants with cyanotic congenital heart disease. Am J Dis Child 1991;145:200–3.

[31] Shohat M, Reisner SH, Krikler R, et al. Retinopathy of prematurity: incidence and risk factors. Pediatrics 1983;72:159–63.

[32] Katzman G, Satish M, Krishnan V, et al. Comparative analysis of lower and higher stage retrolental fibroplasia [abstract]. Pediatr Res 1982;16(Suppl 2):294A.

[33] Dorfman AL, Levine JC, Colan SD, et al. Accuracy of echocardiography in low birth weight infants with congenital heart disease. Pediatrics 2005;115:102–7.

[34] Simpson JM, Moore P, Teitel DF. Cardiac catheterization of low birth weight infants. Am J Cardiol 2001;87:1372–7.

[35] Rhodes JF, Asnes JD, Blaufox AD, et al. Impact of low body weight on frequency of pediatric cardiac catheterization complications. Am J Cardiol 2000;86:1275–8.

[36] Baserga MC, Sola A. Intrauterine growth restriction impacts tolerance to total parenteral nutrition in extremely low birth weight infants. J Perinatol 2004;24:476–81.

[37] Clyman RI. Recommendations for the postnatal use of indomethacin: an analysis of four separate treatment strategies. J Pediatr 1996;128:601–7.

[38] Rossi AF, Seiden HS, Sadeghi AM, et al. The outcome of cardiac operations in infants weighing two kilograms or less. J Thorac Cardiovasc Surg 1998;116:28–35.

[39] Numa A, Butt W, Mee RBB. Outcome of infants with birthweight 2000 g or less who undergo major cardiac surgery. J Paediatr Child Health 1992;28:318–20.

[40] Kecskes Z, Cartwright DW. Poor outcome of very low birthweight babies with serious congenital heart disease. Arch Dis Child Fetal Neonatal Ed 2002;87:F31–3.

[41] Reddy VM, McElhinney DB, Sagrado T, et al. Results of 102 cases of complete repair of congenital heart defects in patients weighing 700 to 2500 grams. J Thorac Cardiovasc Surg 1999; 117:324–31.

[42] Beyens T, Biarent D, Bouton JM, et al. Cardiac surgery with extracorporeal circulation in 23 infants weighing 2500 g or less: short and intermediate term outcome. Eur J Cardiothorac Surg 1998;14:165–72.

[43] Bové T, Francois K, De Groote K, et al. Outcome analysis of major cardiac operations in low birth weight neonates. Ann Thorac Surg 2004;78:181–7.

[44] Reddy VM, Hanley FH. Cardiac surgery in infants with very low birth weight. Semin Pediatr Surg 2000;9:91–5.

[45] Weinstein S, Gaynor JW, Bridges ND, et al. Early survival of infants weighing 2.5 kilograms or less undergoing first-stage reconstruction for hypoplastic left heart syndrome. Circulation 1999; 100(Suppl II):II-167–70.

[46] Pizarro C, Davis DA, Galantowicz ME, et al. Stage I palliation for hypoplastic left heart syndrome in low birth weight neonates: can we justify it? Eur J Cardiothorac Surg 2002;21:716–20.

[47] Ades AM, Wernovsky G, Tabbutt S, et al. Current outcomes of cardiac surgery in the low birth weight infant [abstract]. Pediatr Res 2003;53:183A.

ELSEVIER
SAUNDERS

CLINICS IN
PERINATOLOGY

Clin Perinatol 32 (2005) 1017–1030

Nutrition Care for Newborns with Congenital Heart Disease

Michelle Steltzer, RN, MS, CPNP[a],*,
Nancy Rudd, RN, MS, CPNP[a], Barbara Pick, RD, CSP, CD[b]

[a]*Division of Pediatric Cardiology, Children's Hospital of Wisconsin, Medical College of Wisconsin,*
The Herma Heart Center, 9000 West Wisconsin Avenue, Milwaukee, WI 53226, USA
[b]*Nutritional Services, Children's Hospital of Wisconsin, Medical College of Wisconsin,*
9000 West Wisconsin Avenue, Milwaukee, WI 53226, USA

Nutrition has been recognized as a key determinant of health in infants for centuries. The science of nutrition can be defined in many ways. Simply stated it is the science of nourishing the body properly or the effect of food on the living organism. In 1969 Yudkin, a pioneer in the science of nutrition, defined nutrition as the relationship between man and his food. More recently, the council on Foods and Nutrition of the American Medical Association elaborated further by describing nutrition as "the science of food, the nutrients and other substances therein, their action, interaction, and balance in relation to health and disease." Regardless of the chosen definition of nutrition, the complexity of neonates with congenital heart disease (CHD) requires an understanding of the unique nutritional needs of this population by those entrusted to care for them.

Various terminology is used in the literature to describe inadequate growth in infants with CHD. Malnutrition is one term commonly used to describe a state of poor nutrition and growth failure. Failure to thrive (FTT) is a diagnosis used frequently by health care professionals. It describes a clinical syndrome of growth failure in any infant who fails to grow at the expected rate over a period of months, often with various organic and nonorganic causes. Cardiac cachexia is a syndrome of protein-energy malnutrition seen in some infants with cardiac disease and is most prevalent in infancy. Cachexia can develop over several weeks to months, may range from mild to severe, and is largely amenable to

---

* Corresponding author.
E-mail address: msteltzer@chw.org (M. Steltzer).

0095-5108/05/$ – see front matter © 2005 Elsevier Inc. All rights reserved.
doi:10.1016/j.clp.2005.09.010

medical and surgical therapy [1]. Growth deficiency, undernutrition, and growth failure represent additional terminology used to describe the nutritional condition of an infant whose weight or height is less than the fifth percentile, whose weight or height measurements are static over time (plateau), or whose growth measurements increase more slowly than expected over time (cross percentile lines) on a standardized infant growth chart. Catch-up growth refers to the velocity of growth following a time period of impaired growth caused by undernutrition [2].

Whichever descriptive term is chosen, growth failure is a well-recognized and challenging consequence of CHD. At birth, infants with CHD are usually of appropriate weight for gestational age; however, growth problems frequently become evident early in life. Timely nutritional intervention is necessary to maintain adequate nutritional status. The goals of nutritional support for the at-risk neonate with CHD are to provide adequate nutrition to meet the patient's needs and to correct nutrient deficiency, thus minimizing the physiologic consequences of undernutrition. Providing adequate nutrition to neonates with CHD can be a difficult task. Many variables affect the nutritional intake, energy expenditure and ability to grow in an infant with hemodynamically significant heart disease. Compromised nutritional status may delay surgical intervention and increase the risk for postoperative complications. Further concerns of poor nutrition in neonates with CHD relate to long-term outcomes such as brain development, oral-motor skill attainment, and physical development.

This article defines the congenital, physiologic, and nutritional variables encountered by this population and provides a guide to the care of these infants designed to result in optimal growth and development. It reviews the nutritional needs, multi-factorial sources of undernutrition, and consequences of inadequate nutrition in infants with CHD. In addition, medical and nutritional management strategies intended to optimize growth and reduce morbidity will be discussed [3].

Nutritive needs of infants

Before discussing the numerous nutritional challenges facing neonates with CHD, it is important to review the well-established nutrient needs of healthy infants. There are six classes of nutrients that have an impact on an infant's diet and thus growth. They include carbohydrates, fats, proteins, vitamins, minerals, and water. All six play an important role in maintaining an optimal nutritional state; however, only three yield energy for the body's use. Termed energy nutrients, they include carbohydrates, fats, and proteins. The rapid growth and metabolism of the infant demand ample supplies of these energy nutrients. The normal diet of the infant is either breast milk or commercial formula; it is the only food needed by infants for the first months of life. Breast milk is low in protein (about 6% of calories) and high in fat (about 52% of calories). Infant formula provides slightly more protein (about 9% of calories) and contains similar amounts of fat (about 49%). The chemical components found in breast milk and formula perform two important roles: In addition to supplying energy they promote growth and repair of body tissue.

Information on the precise nutritive needs of healthy infants is available from the National Research Council. The suggested level of intake for energy of 108 to 117 kilocalories (kcal) per kilogram (kg) of body weight per day seems adequate to meet the needs of maintaining body temperature, for growth and for activity for the first six months of life. The needs for protein during early infancy, a time of rapid skeletal and muscular growth, are high. An intake of 2.2 grams (g) of protein per kg of body weight is sufficient to allow normal growth. A neonate weighing <3 kg should have 120 mL/kg/d of fluids and a 3- to10-kg infant should have 100 cc/kg/d of fluids. Immediately after birth infants experience a weight loss resulting from a loss of fluid and from some catabolism. The loss averages 6% of birth weight but occasionally exceeds 10%. Healthy neonates will typically regain their birth weight by 10 to 14 days of age [4]. Expected weight gain in full-term infants during the first 6 months of life averages 20 to 30 g/d. Incremental gain in crown-heel length for full-term infants averages 0.66 cm/wk during the first six months of life. Infants display rapid increases in head circumference, and this head growth correlates well with brain growth. Average gain in head circumference for full-term infants between birth and 6 months of age is 0.33 cm/wk.

In comparison, infants with hemodynamically significant CHD require significantly more nutritional support to sustain growth than their healthy counterparts [5]. Fluid losses in a neonate with congestive heart failure (CHF) are 10% to 15% greater than in a normal neonate because of tachypnea, emesis, diarrhea, and the anti-congestive management with diuretics [6]. Energy intake required in infants with CHD to sustain normal growth is reported to be between 130 and 150 kcal/kg/d [7,8]; and depending on the type of cardiac lesion and catch-up growth needed, some infants can require as much as 175 to 180 kcal/kg/d [1]. Currently there are no established growth parameters for infants with hemodynamically significant CHD. Standard practice includes targeted weight gain of 10 to 20 g/d when adequate calories are provided. Fluid balance is another key factor in the management of most infants with CHD because serum protein imbalance may play a role in the development of edema. It is important to assure protein adequacy in this patient population by monitoring serum albumin, transferrin, or prealbumin levels.

The physical growth of infants is a direct reflection of their nutritional well-being and is the single most important parameter used in assessing their nutritional status. Growth may be defined as an increase in the physical size of the body as a whole or as an increase in any of its parts. Assessments of growth are made by periodic determinations of weight, height, and head circumference; and growth charts for each parameter make it possible to visualize how an infant's growth is proceeding. It is important for persons concerned with an infant's nutritional intake to be aware of how growth progresses. Infants who are undernourished are shorter and weigh less than their well-nourished peers. With undernutrition, the rate of gain in weight is affected more than is the rate of gain in height; but if the nutritional deficit is severe enough and continues long enough, linear growth will be retarded. Weight is affected when energy intake is inadequate, and linear growth is delayed when energy intake is adequate but protein intake is deficient.

Enteral feeding by bottle or at breast is the expected method of nutritional support in full-term infants. Neonates have reflexive behaviors enabling them to suck and swallow and to coordinate sucking bursts with pauses to breath. This pattern of suck, swallow, breathe, is a remarkable and efficient oral motor developmental milestone in the nutritional process. During the first few months of life, as an infant matures, this reflexive feeding is replaced by voluntary, controlled eating. Unfortunately the ability to feed orally is frequently compromised in infants with CHD. Basic motor skills may be delayed by prolonged illness or hospitalization. These infants may not have sufficient energy for feeding; and tachypnea may interfere with their ability to coordinate suck, swallow, and breathe effectively.

Causes of growth failure in congenital heart disease

In 1000 live births, 9 newborns will have CHD. In the United States, 36,000 neonates are born with CHD each year. The severity of the defect seems directly related to likelihood of nutritional implications [9]. Separating cardiac lesions into acyanotic and cyanotic groups helps facilitate a clearer understanding of the nutritional and physiologic issues associated with various congenital cardiac lesions. Depending on the newborns' type of lesion, hemodynamic compromise, and timing of surgical correction or palliation, their nutritional needs and management strategies may vary.

Hemodynamic impairment

A relationship exists between growth failure and abnormal hemodynamics in infancy. The type of cardiac lesion and severity of hemodynamic impairment play a role in undernutrition of infants with CHD [10–12]. A full-term neonate with mild CHD may not need specific intervention other than following the growth curve closely. Unfortunately, growth in neonates with even mild congenital heart lesions is impacted to some degree. Neonates with hemodynamically significant heart disease are at highest risk for becoming nutritionally depleted.

Acyanotic CHD refers to the defects typically associated with increased pulmonary blood flow or obstruction across valves [11–13]. These types of defects have an association with growth disturbances in weight more than height [14]. The type of defect can dictate the potential for growth failure. The obstructive lesions such as aortic stenosis, pulmonary stenosis, and coarctation of the aorta are infrequently associated with poor growth unless they occur in association with CHF [1]. The acyanotic defects that cause left-to-right shunting result in significant volume overload of either the left ventricle, right ventricle, or occasionally both, depending on the specific cardiac abnormality. Invariably pulmonary overcirculation occurs. The acyanotic lesions most prone to pulmonary overcirculation with the accompanying risk for growth failure include ventricular septal defect (VSD), patent ductus arteriosus (PDA), atrial septal defect (ASD), atrial ventricular value (AVV) regurgitation, and less commonly semilunar valve regurgitation [1]. The effect of significant shunting causes height and weight growth disturbances.

Cyanotic CHD refers to those defects associated with right to left shunting and results in hypoxemia. Infants with cyanotic CHD have associated growth disturbances in weight and height [11,14]. The cyanotic lesions include double outlet right ventricle, transposition of the great arteries, tetralogy of fallot with and without pulmonary atresia, tricuspid atresia, and hypoplastic left heart syndrome. There is a direct relationship between hypoxemia and growth. The duration of hypoxemia in years, not severity of hypoxemia, is felt to play a significant factor in growth retardation [1]. If hypoxemia is accompanied by CHF, growth is even more severely affected [1].

Pulmonary hypertension may also play a critical role in growth disturbances in infants with cyanotic and acyanotic CHD. An investigation in 1978 of children with VSD noted that there was significant stunting of height in infants with VSD and pulmonary hypertension [1]. The occurrence of pulmonary hypertension appeared to be the most important factor identified by Varan in growth impairment in infants with CHD. Those infants with cyanosis and pulmonary hypertension had their growth most severely affected [5].

Finally, any hemodynamic impairment resulting in the presence of CHF negatively affects the nutritional status of infants who have CHD [10]. The diagnosis of CHF often correlates with clinical findings of tachypnea, hepatomegaly, and tachycardia [15]. CHF influences growth caused by inadequate caloric intake, increased metabolic rate, alteration in gastrointestinal function and malabsorption [10–12]. Cardiac lesions that commonly result in CHF in the neonate include hypoplastic left heart syndrome, transposition of the great arteries, patent ductus arteriosus, total anomalous pulmonary venous connection, critical valvar aortic stenosis, coarctation of the aorta, and ventricular septal defect [15].

The role of CHF, for example, can be exhibited in the neonate with a large VSD. The larger the left to right shunt across the lesion, the greater the potential for excessive pulmonary blood flow, increased pulmonary artery pressures, increased blood return to the left heart, and elevation of left ventricular end-diastolic volume and pressure. This condition of high output hemodynamics causes hypermetabolism with resulting growth failure [12].

Inadequate caloric intake

Inadequate caloric intake is felt to be the predominant cause of growth failure in infants with CHD. Oral feeding requires large energy expenditure. In the neonate who has symptomatic heart disease, oral feeding is a "stress test." Tachypnea and fatigue may not allow an infant the ability to consume all of the calories and volume needed to maintain growth.

Oral feeding is challenging as the neonate may feel hungry at the start of the feed, feed eagerly initially, then reach early satiety resulting in suboptimal nutrient intake. Other limiting factors include decreased gastric capacity caused by hepatomegaly and delayed gastric emptying secondary to low cardiac output. Respiratory infections and resulting tachypnea may affect the neonate's ability to perform the suck, swallow, and breathe pattern necessary for successful oral feeding. A neonate may start to feed avidly but tire quickly, leading to longer feeding time and increased energy expenditure.

Additional factors leading to an inadequate caloric intake are related to medical management strategies often used to treat CHF. Fluid restriction and anorexia resulting from diuretic use may unintentionally limit caloric intake [1].

Increased metabolic rate

Increased metabolic rate also plays a contributory role in growth failure, particularly when CHF is present [11]. Hypermetabolism is likely related to the increased work of respiratory muscles necessary for adequate ventilation in the presence of decreased lung compliance. The basal metabolic rate (BMR) is elevated in infants with CHD because of cardiac and respiratory work and has been reported three to five times higher compared with an infant who does not have heart disease [6]. The presence of dilated or hypertrophic cardiac muscle also increases oxygen consumption. Hypertrophied cardiac muscle uses 20% to 30% of the body's total oxygen consumption instead of the typical 10%. Finally, overall sympathetic nervous system tone is known to be elevated in infants with hemodynamically significant CHD [1].

Malabsorption

Malabsorption also plays a role in cardiac undernutrition. It can result from CHF and gastrointestinal tissue hypoxia. Malabsorption significantly limits an infant's tolerance of feedings, impinges the neonate's ability to maximize caloric intake, and subsequently decreases nutrient absorption. Altered gastric capacity caused by increased pressure on the stomach as a result of hepatomegaly can play a role in nutrient absorption. In addition, it is speculated that infants with left to right intracardiac shunting resulting in right heart failure and increased systemic venous pressure may develop edema of the intestinal wall and mucosal surfaces leading to malabsorption and impaired nutrient absorption [1,11]. Consequently, the feed volume, caloric concentration, and delivery time of bolus feedings may need to be adjusted.

Perioperative implications

Other contributing factors to growth failure in neonates with CHD may result from prolonged hospital stays or postoperative complications and include fever, sepsis, and chylous effusion. Fever alone can increase the caloric expenditure 12% for each degree Celsius reached above 37°C [16]. Sepsis and its resulting influence on energy consumption and increased autonomic tone can increase caloric expenditure 25% to 50% [16]. The development of chylous effusions may require use of fat-restricted formulas or parenteral nutrition as a treatment strategy. Both options are less than optimal in providing balanced nutrition. Vocal cord issues or airway compromise requiring prolonged intubation can limit enteral feeding, compromise nutrition, and retard growth [6]. Respiratory illnesses can significantly impact a neonate because of increased secretions, tachypnea, wheezing, and desaturations in an infant already compromised by CHD. Gastrointestinal infections such as clostridium difficile and rotavirus can also compromise the nutritional status of a neonate who has CHD.

Noncardiac causes of growth failure

Gastroesophageal reflux (GER) describes the movement of gastric contents back into the esophagus. The reflux can be "silent" or obvious in the form of spit-ups or emesis. GER can occur in up to 65% of healthy infants, and as many as 40% to 50% of 1- to 2- month-old infants have two episodes of reflux per day [17,18]. GER also plays a role in CHD [13]. The role of GER in CHD seems most prevalent when the neonate has a hemodynamically significant lesion and likely results from delayed gastric emptying secondary to malabsorption. The presence of a nasogastric tube (NG) may also contribute to more reflux symptoms [16]. Using an NG to supplement enteral feedings is common practice as neonates advance to full feeds and work on oral feeding skills.

Prematurity, intrauterine growth retardation, presence of associated genetic syndromes, socioeconomic factors, and parental–infant interaction also are contributing factors for inadequate growth in the infant with CHD [12]. Genetic syndromes frequently associated with CHD include trisomy 21, 13, and 18; Turner's syndrome; Williams syndrome; Noonan's syndrome; and DiGeorge syndrome [13]. It is important to identify these noncardiac factors early in life so appropriate interventions may be implemented and the infant's nutritional status optimized.

Strategies to optimize nutrition and growth

With knowledge of the multiple causes of growth deficiency comes the responsibility of the health care team to make nutritional management a high priority in the care of infants with CHD. Necessary therapies should address medical and nutritional risk factors. As cardiac surgical and interventional catheterization procedures have advanced, neonatal defects are being corrected or palliated early in life. Poor nutritional status can negatively impact preoperative and postoperative outcomes. Inadequate protein and calories can reduce skeletal muscle function and increase the risk for postoperative pneumonia [16]. The immune system is also adversely affected by undernutrition, which can result in postoperative infection and impaired wound healing [19,20]. Further concerns of poor nutrition in neonates with CHD relate to long-term outcomes such as brain development, oral-motor skill attainment, and physical development [19]. Several studies have focused on the importance of postsurgical nutrition in infants following repair or palliation.

Boctor in 1999 noted that nutrition and growth after cardiac surgery in infants with CHD varied and that growth was best promoted by bottle-feeding infants [21]. Bottle-fed infants gained a median of 20 g/d, combination breast-fed and bottle-fed infants gained a median of 5 g/d, and exclusively breast-fed infants lost a median of 49 g/d [21]. Pillo-Blocka and Boctor suggested that weight gain following neonatal surgery is often sub-optimal and that greater attention should be focused on nutrition postoperatively, including rapid advancement of feedings to promote optimal growth and nutritional status [21–23]. Pillo-Blocka demonstrated that rapid advancement of calories to higher concentrations significantly improved energy intake and weight gain (20 g/d gain in a control group versus 35 g/d loss in the usual care group) [23]. In this study, feeds were advanced from 20 to 30 calories per ounce over just a 3-day span. Additionally, postoperative hospital stay for the intervention population of infants was significantly decreased [23].

With the above as background, an extensive discussion of the treatment options for optimization of nutritional support follows.

Medical management

Medical management of growth disturbances in infants with CHF focuses on symptomatic improvement of CHF. Traditional anticongestive therapy uses a combination of digoxin and diuretics. Afterload-reducing agents are also used in patients with diminished myocardial function or significant atrioventricular valve regurgitation. Pulmonary vasodilator drugs or oxygen therapy is also used in patients with pulmonary hypertension and pulmonary vascular disease [1]. FTT and a lack of response to standard medical therapy and nutritional support together are an indication for surgical correction or palliation of a congenital heart defect, if it is amenable to such.

Several treatment modalities have been used for the treatment of gastroesophageal reflux. Reflux precautions used include smaller, frequent feedings; upright positioning; thickening of the feeds; antiemetics; and histamine 2 antagonist therapies as indicated. On occasion, despite these interventions, infants may struggle with emesis and poor growth. If the infant is unable to achieve adequate caloric intake and demonstrate reasonable growth over time, other interventions may need to occur. Nutritional supplementation by way of NG, gastrostomy tube (GT), and jejunostomy tube (JT) may be in order. This approach will be discussed in more detail later in this article.

The role of thickened feeds in patients with gastrointestinal reflux is controversial. Some studies have noted fewer episodes of emeses when the feeds are thickened; other studies have shown an increase in the duration of the reflux episode. Commercial formulas with rice added are currently on the market.

Prokinetic agents such as metoclopromide have been used to treat gastroesophageal reflux in infancy; however, there is also debate over its effectiveness. In addition, the use of an antisecretory or acid-neutralizing agent may help prevent erosive esophagitis.

Surgical treatment options for reflux include placement of a JT, which allows enteral feeds to bypass the stomach. The Nissen fundoplication (operation) is reserved for severe cases of reflux that do not respond to the above measures.

Additional medical strategies also focus on preventing infection, particularly respiratory illnesses that can further compromise the nutritional well-being of an infant with symptomatic CHD. Routine immunizations per the American Academy of Pediatrics guidelines are recommended in most patient populations [1,13]. Palivizumab is indicated in high-risk patient with CHD to prevent respiratory syncytial virus infections. A pneumococcal vaccine and continuous antibiotic prophylaxis is needed in patients with asplenia [1].

Primary nutritional interventions

Parenteral nutrition is indicated in infants with CHD when the projected time to establish adequate enteral support exceeds the infant's metabolic reserves. Such instances include postoperative patients in whom oral feedings are not anticipated to commence for more than 3 to 5 days. Infants requiring prolonged intubation, exhibiting marked malnutrition before surgery or gastrointestinal abnormalities such as duodenal atresia and gastroschisis, as well as low birth weight infants may also fall into this category [1]. If enteral nutrition cannot be obtained in longer than 1 week, a central line should be obtained to maximize the dextrose and protein in the total parenteral nutrition (TPN) in addition to intralipids at 20% to prevent fatty acid deficiency and promote optimal nutrition [6].

The use of trophic feeds is important to prevent gastrointestinal complications such as atrophy and infection, which may be associated with disuse of the gastrointestinal tract [6]. The use of formula or breast milk at a rate of 0.5 to 1.0 cc/kg/hr continuous drip uses the gastrointestinal tract and can lessen the risk for systemic bacterial infection by preventing complications related to intestinal mucosal atrophy and loss of the functional intestinal barrier [16].

Enteral feeds are preferable to parenteral nutrition when gastrointestinal function is adequate [16]. Enteral feeds are more physiologic, safer, more accessible, and cost-effective. If full enteral feedings are an option, they should be provided.

Advancement of feedings to a goal volume and calories of 150 cc/kg/d and 120 kcal/kg/d on a neonate with significant CHD, such as shunt dependant single ventricle, is common. Various parameters are watched closely during the advancement of enteral feedings, including daily assessment of weight change, tolerance of feeds, and progress with oral feeds. Adjustment in feeds is then done accordingly under direction of the health professionals.

The goal of nutritional management is to sustain or enable catch-up growth without overburdening circulation or disturbing water balance. The nutritional needs to sustain catch-up growth can be as high as 1.5 to 2 times the daily allowances for age [2]. Gain in weight proceeds rapidly until the infant reaches the correct weight for height, then proceeds at a slower rate as height and weight increase together.

Optimizing enteral caloric intake to meet increased caloric needs may be met by increasing quality or volume of feeds, increasing density of formula, and reducing metabolic demands [1]. In infants with symptoms of CHF, it is usually not necessary to restrict enteral intake if the infant feeds on demand. If volume is tolerated, then standard formula at 20 cal/oz or 0.67 kcal/mL is preferable with no fluid restriction. Breast milk contains 20 kcal/oz and provides an excellent nutritional and immunologic advantage over infant formula [6]. The caloric and protein content, however, is often insufficient to sustain growth in a neonate with CHD, particularly with symptoms of CHF.

Increasing caloric density of the formula may be necessary if tolerance to volume is a limiting factor in meeting caloric requirements. Increasing caloric density may lead to decreased free water, increase in osmolality, and increased solute load including electrolytes and minerals [1,6]. Density can be increased by many methods from standard 20 cal/oz formula or breast milk to 24 to 27 or even 30 cal/oz. The simplest method of increasing calories is adding more powder to water and thus increasing the calories per ounce. For infants who are being breast-fed, it may be necessary to use expressed breast milk if volumes are a question [1]. In a hospital setting, breast milk can be fortified with human milk fortifier (HMF) or a commercial powdered formula to densities of 22, 24, 27, or 30 cal/oz based on nutritional needs. Hind milk is also preferred, as the caloric density is greater than fore milk. There are multiple recipes based on the various formulas commercially available. It is important to check with a nutritionist for an appropriate recipe for home use.

Additionally, fortification may be done by the use of glucose polymers, microlipid or MCT oil, and protein supplements can be added to optimize caloric intake. Glucose polymers such as polycose (2 kcal/mL as liquid and 23 kcal/tbsp as a powder) can increase carbohydrates. Medium chain triglycerides such as microlipid (4.5 kcal/mL) or MCT oil (7.7 kcal/mL) can be used to increase the fat content [1,16]. Lastly, Promod, a protein supplement, can increase the protein content by 3 g/tbsp [16]. Some recipes are simpler for families to prepare such as increasing the formula powder per water ratio, whereas other methods may be more complex. The level of complexity can be a deciding factor in the choice of a fortification for patients and their families. Families must be educated by a nutritionist to ensure that the appropriately prescribed concentration of feedings is provided to the infant.

When the concentration of formula or breast milk is altered, renal solute load issues must be considered. Renal solute load refers to excess nitrogen (the metabolic end product of protein metabolism), sodium, chloride, and potassium that are excreted by the kidneys in the urine with water. This excretion may in turn cause dehydration as the kidneys react to the excessive load and draw too much water from the body into the urine [2].

Delivery modes for enteral nutrition

After surgical palliation or repair, an appropriate enteral feeding regimen must be selected for the neonate. The preferred route is oral; however, fatigue, anorexia, or swallowing problems may make exclusive oral feedings unachievable. Initially, enteral feeds may be best managed as a combination of oral (PO) and nasogastric tube (NG) feedings, allowing the infant to work on oral feeding skills but also receive the necessary energy required for catch-up growth. The advantages of the NG route include delivery of more nutrients, minimal invasiveness, and shortness of term. The disadvantages are interference with PO feeds resulting from a tube in one nare and the esophagus making swallowing and breathing a little more challenging. The NG may also make reflux more prevalent and contribute to esophagitis [12,16]. Nasojejunal (NJ) delivery of nutrients is an option when delayed gastric emptying or GER is present. Oralgastric (OG) tubes are sometimes used in neonatal feeding strategies. An OG tube may be preferred in infants with respiratory distress as neonates are primarily nose breathers. Disadvantages of OG tubes include difficulty securing the tube and need for removal or replacement with oral feed attempts.

The feeding tube chosen is typically the smallest possible to deliver feedings safely, and typically a size 6.5 French would be used in a 2.5- to 3.5-kg neonate. Long dwelling tubes are preferred because they remain soft and flexible up to 30 days. Initially infants are allowed to feed orally for no longer than 20 to 30 minutes to maximize the calories delivered and minimize the calories used during prolonged feedings. The remainder of volume to be given by way of NG is given slowly by gravity or on a feeding pump. The entire oral plus nasogastric feed needs to be delivered over less than 60 minutes to allow adequate gastric emptying before the next feed is started. At the authors' institution, current feeding regimens for neonates with CHD post surgical intervention include PO + NG supplementation. Once the infant has tolerated goal calories for 2 or more days, and is taking greater than 50% of volume needed to meet goal calories, the NG is removed for a 24-hour trial of all PO feedings. In the majority of these patients, there is no need to supplement ever again with tube feedings.

Longer-term supplemental feeds via tube may be required in patients unable to meet the adequate caloric and volume needs via the oral route. Tube feedings may be given via nasogastric tube, gastrostomy tube, or gastrojejunal tube. They may be continuous drip (nasogastric, gastrostomy, or gastrojejunal) or bolus feeds (nasogastric or gastrostomy). Studies suggest [1] that continuous feeds require less energy expenditure than bolus feeds and that continuous 24-hour feeds are a safe and effective way to increase nutrient intake and improve overall nutritional status [24,25]. At the authors' institution, nasogastric tubes are reserved for in-patient use only. Concerns about placement, dislodgement, and vasovagal response with cardiac decompensation are particularly worrisome, especially in the group of patients with single ventricle anatomy and parallel circulations.

If prolonged nutrition via tube feeding is required, a surgical gastrostomy or percutaneous endoscopic gastrostomy (PEG) tube may be inserted to maintain growth and development [16]. Enteral feedings at home can then be adjusted from intermittent boluses, continuous infusion, or a combination of the two. Continuous infusions may be tolerated more than bolus feedings [16]. Practically, to help maximize oral motor skills, normal infant feeding patterns, and ease of delivery at home, bolus feedings during the day, for four to five feeds, and a continuous drip feed at night may be used.

Oral motor and positioning

Infants with tachypnea, weak muscle status, prolonged intubation, or potentially impaired vocal cord function often need specific strategies to optimize oral feedings. Simpler supportive strategies include provision for chin support or use of a low-flow nipple as the infant learns how to sequence and coordinate sucking, swallowing, and breathing. As the infant gets stronger with skills, transition to standard nipples can occur. Although a little more challenging to use, the Haberman feeding system may be helpful in infants with CHD who have a weak suck. This one-way valve feeder system allows for control of flow (low, medium, and high) when concerns exist regarding an infant's ability to handle fluids and regulate breathing pauses without breaking its seal on the nipple.

Some specific positioning strategies include feeding with the right side down if there is documented or concern of left vocal cord dysfunction. In general, using the speech and feeding specialist is necessary in meeting the feeding challenges presented by infants with CHD. These professionals are skilled with feeding assessment and the development of infant-specific feeding strategies designed to promote positive oral feeding outcomes.

Summary

It is apparent that, though challenging, it is possible to meet the metabolic and nutritional needs of neonates with CHD in a manner sufficient to sustain life and promote optimal growth and development. Though complex, the management strategies described are useful. A careful analysis of the details is important. In complex infants, the assistance of the speech and feeding team is beneficial.

References

[1] Rosenthal A. Nutritional considerations in the prognosis and treatment of children with congenital heart disease. In: Suskind RM, Lewinter-Suskind L, editors. Textbook of pediatric nutrition. 2nd edition. New York: Raven Press, Ltd.; 1993. p. 383–91.

[2] Cunningham KF, McLaughlin M. Nutrition. In: Kessler DB, Dawson P, editors. Failure to thrive and pediatric undernutrition: a transdisciplinary approach. Baltimore (MD): Paul H. Brookes Publishing; 1999. p. 99–120.

[3] Greecher C. Congenital heart disease. In: Groh-Wargo S, Thompson M, Hovasi Cox J, editors. Nutritional care for the high-risk newborns. Chicago: Precept Press, Inc; 1994. p. 266–75.

[4] Story M, Holt K, Sofka D. Infancy. In: Bright futures in practice: nutrition. 2nd edition (National Center for Education in Maternal and Child Health). Arlington (VA): National Center for Education in Maternal and Child Health; 2002. p. 23–59.

[5] Varan B, Tokel K, Yilmaz G. Malnutrition and growth failure in cyanotic and acynaotic congenital heart disease with and without pulmonary hypertension. Arch Dis Child 1999; 81:49–52.

[6] Abad-Sinden A, Sutphen JL. Growth and nutrition. In: Allen HD, Gutgesell HP, Clark EB, et al, editors. Heart disease in infants, children, and adolescents including the fetus and young adult. Philadelphia: Lippincott Williams and Wilkins; 1991. p. 325–32.

[7] Gaedeke Norris MK, Hill CS. Nutritional issues in infants and children with congenital heart disease. Crit Care Nurs Clin N Am 1994;6(1):153–63.

[8] Barton JS, Hindmarsh PC, Scrimgeour CM, et al. Energy expenditure in congenital heart disease. Arch Dis Child 1994;70:5–9.

[9] American Heart Association. Website 2005. Available at: http://www.americanheart.org. Accessed May 15, 2005.

[10] Dooley KJ, Bishop L. Medical management of the cardiac infant and child after surgical discharge. Crit Care Nurs Q 2002;25(3):98–104.

[11] Forchielli ML, McColl R, Walker WA, et al. Children with congenital heart disease: a nutrition challenge. Nutr Rev 1994;52(10):348–53.

[12] Norris MK, Hill CS. Nutritional issues in infants and children with congenital heart disease. Crit Care Nurs Clin North Am 1994;6(1):153–63.

[13] Smith P. Primary care in children with congenital heart disease. J Pediatr Nurs 2001;16(5): 308–19.

[14] Linde LM, Dunn OJ, Schireson R, et al. Growth in children with congenital heart disease. J Pediatr 1967;70(3):413–9.

[15] Park M. Congestive heart failure. In: Craven L, editor. Pediatric cardiology for practitioners. 3rd edition. St. Louis (MO): Mosby-Year Book, Inc; 1996. p. 401–11.

[16] Marchand V, Baker SS, Baker RD. Enteral nutrition in the pediatric population. Gastrointest Endoscopy Clin N Am 1998;8(3):669–703.

[17] Krebs N. Gastrointestinal problems and disorders. In: Kessler D, Dawson P, editors. Failure to thrive and pediatric undernutrition: a transdisciplinary approach. Baltimore (MD): Paul H. Brookes Publishing Co.; 1999. p. 215–26.

[18] Jung AD. Gastroesophageal reflux in infants and children. Am Fam Physician 2001; 64(11):1853–60.

[19] Kessler DB. Failure to thrive and pediatric undernutrition; historical and theoretical context. In: Kessler DB, Dawson P, editors. Failure to thrive and pediatric undernutrition: a transdisciplinary approach. Baltimore (MD): Paul H. Brookes Publishing; 1999. p. 3–17.

[20] Mitchell I, Davies P, Day J, et al. Energy expenditure in children with congenital heart disease, before and after cardiac surgery. J Thorac Cardiovasc Surg 1994;107:374–80.

[21] Boctor DL, Pillo-Blocka F, McCrindle BW. Nutrition after cardiac surgery for infants with congenital heart disease. Nutr Clin Pract 1999;14(3):111–5.

[22] Pillo-Blocka F, Miles C, Beghetti M, et al. Nutrition after surgery for hypoplastic left heart syndrome. Nutr Clin Pract 1998;13(2):81–3.

[23] Pillo-Blocka F, Adatia I, Sharieff W, et al. Rapid advancement to more concentrated formula in infants after surgery for congenital heart disease reduces duration of hospital stay: a randomized clinical trial. J Pediatr 2004;145:761–6.

[24] Schwarz SM, Gewitz MH, See CC, et al. Enteral nutrition in infants with congenital heart disease and growth failure. Pediatrics 1990;86(3):368–73.

[25] Schuurmans FM, Pulles-Heintzberger CF, Gerver WJ, et al. Long-term growth of children with congenital heart disease: a retrospective study. Acta Paediatr 1998;87(12):1250–5.

CLINICS IN
PERINATOLOGY

ELSEVIER
SAUNDERS

Clin Perinatol 32 (2005) 1031–1042

Discharging Neonates with Congenital Heart Disease After Cardiac Surgery: A Practical Approach

Kathryn M. Dodds, RN, MSN, CRNP[a],*,
Christine Merle, RN, MSN, PNP[b,c]

[a]The Cardiac Center, Children's Hospital of Philadelphia, 34th and Civic Center Boulevard,
Philadelphia, PA 19041–4399, USA
[b]Morgan Stanley Children's Hospital of New York Presbyterian Hospital, 3959 Broadway, 2 North,
New York, NY 10032–3784, USA
[c]Columbia University, New York, NY, USA

Neonates with critical congenital heart disease (CHD) undergo surgery in the first few days and weeks of life. Even low-birth-weight and preterm neonates are now candidates for surgery when the morbidity and mortality of waiting exceed that of pursuing early corrective or palliative repair [1]. Providing expert care to this population of children begins at diagnosis continuing through surgery, postoperative care, hospital discharge, and ongoing follow-up. Transitioning neonates with CHD safely home after surgical repair requires a coordinated and organized multidisciplinary approach that recognizes discharge as a process rather than a single event.

In 1975, the American Nurses Association defined the discharge planning of any patient as that part of the continuity of care process designed to prepare the patient for the next phase of care and to assist in making arrangements for that phase of care [2]. Thirty years later, this definition of discharge planning is still appropriate; when combined with elements of the nursing process, it can provide a framework for effective discharge planning efforts. The hospital discharge of infants with CHD after surgical repair or palliation has multiple

---

* Corresponding author.
E-mail address: dodds@email.chop.edu (K.M. Dodds).

0095-5108/05/$ – see front matter © 2005 Elsevier Inc. All rights reserved.
doi:10.1016/j.clp.2005.09.009

phases; including assessment, planning, and implementation and concluding with evaluation. This article describes these phases and outlines a practical approach toward discharging these infants.

Multidisciplinary team

"Providing parents with the knowledge and skills to care for their infant during this stressful time requires the concerted effort of a multidisciplinary team who can provide clear, concise and consistent communication" [3]. The patient is the center of the discharge process, requiring participation from each vital member of the team to provide optimal care (Fig. 1). The multidisciplinary team includes the family, the nursing team, and the medical team as well as social workers, nutritionists, therapists, and community agencies [4].

The discharge team may vary between institutions; therefore it is important to identify the roles and responsibilities of each team member throughout the discharge process so as to provide optimal care. The family consists of the immediate and extended family. It is important to determine the immediate family's support systems to assess accurately the family's needs on discharge. The nursing team may include a discharge planner, bedside nurses, advance practice nurses, and home care nurses. The nursing team is responsible for teaching the family, coordinating care, and providing emotional support to the family. The medical team includes specialists in cardiology, cardiothoracic surgery, neonatology, and pediatrics. The cardiology members consist of the referring cardiologist in addition to the cardiologist who cared for the infant during hospitalization. Optimizing nutritional support for these patients is imperative. Nutritionists and feeding therapists are needed to participate in the discharge plan. Early intervention, including occupational therapy and physical therapy, begins during hospitalization and needs to be continued after discharge. Dependent on insurance and state and local resources, these therapists may provide home care or outpatient services. The social worker coordinates the discharge plan incorporating government and community resources. These resources

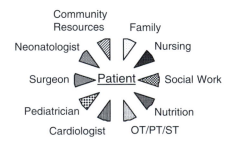

Fig. 1. Multidisciplinary team.

may vary depending on geographic location and insurance coverage. Other essential resources. These resources are pharmacies, durable medical equipment (DME) companies, transportation services, utility companies, and local hospitals.

Assessment and planning

The American Academy of Pediatrics (AAP) guidelines for the hospital discharge of high-risk neonates suggest that discharge occurs when readiness is achieved. Four areas of readiness are assessed: the infant, the family and home environment, the home care plan, and the community health system [5].

Infant readiness

The assessment process begins with determining when an infant is ready for discharge. Elements of this include consistent weight gain; the ability to maintain body temperature without an exogenous heat source; and the ability to maintain stable cardiorespiratory function not only at rest but with feeding, crying, and during times of stress [5]. For infants with CHD, many factors can affect this readiness. The details of the diagnosis, surgery, and hospital course of the infant need to be investigated. The discharge team must identify the ongoing medical issues that follow the infant home and address these issues in the discharge plan.

Gestational age and birth weight are important to consider. Prematurity and low birth weight in neonates with CHD are associated with a longer length of hospital stay and increased morbidity [1]. Premature infants also have additional evaluations that are required before discharge, such as an evaluation for retinopathy of prematurity (ROP).

The complexity of the infant's diagnosis influences the assessment and plans that need to be pursued. Patients with single-ventricle physiology are at risk for interstage mortality, and a home monitoring program that involves arrangements for pulse oximetry and an infant scale may need to be initiated [6]. Infants requiring supplemental oxygen at discharge need to be identified. Other congenital anomalies or associated genetic syndromes can have implications for discharge planning, such as completing any associated medical evaluations.

Preoperative and postoperative complications affect the discharge plan. Neurologic complications, gastroesophageal reflux, and parenchymal lung disease may imply additional needs. Home equipment, specialized medical testing, and the ongoing involvement of other medical and surgical subspecialists may be necessary.

After surgery, neonates with CHD frequently have feeding and nutritional issues that delay discharge readiness [3]. Early identification of those infants and early involvement of a specialized team of therapists are important. Infants being discharged with supplemental gastric feeding tubes pose additional challenges. All feeding supplies need to be ordered and delivered to the home, caregivers need to be instructed, and a strategy for determining who is going to manage the child's feeding issues at home needs to be discussed.

The thoughtful assessment of infant readiness by a multidisciplinary team identifies essential components of an individualized plan early in the discharge process.

Primary care issues

There are state requirements and institutional guidelines about newborn discharge. The discharge team should know the requirements, participate in ensuring compliance with the requirements, include them in the discharge plan, and communicate results to the pediatrician. The primary care of these infants begins in the hospital and is transitioned to the pediatrician at home.

Newborn metabolic and genetic screening

Metabolic screening of newborns is required by all states, and many states require additional genetic screening. Initial screening should be performed at the time of admission and before any surgical procedure. The sample needs to be obtained before any blood products are administered to the patient and as close to 24 hours of age as possible. The team is responsible for tracking results, identifying if additional testing is required, and communicating results to the pediatrician.

Hearing screening

AAP guidelines suggest universal hearing screening for all newborns before discharge [5]. Many states have now mandated a hearing screen before discharge. Neonates with CHD may be at particularly high risk for hearing deficits secondary to severity of illness, associated genetic syndromes, congenital anomalies involving malformations of the head or auditory canal, and the use of ototoxic medications. Brain auditory evoked response (BAER) screening is a noninvasive study easily performed by an audiologist at the bedside. Repeat testing may be warranted for those infants considered to be at extremely high risk or for those infants who fail the initial screen.

Car seat evaluation

Car seat evaluations may vary between states and institutions. Completing this requirement presents an opportunity to assess if the family has a car seat, knows how to use it, and understands infant safety restraint. Newborns less than 37 weeks of gestational age or weighing less than 2500 g at birth and those at risk for apnea or episodes of hemoglobin desaturation should be evaluated. Some might argue that all neonates with CHD, especially postoperative neonates, should be evaluated. A typical test takes approximately 60 minutes, or as long as the drive home. Oxygen saturation, heart rate, and respiratory rate are monitored during the evaluation. A change of 10% or greater is considered a failure, and the test should be repeated after repositioning. Failure at the second attempt requires discharge in a car bed.

Immunizations

CHD is not a contraindication to maintaining the recommended immunization schedule, except after heart transplantation. Children with CHD should receive additional immunizations, such as influenza and pneumococcal vaccines [7]. The newborn hepatitis B vaccination should be administered before discharge. Side effects associated with this vaccine are rare, but it is always a good idea to administer any immunization a few days before the actual discharge date rather than on the day of discharge so as to observe any untoward effects. Parental consent should be obtained before administering any vaccination; known side effects should be discussed with the parents.

Respiratory syncytial virus (RSV) bronchiolitis is one of the most common diseases of childhood. In vulnerable children, RSV can progress to severe bronchiolitis and pneumonia, with an increased chance of morbidity or even death [8]. Synagis is a manufactured monoclonal antibody to RSV that provides temporary protection against RSV. The AAP recommends that it be administered as a standard of care to premature infants and to infants with hemodynamically significant cyanotic and acyanotic CHD until the age of 2 years [8,9]. Neonates, even those with a two-ventricle repair, often qualify for the vaccine. Synagis should be administered before discharge during the RSV season. Because there have been documented cases of nosocomial transmission of RSV in hospital critical care units, it is never too early to immunize at-risk neonates with synagis. Families and pediatricians need to know the hospital administration date. This is a monthly injection during the RSV season. The drug is expensive, so insurance companies may ask for written justification.

Other requirements

Additional primary care–related state or institutional requirements need to be assessed and investigated. This may include the distribution of educational materials about child abuse, shaken baby syndrome, car seats, and restraints.

A developmental assessment of the infant and an evaluation for early intervention should be completed before discharge. Existing evidence suggests that global developmental deficits are common across the developmental spectrum in children with CHD. Defining these developmental deficits is a critical step toward targeting which rehabilitation services are needed to maximize any individual child's neurodevelopmental outcomes [10].

Family readiness

Family consists of those who dwell within the same household and extended family who provide additional support. "The psychosocial characteristics of each family should be reviewed, noting those risk factors that may contribute to an adverse infant outcome" [5].

To assess the family, it becomes essential to evaluate the physical layout of the home environment, including geographic location, description of the dwelling, and number of inhabitants. Accessibility to vital resources, such as electricity, heat, water, and telephone services, needs to be determined. Follow-up care requires traveling to physicians' offices; therefore, it is important to address transportation accessibility. The location of the home may limit follow-up options and present an issue during adverse weather conditions. Geographic limitations may present a problem in arranging home care services.

The needs of the family may depend on whether the home is an apartment or a single family home. It is important to assess the physical layout of the home, including rooms, number of inhabitants, and provisions for the infant's necessities.

The family's financial situation needs to be assessed, including income, insurance, and government assistance. The infant's care may cause significant financial difficulties for a family.

The family dynamics include the number of parents involved in the care of the infant as well as the number of siblings and other caregivers. Important factors to consider include the primary caregiver's work schedule and day care requirements. These issues may necessitate identifying multiple caregivers and instructing each on how to care for an infant with CHD.

Once the caregivers have been identified, assess their educational level, including reading, writing, and language skills. Determine the barriers to learning, and provide solutions to minimize those barriers, including interpreters and translated literature if necessary. Cultural and spiritual diversity exists in many clinical encounters. These issues may cloud other concerns, contribute to inadequate or misleading communication, and affect lifestyle and therapeutic choices [11].

Home medical needs and supplies readiness

Neonates with CHD who undergo surgical repair may have many ongoing medical needs at the time of discharge. A thorough assessment of the infant's medical condition can identify what medical care and supplies are needed at home. All medical supplies need to be identified as early in the discharge process as possible so that timely arrangements can be made and waiting for supplies does not delay the discharge. The discharge team needs to identify who is responsible for all these arrangements. This is usually the role of a discharge planning nurse or social worker.

The discharge team needs to identify the infant's requirement for DME, supplies, nursing care, and therapies. The equipment could include feeding supplies, feeding pump, wound care supplies, oxygen, and pulse oximetry. Those patients with single-ventricle physiology who are at risk for interstage mortality may require extensive home monitoring, including pulse oximetry and an infant scale for daily weight measurement [6,12].

Community resources readiness

All neonates with CHD need a local pediatrician, cardiologist, pharmacist, and emergency plan [5,13]. The family may need assistance and advice in identifying these providers, who should be chosen early in the discharge process. Discovering on the day of discharge that these providers are not yet identified may cause needless delays.

The local pharmacy should be notified when discharge medications are required. Liquid preparations of medications, such as digoxin or lasix, may need to be ordered. The pharmacy may need to obtain preparation instructions and order ingredients necessary to compound medications, such as captopril or enalapril suspensions.

The family, the cardiologist, and the pediatrician should have an emergency plan. In the event of an emergency, the family needs to know whom to call and how to obtain treatment for the infant. This process may require identification of the local fire department, including the emergency response team and local emergency room [5]. Geographic limitations and language barriers may need to be considered when formulating this emergency plan.

Implementation

A collaborative team approach and implementation of the discharge plan begin at admission. When the infant is approaching medical readiness, weekly or even daily meetings of the team may facilitate communication and efficient delivery of services. A checklist of essential items required for discharge aids in communication between team members (Figs. 2 and 3).

On assessment of the family's learning needs, the nurse can begin instructing the family. According to nursing research, "Mothers recommended that information be given gradually during the infants' recuperation and that mothers be encouraged to assume responsibility for their infant's care before discharge. They emphasized that information should not be given in one session, just before discharge or in a noisy or stressful environment" [14]. The family should be taught over a set period, ensuring that they are competent in these necessary skills. Each family requires an individual plan with realistic goals.

The following interventions need to be completed and documented before discharge: newborn screen, hearing screen, car seat evaluation, early intervention referral, shaken baby syndrome education distribution, and administration of immunizations. The family should be taught about bacterial endocarditis (BE) prophylaxis and future requirements. Parents should be supplied with a wallet-sized BE prophylaxis card and instructed on when to present it [15,16].

The bedside nurse should encourage the family to assume increasing responsibility in providing care while the patient is in the hospital. The parents can assist with bathing, feeding, and wound care if necessary. The parents may choose to go to well baby care classes if they are provided at the hospital. The caregivers should attend a cardiopulmonary resuscitation (CPR) class given by the American Red Cross or held within the institution if available. Materials are distributed at the classes as a reference for the families.

PATIENT NAME:
DIAGNOSIS:

DATE COMPLETED

Newborn Screen   _____

Hearing Screen   _____

Car Seat Evaluation   _____

Early Intervention Referral   _____

Shaken Baby Syndrome Education (State Dependent)   _____

Immunizations
   Hep B   _____
   Synagis(during season)   _____

Infant CPR   _____

Education Materials   _____
Defect, Medications, CHF

Medication Teaching   _____

Prescriptions given to parents   _____

Local pharmacy to fill prescriptions identified   _____
(Home medication concentrations verified)

Well Baby Care (bathing instructions, cord care)   _____

Formula Preparation   _____

NG/G/J Tube Teaching   _____

Breast milk Information

Lactation Consultant   _____

Home Care Needs/Supplies
   Nursing Visits   _____
   NG Supplies   _____
   Wound Care Supplies   _____
   DME Equipment Teaching (if applicable)   _____
      Oxygen   _____
      Pulse Oximetry   _____
      Feeding Pump   _____
      Infant Scale   _____
BE Prophylaxis Education   _____
Follow-up Appointments Scheduled
Cardiologist   _____
Pediatrician   _____
Other   _____

Fig. 2. Discharge checklist. BE, bacterial endocarditis; CHF, congenital heart failure; CPR, cardio-pulmonary resuscitation; DME, durable medical equipment; Hep B, hepatitis B; NG/G/J, nasogastric/gastrostomy/jejunostomy.

Patient Name : _____

Diagnosis: _____

Date of Birth: _____

Date of Discharge/Transfer: _____

Discharge Weight: _____

Procedures: _____

Medications (Drug, Dose, Route, Schedule):

Diet/Feeding Instructions:

Immunization Documentation (Date administered):

Hep B   Synagis

Wound Care Instructions:

****

Pediatrician: **Phone**   **Appointment**

Cardiologist: **Phone**   **Appointment**

Surgeon: **Phone**

Other Resources: **Phone**
(Home Care Agency, DME company, Therapists/Special Services, Emergency Numbers)

Fig. 3. Family discharge information. DME, durable medical equipment; Hep B, hepatitis B.

The medical and nursing teams need to teach the family about their child's diagnosis and treatment. Teaching begins when the infant is diagnosed with CHD and continues throughout the hospitalization. It is essential that the family understands the defect and surgical repair. Printed education materials and booklets provided by organizations, such as the American Heart Association (AHA), can aide in the learning process [16,17]. The team needs to provide translated educational materials when language barriers exist.

The therapeutic implications of medical treatment need to be discussed with the family. A medication's action and its side effects are to be included in the discharge teaching. Educational materials describing the medications can also assist the family. The family needs to be aware of each medication concentration and dosages. Prescriptions are to be distributed to the family before discharge. Once the prescriptions have been obtained, the nurse should review the formulation and any changes in the dosage. Families need to demonstrate competency in drawing up doses and in administration of each required medication.

Parents are instructed regarding the feeding plan and the goals for weight gain. Breastfeeding mothers are given the opportunity to meet with a lactation consultant. The mothers are instructed in the use of the breast pumps, storage of breast milk, and cleaning of the equipment. Parents are instructed regarding formula preparation and formulations to increase the caloric density of formula or breast milk as necessary.

Many infants with CHD require supplemental enteral feedings other than by mouth to increase the caloric intake and optimize weight gain. Family members are instructed on placement of nasogastric, gastrostomy, or jejunostomy tubes. Ample time should be allotted when instructing the family regarding supplemental enteral feeding therapy. Once the family members are able to place the feeding tube, they are taught to administer the formula and/or breast milk via gravity or with the assistance of a feeding pump [18].

The family needs to assume care of the infant and become independent from the hospital nursing staff. There are many ways to acclimate the family to caring for the infant. The family can "room in" to provide all the care that the infant needs, including administering medications, feeding, and monitoring. Some institutions may provide separate accommodations for the family to assume all care, with the nursing staff available as a resource [19].

During the preparation for discharge, community resources, including a nursing agency, DME company, and other vendor agencies, are to be arranged for home services. The home care follow-up plan includes intermittent nursing services and early intervention. Geographic limitations may limit these services, requiring outpatient therapy. The infant may require frequent nursing visits after discharge to assess medical status and monitoring equipment while providing support to the family. The family's insurance company may designate specific community resources to be used by the family. The family is instructed as to the operation of the equipment and oxygen therapy. Safety concerns regarding the delivery of oxygen and storage are conveyed to the family. The local electric company should be notified of the child's presence in the community so as to formulate a plan for providing electricity to the home in the event of a power outage.

The family should be instructed as to the signs and symptoms of congestive heart failure. Early recognition of clinical changes can aid in medical therapy. All caregivers should be taught physical assessment skills, including recognition of respiratory distress. A medical emergency plan is formulated that identifies local services. Medical information should be available, including diagnosis, surgical history, baseline vital signs, and medications to aid the medical response team. The local emergency squad can be provided with a diagram of the home, list of vital equipment, and written information about the history [19]. The family should keep all vital information in a file or binder readily available to the emergency medical team.

When the discharge team has determined the date of discharge, follow-up appointments need to be arranged with the pediatrician and cardiologist. On discharge, the family is given the appointments and telephone numbers. The discharge team needs to provide the pediatrician and cardiologist with a discharge summary, operative report, diagnostic test results, medications, and feeding plan. In addition, the pediatrician is forwarded documentation of immunizations and the results of the newborn screen. Ideally, these babies are seen within 1 to 3 days of discharge. The information should arrive at the office, preferably via telefax, before the baby and the family are seen [20].

The family discharge information sheet is completed and given to the family (see Fig. 3). The multidisciplinary team ensures that all discharge requirements are fulfilled (see Fig. 2). The infant with CHD is discharged home with the family.

Evaluation

After discharge, there should be a method to evaluate the process. If the family, pediatrician, cardiologist, or agencies providing services in the home have any questions or issues, a system needs to be in place to address those issues. Pediatricians and referring cardiologists often need to continue dialogue with the institution about management and future surgical procedures.

Many neonatal intensive care units, the truly experienced experts in discharging neonates, have already formalized follow-up programs. These same follow-up services can be tailored to meet the special needs of the baby with CHD. Programs can also objectively evaluate the effectiveness of the discharge plan by investigating rehospitalization statistics and emergency room visits within 30 days of discharge. Programs can determine if these early and unexpected visits are related to inadequate teaching or perhaps to other aspects of the discharge plan [19].

The Children's Hospital of Wisconsin has developed a successful outpatient home monitoring program for infants with single-ventricle heart disease. Despite improved surgical and hospital survival rates, infants at home between the Stage 1 and Stage 2 palliation operations remain vulnerable to interstage mortality [12]. The Children's Hospital of Wisconsin decided to address this issue. Stage 1 infants are discharged to home with a pulse oximeter, infant scale, and standardized data recording sheets with parameters for when to call and report events. Families monitor weight gain and oxygen saturations daily. The nurse practitioners and cardiology staff provide 24-hour and 7-day per week parent support for these infants. Families are given detailed written and verbal instructions about the equipment, feeding, growth parameters, data recording, and reasons to call. Families room in before discharge. Interstage mortality has decreased from 15% to 0% since the initiation of this program [12].

Summary

Discharging neonates to home after cardiac surgery takes time, effective communication, and a commitment to continuity of care. The efforts of all members of a multidisciplinary team are necessary and valuable to ensure success. The discharge process involves many steps beginning at the time of admission and continuing past the actual discharge date. Discharge planning needs to be an evolving process, not a single event.

References

[1] Wernovsky G, Rubenstein S, Spray T. Cardiac surgery in the low-birth neonate new approaches. Clin Perinatol 2001;28(1):249–64.

[2] American Nurses' Association. Continuity of care and discharge planning programs in institutions and community agencies. Kansas City, MO: American Nurses Association; 1975. p. 1–6.

[3] Pye S, Green A. Parent education after newborn congenital heart surgery. Adv Neonatal Care 2003;3(3):147–56.

[4] Robison M, Pirak C, Morrell C. Multidisciplinary discharge assessment of the medically and socially high-risk infant. J Perinat Neonatal Nurs 2000;13(4):67–86.

[5] American Academy of Pediatrics, Committee on Fetus and Newborn. Hospital discharge of the high-risk neonate proposed guidelines. Pediatrics 1998;102(2):411–7.

[6] Soetenga D, Mussatto K. Management of infants with hypoplastic left heart syndrome integrating research into nursing practice. Crit Care Nurse 2004;24(6):646–65.

[7] Smith P. Primary care in children with congential heart disease. J Pediatr Nurs 2003;16(5): 308–19.

[8] Polak M. Respiratory syncytial virus: overview, treatment and prevention strategies. Newborn Infant Nursing 2004;4(1):15–23.

[9] Pickering, editor. Red book report of the Committee on Infectious Disease. Elk Grove Village: American Academy of Pediatrics; 2003. p. 523–8.

[10] Limperopoulos C, Majnemer A, Shavell M, et al. Functional limitations in young children with congenital heart defects after cardiac surgery. Pediatrics 2001;108(6):1325–31.

[11] Kemper K, Barnes L. Considering culture, complementary medicine, and spirituality in pediatrics. Clin Pediatr (Phila) 2003;42(3):205–8.

[12] Ghanayem N, Hoffman G, Mussatto K, et al. Home surveillance program prevents interstage mortality after the Norwood procedure. J Thorac Cardiovasc Surg 2003;126(5):1367–77.

[13] Dooley K, Bishop L. Medical management of the cardiac infant and child after surgical discharge. Crit Care Nurs Q 2002;25(3):98–104.

[14] Stinson J, McKeever P. Mother's information needs related to caring for infants at home following cardiac surgery. J Pediatr Nurs 1995;10(1):48–57.

[15] Bulat D, Kantoch M. How much do parents know about their children's heart condition and prophylaxis against endocarditis? Can J Cardiol 2003;19(5):501–50.

[16] American Heart Association. If your child has a congenital heart defect. Dallas, TX: American Heart Association; 2000–2002.

[17] Merle C. Nursing considerations of the neonate with congenital heart disease. Clin Perinatol 2001;28(1):223–33.

[18] Hofner G, Behrens R, Koch A, et al. Enteral nutritional support by percutaneous endoscopic gastrostomy in children with congenital heart disease. Pediatr Cardiol 2000;21(4):341–6.

[19] Damato E. Discharge planning from the neonatal intensive care unit. J Perinat Neonatal Nurs 1991;5(1):43–53.

[20] Berger S, Holt-Turner I, Cupoli J, et al. Caring for the graduate from the neonatal intensive care unit. Pediatr Clin North Am 1998;45(3):701–12.

CLINICS IN
PERINATOLOGY

ELSEVIER
SAUNDERS

Clin Perinatol 32 (2005) 1043–1057

Long-Term and Developmental Outcomes of Children with Complex Congenital Heart Disease

Matthew D. Brown, MD[a,b],*, Gil Wernovsky, MD[c,d],
Kathy A. Mussatto, BSN[a,b], Stuart Berger, MD[a,b]

[a]*Division of Cardiology, Children's Hospital of Wisconsin, 9000 West Wisconsin Avenue,
Milwaukee, WI 53226, USA*
[b]*Department of Pediatrics, Medical College of Wisconsin, Milwaukee, WI, USA*
[c]*Pediatric Cardiology, The Children's Hospital of Philadelphia, 34th Street and Civic Center,
Boulevard,
Philadelphia, PA 19104, USA*
[d]*Department of Pediatrics, University of Pennsylvania School of Medicine, Philadelphia, PA, USA*

Advances in the medical and surgical management of congenital heart disease (CHD) in the recent past have shifted the focus from mortality to an increasing emphasis on other measures of long-term outcomes, particularly neurodevelopment and quality of life. Outcomes are dependent on a multitude of factors, including the complexity of the lesion, comorbid syndromes, and other diseases as well as other preoperative, intraoperative, and postoperative factors. Studying long-term outcomes is difficult, because "accepted" therapies are ever evolving and multiple decades are required to assess meaningful outcomes in a child. Many surgical techniques are still new enough that long-term follow-up is not yet possible. Many studies have been performed to attempt to delineate outcomes, particularly of various surgical corrections and palliations for CHD in its various forms. This article briefly discusses late outcomes in general and focuses on neurodevelopmental outcomes in children with CHD.

* Corresponding author. Herma Heart Center, MS 713, Children's Hospital of Wisconsin, 9000 West Wisconsin Avenue, Milwaukee, WI 53226.
E-mail address: mdbrown@chw.org (M.D. Brown).

0095-5108/05/$ – see front matter © 2005 Elsevier Inc. All rights reserved.
doi:10.1016/j.clp.2005.09.008   *perinatology.theclinics.com*

Late outcomes

Measures of late outcomes

Although early mortality in patients with CHD has declined over the past several decades [1], the risk of sudden death late after surgery for common CHD has been shown to be 25 to 100 times greater than that in age-matched controls, with the highest risk for aortic stenosis, coarctation of the aorta, D-transposition of the great arteries (D-TGA), and tetralogy of Fallot [2].

Other measures of outcomes include but are not limited to the incidence of planned and unplanned reoperations, ventricular dysfunction and heart failure, rhythm disturbances, endocarditis, exercise limitations (physician imposed and attributable to patient inability), ability to tolerate the stresses of pregnancy, functional status and quality of life, and neurodevelopmental outcomes [3].

Functional status and quality of life may be difficult to measure and interpret but are recognized as important long-term outcomes. In patients with D-TGA, parent questionnaires and psychometric testing have revealed an increased incidence of problems with attention, learning, speech, and developmental delays at 8 years of age after the arterial switch procedure; however, parents reported physical and psychosocial quality of life that was not different from healthy controls [4]. In a similar follow-up study of teenaged patients with hypoplastic left heart syndrome (HLHS), most parents had the perception that their children were doing well or excellent. One third were receiving some form of special education, the median full-scale IQ was 86, and 18% were in the range of mental retardation, however [5].

Examples of individual lesions

Tetralogy of Fallot

Because tetralogy of Fallot was one of the first complex lesions to undergo successful palliation and eventual repair, follow-up studies are quite prevalent in the literature. Murphy and colleagues [6] studied 163 patients at the Mayo Clinic who underwent surgical repair and followed them for 29 to 34 years. Thirty-year actuarial survival rates were similar to those of aged-matched controls for patients operated on at less than 12 years of age but decreased from 91% to 76% if the surgery was performed later in life. Other factors associated with a higher risk of mortality included a prior Waterston or Potts shunt and a right ventricular (RV)/left ventricular (LV) systolic pressure ratio greater or equal to 0.5. Factors like a Blalock-Taussig shunt or the necessity of a transannular patch did not carry an increased risk of mortality. Other potential long-term issues identified included late conduction abnormalities, the need for pacemaker implantation, and reoperation. In another long-term study, Cesnjevar and coworkers [7] studied 411 patients with tetralogy of Fallot repaired over a 42-year period and found that 11.4% underwent a late pulmonary valve replacement. Of these patients, 76.6% had RV dilatation and 34% had impaired RV function.

Physiologically corrected transposition of the great arteries

A long-term study of patients with corrected TGA from 1963 through 1996 was recently reported by Hraska and colleagues [8] from the Children's Hospital in Boston. In this series, it was suggested that long-term outcomes with the classic surgical approach are unsatisfactory by the third decade after surgery, with the poorest outcomes in patients with tricuspid insufficiency requiring tricuspid valve replacement; interestingly, patients undergoing the Fontan procedure had the best survival overall in the group.

Single ventricle

Perhaps the lesions that have received the most attention in recent years are those with a functionally univentricular heart in which the Fontan operation is used for palliation. One of the difficulties in interpreting the literature for this group of patients is the rapidity with which intervention philosophy (eg, timing of surgery) and surgical modifications have changed in the past couple of decades, including the widespread adoption of Norwood palliation for a hypoplastic left heart, an interim superior cavopulmonary anastomosis, baffle fenestration, extracardiac baffles, and technical modifications of cardiopulmonary bypass (CPB) to accomplish these procedures. Late-outcome studies in this patient population demonstrate that mortality has improved dramatically over the past decade. In addition, hospital length of stay has been dramatically reduced, mostly because of a reduction in the severity and duration of pleural effusions. Late morbidity can be compartmentalized into neurodevelopmental outcomes [9,10], abnormal hemodynamics with systolic and diastolic myocardial dysfunction [11,12], decreased exercise capacity [13,14], arrhythmias, protein-losing enteropathy [15], somatic growth retardation, neoaortic root dilatation and valve insufficiency, and thrombotic complications [16].

A recent report from Gaynor and colleagues [17] at the Children's Hospital of Philadelphia evaluated 332 patients who underwent a lateral-tunnel or extracardiac conduit Fontan operation between 1992 and 1999. Mortality decreased over the duration of the study period, and in multivariate analysis, factors associated with a decreased mortality risk included a single-punch fenestration in a lateral-tunnel Fontan operation and the use of modified ultrafiltration. These two improvements also were associated with a shorter duration of pleural effusions and decreased hospital stay. Other studies have shown similar benefits with the use of baffle fenestration, but "routine" use remains center specific [18–20].

Neurodevelopmental outcomes

Neurodevelopmental sequelae in survivors of CHD are varied and include motor delays, problems with visual-motor integration, mental retardation, and learning disabilities as well as behavioral abnormalities, including inattention and hyperactivity. A multitude of factors contribute to long-term neurodevelopmental outcomes and can be separated to some extent into preoperative, intraoperative, and postoperative events.

Preoperative factors

The incidence of structural central nervous system (CNS) abnormalities among patients with CHD is higher than in the general population. Licht and colleagues [21] at the Children's Hospital of Philadelphia studied 25 term infants with CHD and found that 53% had structural brain abnormalities, with periventricular leukomalacia being the most common (28%), followed by microcephaly (24%) and incomplete closure of the operculum (16%). This may in part be caused by abnormal fetal flow patterns in children with complex CHD. In addition, postnatal cerebral blood flow is dramatically reduced in some patients [22,23].

In a study of necropsies, Jones [24] compared 52 patients with CHD with 52 controls and found brain anomalies in 67.8% cases without and 75% of cases with "multimalformative syndrome" in the CHD cohort.

Most named chromosomal syndromes, which have a higher incidence of CHD, are associated with structural and functional CNS abnormalities [25]. Trisomy 21 is commonly associated with CHD (40%–50%) and is universally associated with neurodevelopmental delay. After 1 year of age, brain weight increase in patients with Down syndrome is less than normal (suggestive of a failure of brain growth). Cerebral calcifications are fairly common in patients with Down syndrome and atrioventricular septal defects [26]. Trisomy 21 is also associated with structural changes that include a narrow superior temporal gyrus, disproportionately small cerebellum and brain stem, and other morphologic abnormalities imposed by the altered bony structure of the cranial cavity [25].

Velocardiofacial syndrome, associated with a microdeletion of 22q11.2, is associated with conotruncal defects, neurocognitive deficits, hypocalcemia, mild conductive hearing loss, velopharyngeal insufficiency, and cleft palate. There are a wide variety of neuroanatomic anomalies, including corpus callosum sizes, that are larger than those of controls [27]. According to Miller and Vogel [25], velocardial facial syndrome is associated with microcephaly in 40% of cases; learning difficulties in 100%; psychiatric disorders in 10% to 22%; and brain anomalies, including small vermis and posterior fossa cysts adjacent to the anterior horns.

Williams syndrome is a multisystem disorder associated with CHD in 60% to 80% of patients, most commonly supravalvar aortic stenosis, followed in frequency by peripheral pulmonary stenosis [28]. Typical dysmorphic facies and infantile hypercalcemia are common. Cognitive abnormalities include hypersociability, attention deficit and hyperactivity, hyperacusia, deficient visuocon-structive abilities, and mental retardation [29]. Structurally, Williams syndrome is associated with microcephaly, abnormal neuronal cytoarchitecture, cerebrovas-cular stenosis [25], and cerebellar enlargement [30].

Neurodevelopmental abnormalities were found in 25% of patients with CHD before open-heart surgery was common, secondary to severe cyanosis and poly-cythemia with increased risk of stroke or abscess [25]. Other preoperative find-ings include tone abnormalities, jitteriness, poor oromotor coordination, and feeding difficulties. Abnormal hemodynamics create a higher risk of neurologic insult. Hypoxemia, poor feeding, congestive heart failure, and ductal-dependent flow may present as hypoxic-ischemic brain injury. Prolonged hypoxemia, congestive heart failure, and failure to thrive are likely to affect development, because 50% of brain growth occurs during the first year of life [31].

Mild ischemic lesions occur, particularly in the form of periventricular leukomalacia, in some patients with CHD before surgery, with similar changes in more than 50% of patients after surgery. Although these lesions often resolve by 4 to 6 months after surgery, the long-term effects remain unknown [32].

Apolipoprotein E genotype is an independent risk factor for adverse develop-mental outcomes after a variety of neurologic injuries, including ischemia, intra-cerebral hemorrhage, and traumatic brain injury. Apolipoprotein E is important in the regulation of cholesterol metabolism and is thought to affect neurologic recovery. Recently, Gaynor and coworkers [33] demonstrated that patients carry-ing genetic variations of the apolipoprotein allele had smaller head circum-ferences as well as lower scores on the Bayley Scales of Infant Development 1 year after cardiac surgery in infancy. The effect of the genotype was inde-pendent of ethnicity, socioeconomic status, cardiac defect, and the use of deep hypothermic circulatory arrest (DHCA).

In studying a group of newborns and a group of infants with CHD, Limp-eropoulos and colleagues [34] found that greater than 50% of newborns and 38% of infants had neurobehavioral abnormalities before surgery, such as hypotonia, hypertonia, jitteriness, motor asymmetries, or absent suck. There was a strong association between preoperative and postoperative neurodevelopmental status, which was generally unchanged in most patients. These investigators also found that an oxygen saturation of less than 85% was significantly associated with an abnormal finding [35].

Intraoperative factors

Cardiopulmonary bypass

CPB is necessary in many cardiac operations for CHD and is not without risk. Potential deleterious effects include embolic complications, activation of a va-riety of inflammatory pathways, and short- and long-term cognitive defects [25,31]. Prolonged CPB is an important risk for infants [35] and is related to neurologic and speech dysfunction [36]. Compared with DHCA, more prolonged periods of low-flow CPB (50 mL/kg/min) have been associated with a more impulsive response and worse behavior [37].

Deep hypothermic circulatory arrest

DHCA, essentially planned total-body ischemia-reperfusion, is frequently used during the repair of some complex forms of CHD. During CPB, the patient is cooled to 16°C to 18°C, blood is drained to the venous reservoir, and circulation is arrested. The process is reversed by de-airing the heart, restoring circulation, and rewarming blood by CPB. This technique is also not without risk and has been associated with cognitive defects, particularly with prolonged duration.

Perhaps the best-characterized study of DHCA is the Boston Circulatory Arrest Study, which originally enrolled 171 patients with D-TGA between 1988 and 1992 and randomized them to predominantly DHCA or low-flow CPB. It is important to emphasize that other lesions and their repairs have not been studied in such a comprehensive manner, making generalizability an important limitation. In addition, the results of similar periods of DHCA in the current era are likely to be better, with ongoing improvements in CPB and perioperative care.

At 1 year of age, Bellinger and colleagues [38] reported a lower mean score on the Psychomotor Development Index in the DHCA group, which was inversely related to duration of DHCA. The groups were similar in the incidence of MRI changes, scores on the Mental Development Index, and tests of visual recognition.

At 4 years of age, Bellinger and colleagues [37] reported that the DHCA group had decreased motor function, more apraxia of speech, problems with visual-motor tracking, and phonologic awareness. The mean IQ for both groups was significantly lower than expected.

Finally, in the most recent report at 8 years of age, neurodevelopmental outcomes were generally similar between the groups unless the duration of circulatory arrest exceeded a threshold of 41 minutes. The association was non-linear, with little influence at shorter durations and steadily worsening outcomes after longer durations [39].

Postoperative factors

In the same group of patients, Rappaport and coworkers [40] demonstrated that at the age of 1 and 2.5 years, patients with transient postoperative clinical and electroencephalographic (EEG) seizures had worse neurodevelopmental outcomes.

Rosenblatt [41] has recently shown the benefits of monitoring EEG and evoked potentials as a measure of postoperative neurologic integrity in patients with complex congenital heart lesions. Finally, in the Boston Circulatory Arrest Study, Newburger and colleagues [42] demonstrated that longer postoperative length of stay in the cardiac intensive care unit was associated with worse cognitive function, even when adjusted for perioperative events, perfusion times, and sociodemographic variables.

New strategies

The use of new strategies in the operative and early postoperative period is promising. Shaaban Ali and coworkers [43] demonstrated the utility of near-infrared spectroscopy (NIRS) compared with S100β during warm or cold CPB and found that although there was no significant difference for S100β protein, data obtained via NIRS was useful. These investigators demonstrated that cerebral oxygenation was significantly impaired during rewarming from cold CPB.

Hayashida and coworkers [44] studied cerebral ischemia during cardiac surgery with the use of bispectral index (BIS) and NIRS and found that there were many more than expected episodes of cerebral ischemia. Ischemia was more common in children less than 4 years of age.

Hoffman and colleagues [45] followed changes in cerebral and somatic oxygenation via NIRS in patients undergoing stage 1 palliation of HLHS while using continuous cerebral perfusion via the innominate artery in conjunction with whole-body cooling. These investigators found that the risk of cerebral desaturation was significantly increased after CPB, even with continuous perfusion techniques, likely because of increased cerebrovascular resistance after surgery.

Nagdyman and coworkers [46] compared cerebral tissue oxygenation via NIRS with central venous oxygen saturation and found a significant correlation. Although the values are not interchangeable, the cerebral tissue oxygenation index reflects the hemodynamic influence on cerebral oxygenation.

Hoffman and colleagues at the Children's Hospital of Wisconsin investigated the relation between perioperative physiologic data after the Norwood procedure as they relate to neurodevelopmental outcome after the Fontan procedure in patients 3.5 to 6 years of age. The subjects evaluated had delays in motor skills and visual-motor integration and a composite neurodevelopmental outcome score. Patients with abnormal neurodevelopmental outcomes were found to have had significantly lower postoperative systemic venous oxygen saturation values during the first 48 hours after the Norwood operation as compared with those patients with a normal neurodevelopmental outcome. Systemic venous oxygen saturation was related to poorer developmental outcome, with a breakpoint at values less than 40%. Using multivariate analysis, circulatory arrest time, systemic venous oxygen saturation, blood pressure, and carbon dioxide tension accounted for 79% of the variance in outcome scores. Arterial oxygen saturation values were not predictive of outcomes [47]. This indicates that inadequate postoperative oxygen delivery can result in adverse long-term neurodevelopmental outcome.

Review of the literature

D-transposition of the great arteries

In addition to the Boston Circulatory Arrest Trial described previously, various studies have been performed in this patient population. Ellerbeck and coworkers

[48] studied 57 of 60 survivors of surgical correction of d-TGA, along with 35 siblings in a control group. Children who underwent surgery were more likely to have learning disabilities, abnormal neurologic evaluations, and behavioral disorders. Compared with their siblings, they had more disabilities and abnormal findings. Interestingly, the siblings had more learning problems than was expected in the general population.

Karl and colleagues [49] evaluated 74 patients who underwent an arterial switch operation for D-TGA as well as an equal number of "best friend" controls nominated by the patients or their families and found to be well matched. Patients were more likely than their controls to have mild neurologic abnormalities and to be perceived by their teachers or parents as having a speech and expressive language or behavioral problem.

A parent questionnaire in the same patient population at 8 years old as well as psychometric testing demonstrated mean Physical Health Summary and Psychosocial Summary scores similar to normal; however, there were more problems with attention, learning, speech, and developmental delay compared with normal. Generally, poor psychosocial health status was associated with lower IQ scores and academic achievement. Additionally, a longer hospital course after the initial surgery was associated with a worse physical health status [4].

Hövels-Gürich and colleagues [36] at the Aachen University of Technology in Germany studied 60 patients with D-TGA undergoing an arterial switch operation with combined DHCA and low-flow CPB and evaluated neurodevelopmental outcomes in school-aged children. They found that neurologic and speech impairments were more frequent than in the general population, although intelligence and socioeconomic status were not different. Motor function, acquired abilities, and language were reduced. The overall rate of developmental impairment in one or more domains was 55%. Severe preoperative acidosis and hypoxia were related to reduced motor function, whereas prolonged CPB duration predicted neurologic and speech dysfunction. Finally, perioperative and postoperative cardiocirculatory insufficiency predicted neurologic and motor dysfunction.

Fontan operation

Du Plessis and coworkers [50] studied cerebrovascular accidents after the Fontan operation. A retrospective study of 645 patients over 15 years in Boston from 1978 through 1993 demonstrated that 17 patients (2.6%) had an identified stroke. The greatest risk of stroke was from the first postoperative day to 32 months after the Fontan operation.

Goldberg and colleagues [10] sought to compare patients with HLHS with other children with single-ventricle lesions who have undergone a Fontan operation. In studying the status of 51 patients after the Fontan operation, these investigators found that the full-scale Wechsler Intelligence scores were generally in the normal range, although patients with HLHS scored lower than patients without HLHS. Socioeconomic status, duration of DHCA, and perioperative seizures were predictive of neurodevelopmental outcomes.

Wernovsky and coworkers [9] studied cognitive development by standardized testing in 133 patients who had undergone the Fontan operation. These investigators found that lower IQ scores were associated with the use of circulatory arrest before the Fontan operation, with the anatomic diagnosis of HLHS, and with prior placement of a pulmonary artery band. Although most of these patients who had undergone the Fontan operation in the 1970s and 1980s had a cognitive outcome and academic function within the normal range, performance was still lower than that of the general population.

Hypoplastic left heart syndrome

In addition to the previous studies, Mahle and colleagues [5] studied 115 school-aged survivors of staged palliation for HLHS by questionnaires, 32 of whom also underwent formal evaluation with standardized testing and neurologic examinations. In this group, preoperative seizures were the only factor in multivariable modeling that predicted lower full-scale IQ scores. Duration of DHCA, hospital length of stay, and socioeconomic status were not related to outcome. By clinical evaluation, two thirds had problems with attention or hyperactivity.

Total anomalous pulmonary venous return

Similar to the reports in TGA and HLHS, Kirshbom and coworkers [51] studied school-aged survivors of infant total anomalous pulmonary venous return. During formalized testing, they found a significant incidence of neurodevelopmental difficulties, including fine motor function, visual motor function, and attention deficits.

Studies evaluating heterogeneous forms of congenital heart disease

Dittrich and colleagues [52] studied neurodevelopment at 1 year of age in infants with various forms of CHD. These investigators found that developmental delay was more common after palliative surgery (63%) compared with corrective surgery (19%).

Forbess and coworkers [53] studied the results of 243 5-year-old children who had undergone surgical repair or palliation for various forms of CHD. On the whole, children with CHD performed within the average range for intellectual abilities. Lower socioeconomic status and velocardiofacial syndrome were associated with a lower IQ. There were trends toward worse outcomes for patients with a single ventricle, biventricular repair with longer postoperative intensive care unit (ICU) stays, and longer periods of hypothermic circulatory arrest.

Limperopoulos and colleagues [35] studied 131 patients less than 2 years of age with various forms of CHD, excluding HLHS. These investigators assessed these patients serially, including examinations before and after surgery. Before surgery, they found that more than 50% of newborns and 38% of infants had neurobehavioral abnormalities and that these abnormalities persisted throughout infancy in most cases. After surgery, they found that only 21% were functioning within the expected age range; 37% had a moderate disability, and 6% had severe disability. Functional difficulties in daily living skills were present in 40%. Greater than 50% had poor socialization skills, and 41% had abnormal neurologic examinations. In addition, 42% had gross or fine motor delays, and 23% had global developmental delay. Factors that increased the risk of functional disabilities included abnormal perioperative neurodevelopmental status, microcephaly, length of DHCA, length of ICU stay, age at surgery, and maternal education. Their conclusions were that adverse neurodevelopmental outcomes are multifactorial and include brain injury before, during, and after surgery [54,55].

Wray and Sensky [56] performed a controlled study of children with CHD before and 12 months after surgery, patients awaiting bone marrow transplantation (BMT), and healthy children. Using Ruth Griffiths Mental Developmental Scales, they found mean values in the normal range for all three groups, although preoperative patients with CHD and pre-BMT patients showed deficits. CHD patients with persistent postoperative hypoxemia showed continued developmental deficits, whereas those normal oxygen saturations showed no such deficits.

Quality of life, well-being, and impact on the family

Subjective outcomes, such as health-related quality of life (HRQOL), general well-being or life satisfaction, and impact on the family for subjects and families living with CHD, are difficult to measure but are increasingly recognized as some of the most important outcomes of CHD and its treatment. Research in this area is just beginning to mature. Early investigations of quality of life in subjects with CHD have been rightfully criticized for limits in methodologic rigor and inconsistent definitions of quality of life [57]; however, these descriptive results offer many lessons for future research. It has been difficult to draw broad generalizations from studies representing small heterogeneous samples frequently from one or only a few institutions. Large-scale multicenter research remains needed to begin to identify risk factors for poor psychosocial outcomes in children and their families and to identify opportunities for interventions to improve outcomes [57–59].

Several studies have found that samples of children and adults with CHD have reported quality of life that was not significantly different from healthy peers [4,60–62], although others have found that parental and child reports of HRQOL have been lower than in healthy controls, especially as related to physical, social, and school functioning [58,59,63–65]. Results from these studies are likely influenced by the type of subjects assessed (ie, age, state of repair or palliation, methods used in the study [research instruments chosen]).

The diagnosis of CHD also has important implications for parents and the family unit as a whole. Parents of children with CHD have reported more social problems, less leisure activity [66], greater feelings of distress and hopelessness

[67], and higher levels of overall stress [68,69] than parents of healthy children or those of children with other chronic conditions. With large cohorts of patients with some of the most severe forms of CHD surviving for the first time in history and increasing numbers of children with CHD reaching adulthood, further investigation of family stress and adaptation is warranted.

Results of investigations into quality of life and family impact have been inconsistent to date, and no reliable predictor of outcomes has been identified; however, functional disabilities, activity limitations, and altered social interactions seem to be the most significant variables influencing subject and family perceptions of the impact of CHD [61,63,70–72]. One of the important lessons to be learned from existing research is that severity of illness has not been shown to be a reliable predictor of HRQOL, well-being, or parenting stress [4,70–72]. It is possible for someone to have relatively poor health but generally good quality of life, satisfaction, and family outcomes. The most important predictor of subjective psychosocial outcomes has remained the subject's and family's perception of the impact of the disease, which does not always equate with the perception held by health care professionals [71]. Given this fact, we must take care to provide accurate and timely anticipatory guidance for children and families regarding the role that CHD is likely to play in their lives. Ongoing attempts to reduce morbidity and functional and social limitations and the provision of counseling for subjects and parents to facilitate healthy adjustment to the diagnosis and treatment of CHD are likely to have a positive influence on these important outcomes.

Summary

As short-term survival of complex CHD continues to improve dramatically with advances in medical and surgical treatment, further efforts must be made to understand the long-term outcomes of our efforts. As survival continues to improve, cardiovascular morbidity and, equally importantly, neurodevelopmental and social outcomes must be a continual focus in our treatment of these complex patients. Further study of these effects is underway, and more is certainly warranted. Understanding should lead to modification of current techniques and management strategies, all with the ultimate goal of improving our patients' quality of life.

References

[1] Boneva RS, Botto LD, Moore CA, et al. Mortality associated with congenital heart defects in the United States: trends and racial disparities, 1979–1997. Circulation 2001;103:2376–81.
[2] Silka MJ, Hardy BG, Menashe VD, et al. A population-based prospective evaluation of risk of sudden cardiac death after operation for common congenital heart defects. J Am Coll Cardiol 1998;32:245–51.

[3] Schultz AH, Wernovsky G. Late outcomes in patients with surgically treated congenital heart disease. Semin Thorac Cardiovasc Surg Pediatr Card Surg Annu 2005;8:145–56.

[4] Dunbar-Masterson C, Wypij D, Bellinger DC, et al. General health status of children with D-transposition of the great arteries after the arterial switch operation. Circulation 2001; 104(Suppl 1):I-138–42.

[5] Mahle WT, Clancy RR, Moss EM, et al. Neurodevelopmental outcome and lifestyle assessment in school-aged and adolescent children with hypoplastic left heart syndrome. Pediatrics 2000; 105:1082–9.

[6] Murphy JG, Gersh BJ, Mair DD, et al. Long-term outcome in patients undergoing surgical repair of tetralogy of Fallot. N Engl J Med 1993;329:593–9.

[7] Cesnjevar R, Harig F, Raber A, et al. Late pulmonary valve replacement after correction of Fallot's tetralogy. Thorac Cardiovasc Surg 2004;52:23–8.

[8] Hraska V, Duncan BW, Mayer Jr JE, et al. Long-term outcome of surgically treated patients with corrected transposition of the great arteries. J Thorac Cardiovasc Surg 2005;129:182–91.

[9] Wernovsky G, Stiles KM, Gauvreau K, et al. Cognitive development after the Fontan operation. Circulation 2000;102:883–9.

[10] Goldberg CS, Schwartz EM, Brunberg JA, et al. Neurodevelopmental outcome of patients after the Fontan operation: s comparison between children with hypoplastic left heart syndrome and other functional single ventricle lesions. J Pediatr 2000;137:646–52.

[11] Senzaki H, Masutani S, Kobayashi J, et al. Ventricular afterload and ventricular work in Fontan circulation: comparison with normal two-ventricle circulation and single-ventricle circulation with Blalock-Taussig shunts. Circulation 2002;105:2885–92.

[12] Cheung YF, Penny DJ, Redington AN. Serial assessment of left ventricular diastolic function after Fontan procedure. Heart 2000;83:420–4.

[13] Fredriksen PM, Therrien J, Veldtman G, et al. Lung function and aerobic capacity in adult patients following modified Fontan procedure. Heart 2001;85:295–9.

[14] Mahle WT, Wernovsky G, Bridges ND, et al. Impact of early ventricular unloading on exercise performance in preadolescents with single ventricle Fontan physiology. J Am Coll Cardiol 1999;34:1637–43.

[15] Mertens L, Hagler DJ, Sauer U, et al. Protein-losing enteropathy after the Fontan operation: an international multicenter study. PLE Study Group. J Thorac Cardiovasc Surg 1998;115: 1063–73.

[16] Mair DD, Puga FJ, Danielson GK. The Fontan procedure for tricuspid atresia: early and late results of a 25-year experience with 216 patients. J Am Coll Cardiol 2001;37:933–9.

[17] Gaynor JW, Bridges ND, Cohen MI, et al. Predictors of outcome after the Fontan operation: is hypoplastic left heart syndrome still a risk factor? J Thorac Cardiovasc Surg 2002;123:237–45.

[18] Lemler MS, Scott WA, Leonard SR, et al. Fenestration improves clinical outcome of the Fontan procedure: a prospective, randomized study. Circulation 2002;105:207–12.

[19] Hsia TY, Khambadkone S, Redington AN, et al. Effect of fenestration on the sub-diaphragmatic venous hemodynamics in the total-cavopulmonary connection. Eur J Cardiothorac Surg 2001;19: 785–92.

[20] Hsu DT, Quaegebeur JM, Ing FF, et al. Outcome after the single-stage, nonfenestrated Fontan procedure. Circulation 1997;96(Suppl 2):II-335–40.

[21] Licht DJ, Wang J, Silvestre DW, et al. Preoperative cerebral blood flow is diminished in neonates with severe congenital heart defects. J Thorac Cardiovasc Surg 2004;128:841–9.

[22] Kaltman JR, Di H, Tian Z, et al. Impact of congenital heart disease on cerebrovascular blood flow dynamics in the fetus. Ultrasound Obstet Gynecol 2005;25:32–6.

[23] Donofrio MT, Bremer YA, Schieken RM, et al. Autoregulation of cerebral blood flow in fetuses with congenital heart disease: the brain sparing effect. Pediatr Cardiol 2003;24:436–43.

[24] Jones M. Anomalies of the brain and congenital heart disease: a study of 52 necropsy cases. Pediatr Pathol 1991;11:721–36.

[25] Miller G, Vogel H. Structural evidence of injury or malformation in the brains of children with congenital heart disease. Semin Pediatr Neurol 1999;6:20–6.

[26] Mito T, Pereyra PM, Becker LE. Neuropathology in patients with congenital heart disease and Down syndrome. Pediatr Pathol 1991;11:867–77.

[27] Antshel KM, Conchelos J, Lanzetta G, et al. Behavior and corpus callosum morphology relationships in velocardiofacial syndrome (22q11.2 deletion syndrome). Psychiatry Res 2005; 138:235–45.

[28] Zalzstein E, Moes CA, Musewe NN, et al. Spectrum of cardiovascular anomalies in Williams-Beuren syndrome. Pediatr Cardiol 1991;12:219–23.

[29] Carrasco X, Castillo S, Aravena T, et al. Williams syndrome: pediatric, neurologic, and cognitive development. Pediatr Neurol 2005;32:166–72.

[30] Jones W, Hesselink J, Courchesne E, et al. Cerebellar abnormalities in infants and toddlers with Williams syndrome. Dev Med Child Neurol 2002;44:688–94.

[31] Mahle WT, Wernovsky G. Long-term developmental outcome of children with complex congenital heart disease. Clin Perinatol 2001;28:235–47.

[32] Mahle WT, Tavani F, Zimmerman RA, et al. An MRI study of neurological injury before and after congenital heart surgery. Circulation 2002;106(Suppl 1):I-109–14.

[33] Gaynor JW, Gerdes M, Zackai EH, et al. Apolipoprotein E genotype and neurodevelopmental sequelae of infant cardiac surgery. J Thorac Cardiovasc Surg 2003;126:1736–45.

[34] Limperopoulos C, Majnemer A, Shevell MI, et al. Neurologic status of newborns with congenital heart defects before open heart surgery. Pediatrics 1999;103:402–8.

[35] Limperopoulos C, Majnemer A, Shevell MI, et al. Neurodevelopmental status of newborns and infants with congenital heart defects before and after open heart surgery. J Pediatr 2000; 137:638–45.

[36] Hövels-Gürich HH, Seghaye MC, Schnitker R, et al. Long-term neurodevelopmental outcomes in school-aged children after neonatal arterial switch operation. J Thorac Cardiovasc Surg 2002; 124:448–58.

[37] Bellinger DC, Wypij D, Du Plessis AJ, et al. Neurodevelopmental status at eight years in children with dextro-transposition of the great arteries: the Boston circulatory arrest trial. J Thorac Cardiovasc Surg 2003;126:1385–96.

[38] Bellinger DC, Jonas RA, Rappaport LA, et al. Developmental and neurologic status of children after heart surgery with hypothermic circulatory arrest or low-flow cardiopulmonary bypass. N Engl J Med 1995;332:549–55.

[39] Wypij D, Newburger JW, Rappaport LA, et al. The effect of duration of deep hypothermic circulatory arrest in infant heart surgery on late neurodevelopment: the Boston circulatory arrest trial. J Thorac Cardiovasc Surg 2003;126:1397–403.

[40] Rappaport LA, Wypij D, Bellinger DC, et al. Relation of seizures after cardiac surgery in early infancy to neurodevelopmental outcome. Boston Circulatory Arrest Study Group. Circulation 1998;97:773–9.

[41] Rosenblatt B. Monitoring the central nervous system in children with congenital heart defects: Clinical neurophysiological techniques. Semin Pediatr Neurol 1999;6:27–31.

[42] Newburger JW, Wypij D, Bellinger DC, et al. Length of stay after infant heart surgery is related to cognitive outcome at age 8 years. J Pediatr 2003;143:67–73.

[43] Shaaban Ali M, Harmer M, Elliott M, et al. A pilot study of evaluation of cerebral function by S100beta protein and near-infrared spectroscopy during cold and warm cardiopulmonary bypass in infants and children undergoing open-heart surgery. Anaesthesia 2004;59:20–6.

[44] Hayashida M, Kin N, Tomioka T, et al. Cerebral ischaemia during cardiac surgery in children detected by combined monitoring of BIS and near-infrared spectroscopy. Br J Anaesth 2004;92: 662–9.

[45] Hoffman GM, Stuth EA, Jaquiss RD, et al. Changes in cerebral and somatic oxygenation during stage 1 palliation of hypoplastic left heart syndrome using continuous regional cerebral perfusion. J Thorac Cardiovasc Surg 2004;127:223–33.

[46] Nagdyman N, Fleck T, Barth S, et al. Relation of cerebral tissue oxygenation index to central venous oxygen saturation in children. Intensive Care Med 2004;30:468–71.

[47] Hoffman GM, Mussatto KA, Brosig CL, et al. Systemic venous oxygen saturation after the

Norwood procedure and childhood neurodevelopmental outcome. J Thorac Cardiovasc Surg 2005;130:1094–100.

[48] Ellerbeck KA, Smith ML, Holden EW, et al. Neurodevelopmental outcomes in children surviving d-transposition of the great arteries. J Dev Behav Pediatr 1998;19:335–41.

[49] Karl TR, Hall S, Ford G, et al. Arterial switch with full-flow cardiopulmonary bypass and limited circulatory arrest: neurodevelopmental outcome. J Thorac Cardiovasc Surg 2004;127: 213–22.

[50] Du Plessis AJ, Chang AC, Wessel DL, et al. Cerebrovascular accidents following the Fontan operation. Pediatr Neurol 1995;12:230–6.

[51] Kirshbom PM, Flynn TB, Clancy RR, et al. Late neurodevelopmental outcome after repair of total anomalous pulmonary venous connection. J Thorac Cardiovasc Surg 2005;129:1091–7.

[52] Dittrich H, Buhrer C, Grimmer I, et al. Neurodevelopment at 1 year of age in infants with congenital heart disease. Heart 2003;89:436–41.

[53] Forbess JM, Visconti KJ, Hancock-Friesen C, et al. Neurodevelopmental outcome after congenital heart surgery: results from an institutional registry. Circulation 2002;106(Suppl 1): I-95–102.

[54] Limperopoulos C, Majnemer A, Shevell MI, et al. Functional limitations in young children with congenital heart defects after cardiac surgery. Pediatrics 2001;108:1325–31.

[55] Limperopoulos C, Majnemer A, Shevell MI, et al. Predictors of developmental disabilities after open heart surgery in young children with congenital heart defects. J Pediatr 2002;141:51–8.

[56] Wray J, Sensky T. Controlled study of preschool development after surgery for congenital heart disease. Arch Dis Child 1999;80:511–6.

[57] Moons P, Van Deyk K, Budts W, et al. Caliber of quality-of-life assessments in congenital heart disease: a plea for more conceptual and methodological rigor. Arch Pediatr Adolesc Med 2004; 158:1062–9.

[58] Mussatto K, Tweddell J. Quality of life following surgery for congenital cardiac malformations in neonates and infants. Cardiol Young 2005;15(Suppl 1):174–8.

[59] Uzark K, Jones K, Burwinkle TM, et al. The pediatric quality of life inventory in children with heart disease. Prog Pediatr Cardiol 2003;18:141–8.

[60] Connolly D, Rutkowski M, Auslender M, et al. Measuring health-related quality of life in children with heart disease. Appl Nurs Res 2002;15:74–80.

[61] Moyen Laane K, Meberg A, Otterstad JE, et al. Quality of life in children with congenital heart defects. Acta Paediatr 1997;86:975–80.

[62] Saliba Z, Butera G, Bonnet D, et al. Quality of life and perceived health status in surviving adults with univentricular heart. Heart 2001;86:69–73.

[63] Kamphuis M, Ottenkamp J, Vliegen HW, et al. Health related quality of life and health status in adult survivors with previously operated complex congenital heart disease. Heart 2002;87: 356–62.

[64] Lane DA, Lip GY, Millane TA. Quality of life in adults with congenital heart disease. Heart 2002;88:71–5.

[65] Williams DL, Gelijns AC, Moskowitz AJ, et al. Hypoplastic left heart syndrome: valuing the survival. J Thorac Cardiovasc Surg 2000;119:720–31.

[66] Casey FA, Sykes DH, Craig BG, et al. Behavioral adjustment of children with surgically palliated complex congenital heart disease. J Pediatr Psychol 1996;21:335–52.

[67] Lawoko S, Soares JJ. Distress and hopelessness among parents of children with congenital heart disease, parents of children with other diseases, and parents of healthy children. J Psychosom Res 2002;52:193–208.

[68] Goldberg S, Morris P, Simmons RJ, et al. Chronic illness in infancy and parenting stress: a comparison of three groups of parents. J Pediatr Psychol 1990;15:347–58.

[69] Morelius E, Lundh U, Nelson N. Parental stress in relation to the severity of congenital heart disease in the offspring. Pediatr Nurs 2002;28:28–33.

[70] Ternestedt BM, Wall K, Oddsson H, et al. Quality of life 20 and 30 years after surgery in patients operated on for tetralogy of Fallot and for atrial septal defect. Pediatr Cardiol 2001;22: 128–32.

[71] DeMaso DR, Campis LK, Wypij D, et al. The impact of maternal perceptions and medical severity on the adjustment of children with congenital heart disease. J Pediatr Psychol 1991; 16:137–49.
[72] Uzark K, Jones K. Parenting stress and children with heart disease. J Pediatr Health Care 2003;17:163–8.

ELSEVIER
SAUNDERS

CLINICS IN
PERINATOLOGY

Clin Perinatol 32 (2005) 1059–1093

Cumulative Index 2005

Note: Page numbers of article titles are in **boldface** type.

A

Abdomen
  abscess, in radiography in, 797–798
  injury within, 32–33

Abortion, spontaneous, in infections, 526–527

Abruptio placenta, in multiple gestations, 405

Abscess, radiography in
  abdominal, 797–798
  brain, 793
  epidural, 792–793
  psoas, 799–800

Accelerated ventricular rhythm, 900

Accessory pathway, defects of, in
  supraventricular tachycardia, 939

Acidemia, 88

Acidosis
  in asphyxia, measurement of, 62–63
  metabolic, in heart disease, 931

Acute respiratory distress syndrome, in
  pyelonephritis, 759

Acyclovir
  for herpes simplex virus infections,
    634–635, 663–665
  for varicella, 685–687

Adenosine, for arrhythmias, 895, 940,
  980–982

Administration, of drugs, error prevention in,
  116–117

Administrative compensation model, for medical injuries, 218–221

Adrenal gland, injury of, 32–33

Advance care planning, 161

Advance lists of avoidable events, 221–225

Adverse events, in medication errors as. *See*
  Medication errors.

Affymetrix genotyping chip, in heart
  disease, 828

Age, maternal, multiple gestations and, 302,
  311–312, 320

Agency for Health Care Policy and Research,
  National Summit on Patient Safety and
  Medical Errors, on kernicterus, 130–131

Airway, obstruction of, ex utero intrapartum
  treatment for, 936

Alarm systems, effectiveness of, for safety,
  102–103

Alpha-fetoprotein, in triple screen, for Down
  syndrome, in twin pregnancies, 375–382

Altered flow theory, of heart disease, 880–884

Alternate dispute resolution, 243

Amantadine, for influenza, 730–731

American Academy of Pediatrics, on
  kernicterus prevention, 132–134

American Association of Nurse Attorneys, 279

American College of Obstetricians and
  Gynecologists, asphyxia criteria of,
  70–72

Amiodarone, for arrhythmias
  fetal, 893, 900, 902
  neonatal, 983–984

Amniocentesis
  in bacterial culture, 585, 589
  in cytomegalovirus infections, 677
  in multiple gestations, 355–358, 446
    versus chorionic villus sampling,
      359–360

Amnionitis. *See* Intra-amniotic infections.

Amnioreduction, in twin–twin transfusion,
  481–483, 502–503, 871

Amniotic membrane, thickness of, in
  chorionicity determination, 478

Amoxicillin
  for *Chlamydia trachomatis* infections, 639
  for neonatal sepsis prevention, 609

0095-5108/05/$ – see front matter © 2005 Elsevier Inc. All rights reserved.
doi:10.1016/S0095-5108(05)00110-7

Changing Your Address?

Make sure your subscription changes too! When you notify us of your new address, you can help make our job easier by including an exact copy of your Clinics label number with your old address (see illustration below.) This number identifies you to our computer system and will speed the processing of your address change. Please be sure this label number accompanies your old address and your corrected address—you can send an old Clinics label with your number on it or just copy it exactly and send it to the address listed below.

We appreciate your help in our attempt to give you continuous coverage. Thank you.

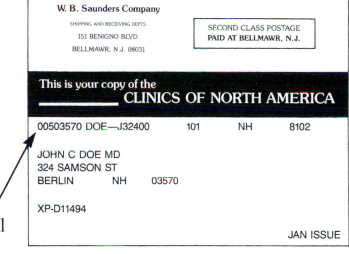

W. B. Saunders Company

SHIPPING AND RECEIVING DEPTS.

151 BENIGNO BLVD.

BELLMAWR, N.J. 08031

SECOND CLASS POSTAGE
PAID AT BELLMAWR, N.J.

This is your copy of the
CLINICS OF NORTH AMERICA

00503570 DOE—J32400   101   NH   8102

JOHN C DOE MD
324 SAMSON ST
BERLIN   NH   03570

XP-D11494

JAN ISSUE

Your Clinics Label Number
Copy it exactly or send your label
along with your address to:
W.B. Saunders Company, Customer Service
Orlando, FL 32887-4800
Call Toll Free 1-800-654-2452

Please allow four to six weeks for delivery of new subscriptions and for processing address changes.

United States Postal Service
Statement of Ownership, Management, and Circulation

1. Publication Title				2. Publication Number										3. Filing Date
Clinics in Permatology				0	0	9	5	-	5	1	0	8		9/15/05

4. Issue Frequency	5. Number of Issues Published Annually	6. Annual Subscription Price
Mar, Jun, Sep, Dec	4	$155.00

7. Complete Mailing Address of Known Office of Publication *(Not printer) (Street, city, county, state, and ZIP+4)*

Elsevier Inc.
6277 Sea Harbor Drive
Orlando, FL 32887-4800

Contact Person
Gwen C. Campbell
Telephone
215-239-3685

8. Complete Mailing Address of Headquarters or General Business Office of Publisher *(Not printer)*

Elsevier Inc., 360 Park Avenue South, New York, NY 10010-1710

9. Full Names and Complete Mailing Addresses of Publisher, Editor, and Managing Editor *(Do not leave blank)*
Publisher *(Name and complete mailing address)*

Tim Griswold, Elsevier Inc., 1600 John F. Kennedy Blvd., Suite 1800, Philadelphia, PA 19103-2899

Editor *(Name and complete mailing address)*

Carin Davis, Elsevier Inc., 1600 John F. Kennedy Blvd., Suite 1800, Philadelphia, PA 19103-2899

Managing Editor *(Name and complete mailing address)*

Heather Cullen, Elsevier Inc., 1600 John F. Kennedy Blvd., Suite 1800, Philadelphia, PA 19103-2899

10. Owner *(Do not leave blank. If the publication is owned by a corporation, give the name and address of the corporation immediately followed by the names and addresses of all stockholders owning or holding 1 percent or more of the total amount of stock. If not owned by a corporation, give the names and addresses of the individual owners. If owned by a partnership or other unincorporated firm, give its name and address as well as those of each individual owner. If the publication is published by a nonprofit organization, give its name and address.)*

Full Name	Complete Mailing Address
Wholly owned subsidiary of	4520 East-West Highway
Reed/Elsevier Inc., US holdings	Bethesda, MD 20814

11. Known Bondholders, Mortgagees, and Other Security Holders Owning or Holding 1 Percent or More of Total Amount of Bonds, Mortgages, or Other Securities. If none, check box ☐ None

Full Name	Complete Mailing Address
N/A	

12. Tax Status *(For completion by nonprofit organizations authorized to mail at nonprofit rates) (Check one)*
The purpose, function, and nonprofit status of this organization and the exempt status for federal income tax purposes:
☐ Has Not Changed During Preceding 12 Months
☐ Has Changed During Preceding 12 Months *(Publisher must submit explanation of change with this statement)*

(See Instructions on Reverse)

PS Form 3526, October 1999

---

13. Publication Title			14. Issue Date for Circulation Data Below
Clinics in Permatology			June 2005

15.	Extent and Nature of Circulation		Average No. Copies Each Issue During Preceding 12 Months	No. Copies of Single Issue Published Nearest to Filing Date
a.	Total Number of Copies *(Net press run)*		4625	4400
b. Paid and/or Requested Circulation	(1)	Paid/Requested Outside-County Mail Subscriptions Stated on Form 3541. *(Include advertiser's proof and exchange copies)*	2761	2700
	(2)	Paid In-County Subscriptions Stated on Form 3541 *(Include advertiser's proof and exchange copies)*		
	(3)	Sales Through Dealers and Carriers, Street Vendors, Counter Sales, and Other Non-USPS Paid Distribution	973	930
	(4)	Other Classes Mailed Through the USPS		
c.	Total Paid and/or Requested Circulation *[Sum of 15b. (1), (2), (3), and (4)]*	▲	3734	3630
d. Free Distribution by Mail *(Samples, complimentary, and other free)*	(1)	Outside-County as Stated on Form 3541	63	78
	(2)	In-County as Stated on Form 3541		
	(3)	Other Classes Mailed Through the USPS		
e.	Free Distribution Outside the Mail *(Carriers or other means)*			
f.	Total Free Distribution *(Sum of 15d. and 15e.)*	▲	63	78
g.	Total Distribution *(Sum of 15c. and 15f.)*	▲	3797	3708
h.	Copies not Distributed		828	692
i.	Total *(Sum of 15g. and h.)*	▲	4625	4400
j.	Percent Paid and/or Requested Circulation *(15c. divided by 15g. times 100)*		98%	98%

16. Publication of Statement of Ownership
☐ Publication required. Will be printed in the **December 2005** issue of this publication. ☐ Publication not required

17. Signature and Title of Editor, Publisher, Business Manager, or Owner

[signature] Date 9/15/05
John Schrefer – Executive Director of Subscription Services

I certify that all information furnished on this form is true and complete. I understand that anyone who furnishes false or misleading information on this form or who omits material or information requested on the form may be subject to criminal sanctions (including fines and imprisonment) and/or civil sanctions (including civil penalties).

Instructions to Publishers

1. Complete and file one copy of this form with your postmaster annually on or before October 1. Keep a copy of the completed form for your records.
2. In cases where the stockholder or security holder is a trustee, include in items 10 and 11 the name of the person or corporation for whom the trustee is acting. Also include the names and addresses of individuals who are stockholders who own or hold 1 percent or more of the total amount of bonds, mortgages, or other securities of the publishing corporation. In item 11, if none, check the box. Use blank sheets if more space is required.
3. Be sure to furnish all circulation information called for in item 15. Free circulation must be shown in items 15d, e, and f.
4. Item 15h., Copies not Distributed, must include (1) newsstand copies originally stated on Form 3541, and returned to the publisher, (2) estimated returns from news agents, and (3), copies for office use, leftovers, spoiled, and all other copies not distributed.
5. If the publication had Periodicals authorization as a general or requester publication, this Statement of Ownership, Management, and Circulation must be published; it must be printed in any issue in October or, if the publication is not published during October, the first issue printed after October.
6. In item 16, indicate the date of the issue in which this Statement of Ownership will be published.
7. Item 17 must be signed.

Failure to file or publish a statement of ownership may lead to suspension of Periodicals authorization.

PS Form 3526, October 1999 *(Reverse)*